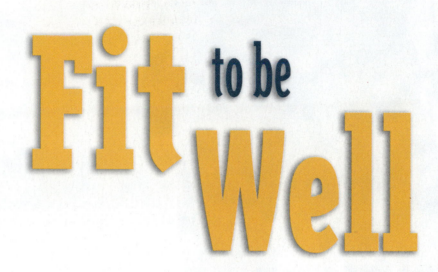

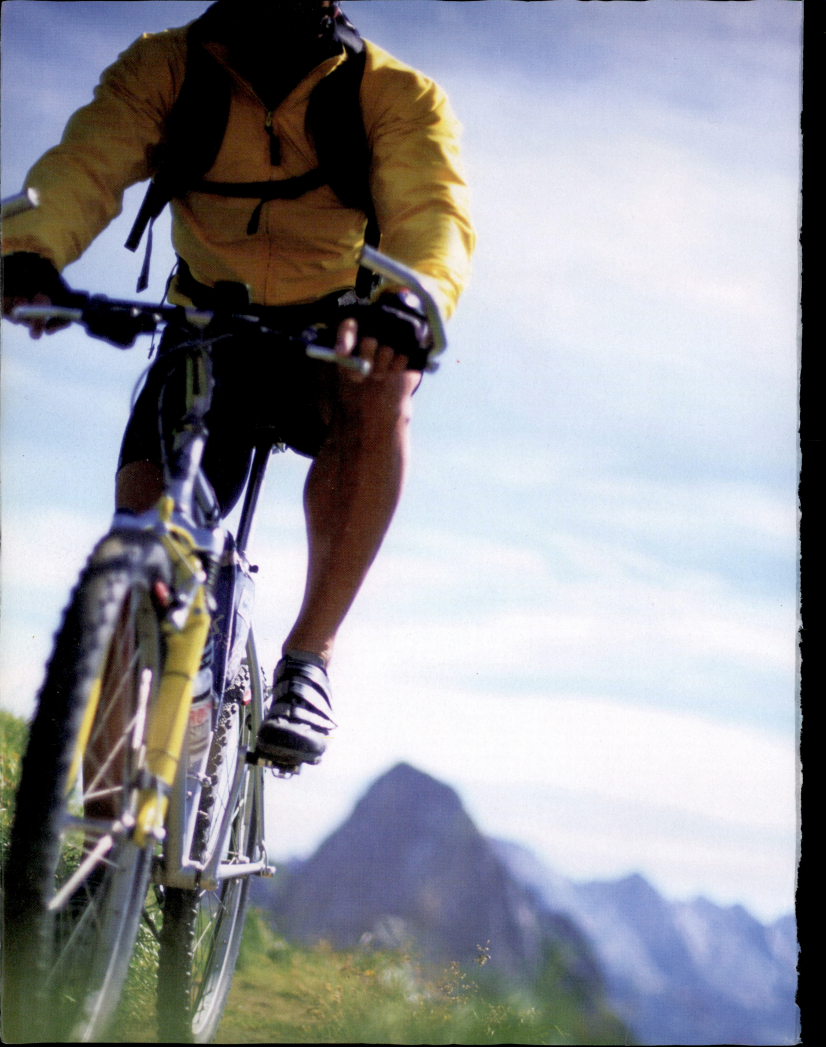

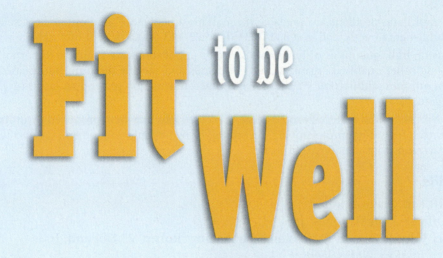

# Fit to be Well

**Alton L. Thygerson**

Brigham Young University

Department of Health Science

**Karl L. Larson**

Gustavus Adolphus College

Department of Health and Exercise Science

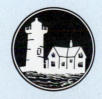

JONES AND BARTLETT PUBLISHERS

*Sudbury, Massachusetts*

BOSTON    TORONTO    LONDON    SINGAPORE

## World Headquarters

Jones and Bartlett Publishers
40 Tall Pine Drive
Sudbury, MA 01776
978-443-5000
info@jbpub.com
www.jbpub.com

Jones and Bartlett Publishers
Canada
2406 Nikanna Road
Mississauga, ON L5C 2W6
CANADA

Jones and Bartlett Publishers
International
Barb House, Barb Mews
London W6 7PA
UK

Copyright © 2006 by Jones and Bartlett Publishers, Inc.

Jones and Bartlett's books and products are available through most bookstores and online booksellers. To contact Jones and Bartlett Publishers directly, call 800-832-0034, fax 978-443-8000, or visit our website www.jbpub.com.

Substantial discounts on bulk quantities of Jones and Bartlett's publications are available to corporations, professional associations, and other qualified organizations. For details and specific discount information, contact the special sales department at Jones and Bartlett via the above contact information or send an email to specialsales@jbpub.com.

## Production Credits

Chief Executive Officer: Clayton Jones
Chief Operating Officer: Don W. Jones, Jr.
President of Higher Education and Professional Publishing: Robert W. Holland, Jr.
V.P., Design and Production: Anne Spencer
V.P., Manufacturing and Inventory Control: Therese Bräuer
V.P., Sales and Marketing: William J. Kane
Acquisitions Editor: Jacqueline Mark-Geraci
Production Editor: Anne Spencer
Associate Editor: Nicole Quinn
Editorial Assistant: Amy Flagg
Associate Marketing Manager: Wendy Thayer
Interactive Technology Manager: Dawn Mahon Priest
Senior Photo Researcher: Kimberly Potvin
Photo Researcher: Christine McKeen
Composition: Graphic World
Cover and Interior Design: Anne Spencer
Cover Image: © Image Source Limited/Index Stock Imagery, Inc.
Printing and Binding: Courier Kendallville
Cover Printing: Courier Kendallville

## Library of Congress Cataloging-in-Publication Data

Thygerson, Alton L.
  Fit to be well / Alton Thygerson, Karl Larson.
      p. cm.
  Includes bibliographical references and index.
  ISBN 0-7637-3547-7 (alk. paper)
  1.  Physical fitness. 2.  Exercise. 3.  Nutrition. 4.  Health behavior. 5.  Health.  I. Larson, Karl. II. Title.
  RA781.T49 2006
  613.7--dc22

                                    2005026420

6048

Printed in the United States of America
09 08 07 06 05  10 9 8 7 6 5 4 3 2 1

# Contents

CHAPTER **4**   **Increasing Flexibility** 52

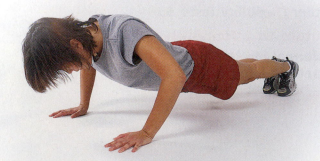

CHAPTER 6

## Choosing a Nutritious Diet  88

CHAPTER **7**  **Maintaining a Healthy Body Composition and Body Weight 124**

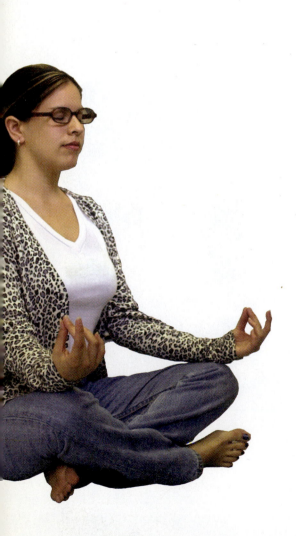

CHAPTER **8** **Managing Stress 152**

The purpose of this book is, first, to introduce you to the extraordinary world of health, wellness, and physical fitness and, second, to help you to change your life.

In a time of high-tech advances, we have lost sight of the fact that the greatest high-tech invention of all time is the human body. What happens to our packaging—our mind and our bodies—as we move through life is primarily the result of the choices we make every day—our lifestyle.

As priceless as good health is, it is paradoxically freely available to us, if we live the right way. When it comes to fitness, the child does not have to be taught to play, but the adult must learn how to exercise because we lose that childhood instinct to run and jump, to skip, and to walk briskly. Our mental and emotional wellness on the other hand, depends entirely on how we interpret the environment in which we function, and the choices we make related to that environment. All people possess the capacity for healthy living, and this book is designed to help you use that capacity by teaching skills in exercising, eating properly, avoiding the onset of chronic disease and managing stress.

The best news is that it is never too late to start living healthfully, regardless of your age or current condition. This book can help you to make changes that will sustain your health, and therefore, make your life a better one.

Attempting to reach the goal of good health and wellness through the practice of positive wellness and physical fitness can be compared with preparing to take a journey. If you were driving from Los Angeles to New York City, you would first obtain a road map to determine the best route to follow. The journey to good health and wellness is very similar, but most people are not familiar with, or do not know where to obtain, a road map leading to good health and wellness. This book represents such a road map. It takes you from your current level of wellness toward increased fitness, as well as helping you to maintain a healthy weight, learn to relax, and avoid chronic disease.

*Fit to be Well* offers a comprehensive look at wellness with simple, workable approaches to a healthy lifestyle.

## Note to Students and Instructors

**No other fitness and wellness book is like this one, despite sharing similar content.**

The content of this book is organized in a succinct, easy-to-navigate manner, with emphasis placed on important concepts and applications. The advantages of this approach include:

- Decreased reading time
- Quicker access to information
- Improved learning
- Less expensive text
- High reader satisfaction
- Creative uses of information (e.g., uses "chunking" to put content into manageable units for better learning)
- No long-winded passages—the content is concise, straightforward information that a person "needs" to know
- Evidence-based medical sources provide the content and latest recommendations

## Special Features

Special features to improve learning include:

**Time-Outs** These boxes explore topics of interest to students such as fad diets, environmental health, relationships, and a health procedure timeline.

**What's the word...** Boxes throughout the text containing target terms offer simple, clear definitions for terms of interest.

**The Inside Track** Here you will find quick and easy guides to important information.

**Tipping Point** These helpful hints and tips explain how to manage your fitness and healthy lifestyle program.

**Knowledge Check** Multiple-choice questions appear at the end of each chapter to test your knowledge of the information covered in the text.

**Modern Modifications** Each chapter contains a section that provides a list of simple suggestions related to that chapter's topic. Each of these suggestions is specifically intended to be easily absorbed into your daily routine. The strategies are realistic and take into consideration "real life" obstacles.

**Critical Thinking**  These sections give you a chance to apply what you learned in each chapter. Questions and scenarios about the work that you will do and the goals to achieve will bring about some critical thoughts. This will help you assimilate what you learn and apply it to your daily life.

**Going Above and Beyond**  At the end of each chapter, this book provides a perfect opportunity for those with a desire to take their research one step further. Complete bibliographies and websites are included so that you can take any of the information you find interesting and learn more.

## Supplements

**Text-Specific Website http://health.jbpub.com/fitness**  This website provides instructors with helpful teaching aids: Instructor's Manual, PowerPoint Slides, and a Test Bank. Students can access flashcards, practice quizzes, crossword puzzles, an interactive glossary and weblinks that help reinforce key concepts in the text.

**Lab Manual**  Every NEW text comes with a student lab manual at no additional cost to your students! By adding self-assessments and related labs to each of the chapters, this text becomes an interactive guide to building and implementing a fitness program that will work with a student's individual needs and schedule.

## Acknowledgments

Any book requires a great deal of effort, and not just on the part of the authors. This book is no exception to that rule.

I am fortunate to have a publisher, Clayton Jones, who believes in this unique project, and who encouraged me to write this textbook. I am very grateful to Jacqueline Mark-Geraci, acquisitions editor, for pushing the project along the way, and Erin Murphy and Nicole Quinn for helping to make it a better book. A strong appreciation goes to the Jones and Bartlett Publishers production staff, including Anne Spencer and Julie Bolduc, for publishing a book of high quality, and to Graphic World for putting it all together.

To all of the reviewers, I express my thanks for their help and many worthwhile suggestions. Finally, I thank my wife for her encouragement and support.

—Aton L. Thygerson

I would like to thank Alton and the folks at Jones and Bartlett, in particular Jacqueline Mark-Geraci for offering me this opportunity. The experience has been great. Like Alton, I would note the tireless efforts of Erin Murphy and Nicole Quinn for helping me through the process of writing my first textbook. I dedicate this book to my wife, Kathy, whose belief in my abilities far exceeds my own, and to the newest member of the Larson clan, Brenden Isaac.

—Karl L. Larson

The authors would also like to thank the following reviewers, whose suggestions and insight provided direction for the development of this text:

Paul Alvarez, Ph.D., ATC
Movement and Sports Science Department
University of La Verne

Matthew D. Beekley, Ph.D.
Director, Center for Physical Development Excellence
Department of Physical Education
United States Military Academy

Megan Franks, M.A.
Health and Human Services, Kinesiology Department
North Harris College

Sandor Helfgott, M.S.
Fitness Coordinator
Department of Physical Education
United States Military Academy

John Knorr, Ph.D.
School of Education, Kinesiology
St. Edward's University

Scott C. Swanson, Ph.D.
Human Performance and Sport Sciences
Ohio Northern University

Susan M. Tendy, Ed.D.
Director of Assessment
Department of Physical Education
Unites States Military Academy

James A. Van Atta, M.S.
Assistant Fitness Testing Officer
Department of Physical Education
United States Military Academy

Jeannette Williams, M.S.
Physical Education Department
Rio Hondo College

Although there are no sure-fire recipes for good health, the mixture of regular exercise and healthy eating comes awfully close. According to the *New England Journal of Medicine* (Myers et al. 2002), poor physical fitness is a better predictor of death than smoking, hypertension, and heart disease. Although tobacco is still the top cause of avoidable deaths, the widespread pattern of physical inactivity combined with unhealthy diets is poised to top the list because of the resulting epidemic of obesity **Figure 1** (Mokdad et al. 2004). Americans are sitting around and eating themselves to death, with obesity closing in on tobacco as the nation's leading underlying preventable killer. The alarming part is that behavior is going in the wrong direction.

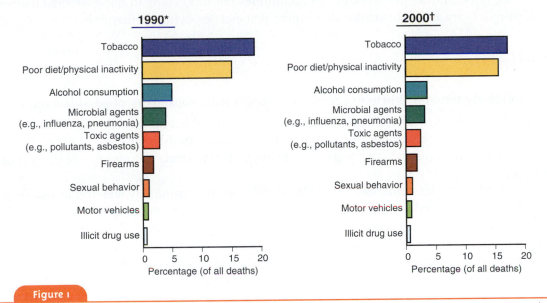

**Figure 1**

Comparing actual causes of death in the United States from 1990 to 2000. (*Sources:* * McGinnis J. M. and Foege W. H. *Journal of the American Medical Association,* 1993; 270(18):2207–2212; † Mokdad A., Marks J., Stroup D., and Gerberding J. Actual causes of death in the United States, 2000. *Journal of the American Medical Association,* March 10, 2004; 291:1238–1245.

Regular exercise, or physical activity, can do everyone a world of good. It helps prevent heart disease, diabetes, osteoporosis, and a host of other diseases. It is also a key ingredient for losing weight or maintaining a healthy weight.

With all these advantages, it is mind boggling that only a minority of Americans get enough exercise or leisure-time physical activity to benefit them. Studies that have followed the health of large groups of people for many years, as well as short-term studies of the physiologic effects of exercise, all point in the same direction: *A sedentary (inactive) lifestyle increases the chances of becoming overweight and developing a number of chronic diseases.*

Exercise or regular physical activity helps many of the body's systems function better and keeps a host of diseases at bay.

According to the U.S. Surgeon General's report, *Physical Activity and Health* (U.S. Department of Health and Human Services 1996) regular physical activity:

- Improves your chances of living longer and living healthier
- Helps protect you from developing heart disease and its precursors, high blood pressure and high cholesterol

- Helps protect you from developing certain cancers, including colon and breast cancer
- Helps prevent or control type 2 diabetes (previously called adult-onset diabetes)
- Helps prevent arthritis and may relieve pain and stiffness in people with this condition
- Helps prevent the insidious loss of bone known as osteoporosis
- Reduces the risk of falling among older adults
- Controls weight

If you do not currently exercise and are not very active during the day, any increase in exercise or physical activity is good for you. Some studies show that walking briskly for even one to two hours per week (15 to 20 minutes per day) starts to decrease the chances of having a heart attack or stroke, developing diabetes, or dying prematurely.

## Definitions

The following terms will help to get you started toward a vocabulary of good health.

**Health**  The 1946 World Health Organization's definition of health has been used as a foundation for the contemporary term of wellness (WHO 1946): "Health is a state of complete physical, mental, and social well-being and not merely the absence of disease or infirmity."

In 1990, the Joint Commission on Health Education terminology stated that health is "an integrated method of functioning which is oriented toward maximizing the potential of which the individual is capable. It requires the individual to maintain a continuum of balance and purposeful direction with the environment where he (sic) is functioning." This definition suggests that health is much more than simply not being sick.

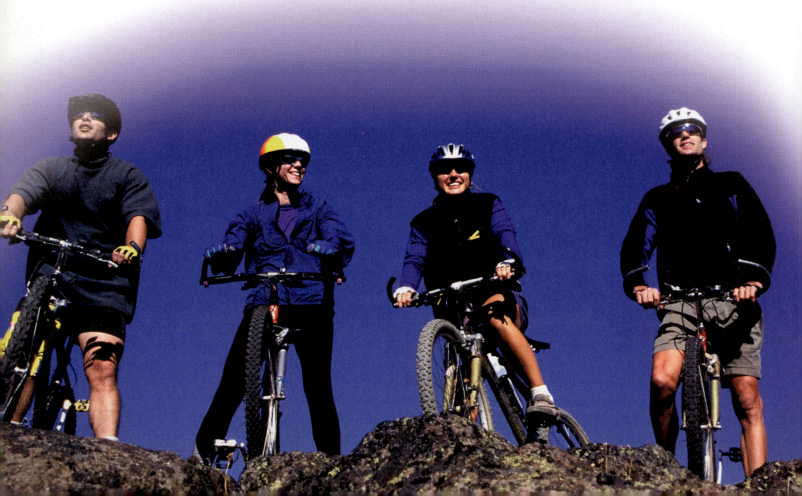

**Wellness** There are many definitions of wellness. All definitions focus on the nature of personal responsibility as being a key to wellness. The National Wellness Institute offers the idea that wellness is an active process of becoming aware of and making choices toward a more successful existence. Wellness is multidimensional consisting of six dimensions: (1) social, (2) occupational, (3) spiritual, (4) physical, (5) intellectual, and (6) emotional. These dimensions are interdependent. Thus, as a person affects one dimension, whether positively or negatively, other dimensions are also influenced.

**Physical activity** Bodily movement produced by skeletal muscles that increases energy expenditure.

**Exercise** Planned, structured, and repetitive physical activity done to improve or maintain one or more components of physical fitness.

**Physical fitness** A set of attributes that people have or achieve that relates to the ability to perform physical activity. Health-related components of physical fitness include:

- Cardiorespiratory endurance
- Muscular strength
- Muscular endurance
- Flexibility
- Body composition

# National Wellness Goals

The U.S. Department of Health and Human Services (DHHS) has launched *Healthy People 2010* (2000), a comprehensive, nationwide health promotion and disease prevention agenda. *Healthy People 2010* serves as a road map for improving the health of all people in the United States during the first decade of the 21st century.

*Healthy People 2010* identifies the leading health indicators intended to help everyone more easily understand the importance of health promotion and disease prevention and to encourage wide participation in improving health in the next decade.

Two of the 10 leading health indicators, (1) physical activity and (2) overweight and obesity, are the major focus of this book. Indicators affecting the health of people also include:

1. Physical activity
2. Overweight and obesity
3. Tobacco use
4. Substance abuse
5. Responsible sexual behavior
6. Mental health
7. Injury and violence
8. Environmental quality
9. Immunization
10. Access to health care

## Physical Activity

Regular physical activity throughout life is important for maintaining a healthy body, enhancing psychological well-being, and preventing premature death. The evidence in favor of this position is growing and is more convincing than ever! People of all ages who are generally inactive can improve their health and well-being by becoming physically active. Despite the proven benefits of physical activity, more than 50% of American adults do not get enough physical activity to provide health benefits. Twenty-five percent of adults are not active at all in their leisure time.

## Overweight and Obesity

Overweight and obesity are major contributors to many preventable causes of death. On average, higher body weights are associated with high death rates.

In the United States, obesity has increased at an epidemic rate during the past 20 years. Research indicates that the situation is worsening rather than improving.

Where do we need to focus our efforts? The answer lies in focusing on individuals changing their health-related lifestyles. That is why Chapter 1, about changing to a healthier lifestyle, forms the foundation of enhancing your health and wellness.

*Fit to be Well* offers simple, workable approaches for being healthy and fit that can easily be added into your lifestyle and schedule. A healthy lifestyle incorporates all facets of fitness. The goal is to introduce simple ways to integrate each of these elements into your daily life. As you progress through the chapters you will find easy-to-follow guidelines for:

- Modifying your lifestyle behaviors
- Increasing your self-esteem and creating a more positive self-image
- Eating a balanced and nutritional diet
- Keeping your body composition and weight at healthy levels
- Improving physical endurance, strength, and flexibility
- Managing stress

*Fit to be Well* aims to increase your awareness of each aspect of a physically fit lifestyle. By adding self-assessments and related labs to each of the chapters, this text becomes an interactive guide to building and implementing a fitness program that will work with your individual needs and schedule.

## Getting Started

Right from the start, Chapter 1: Changing to a Healthy Lifestyle, has you actively participating as you learn how to effectively change your behavior. The nine chapters that follow provide a fitness road map that will guide you through:

- Preparing for Physical Activity and Exercise (Chapter 2),
- Improving Cardiorespiratory Endurance (Chapter 3),
- Increasing Flexibility (Chapter 4),
- Increasing Muscular Strength and Endurance (Chapter 5),
- Choosing a Nutritious Diet (Chapter 6),
- Maintaining a Healthy Body Composition and Body Weight (Chapter 7),
- Managing Stress (Chapter 8),
- Keeping Heart Smart: Preventing Cardiovascular Disease (Chapter 9),
- Preventing Cancer (Chapter 10),
- Avoiding Addictive Behaviors (Chapter 11)
- Preventing Sexually Transmitted Infections (Chapter 12), and
- Responsible Decision Making (Chapter 13).

You are the most important person taking care of your health. The key to taking responsibility for yourself is learning what works for you and then implementing what you have learned into your daily life. Some people view fitness-related goals as impossible dreams. The truth, however, is that everyone is capable of obtaining a healthy lifestyle. Keep in mind that every change you make is significant, no matter how big or small.

## References

Mokdad A., Marks J., Stroup D., and Gerberding J. Actual causes of death in the United States, 2000. *Journal of the American Medical Association,* March 10, 2004; 291:1238–1245.

Myers J., Prakash M., Froelicher V., Do D., Partington S., and Atwood J. E. Exercise capacity and mortality among men referred for exercise testing. *New England Journal of Medicine,* March 14, 2002; 346:793–801.

U.S. Department of Health and Human Services (DHHS). *Healthy People 2010: Understanding and Improving Health.* Washington, DC: DHHS, 2000. http://www.healthypeople.gov/

U.S. DHHS, Centers for Disease Control and Prevention (CDC). *Physical Activity and Health: A Report of the Surgeon General.* Atlanta, GA: DHHS, 1996. http://www.cdc.gov/nccdphp/sgr/sgr.htm.

World Health Organization (WHO). Preamble to the Constitution of the World Health Organization as adopted by the International Health Conference, New York, June 19–22, 1946; signed on July 22, 1946 by the representatives of 61 states (*Official Records of the World Health Organization,* no. 2, p. 100) and entered into force on April 7, 1948.

## CHAPTER 1

# Changing to a Healthy Lifestyle

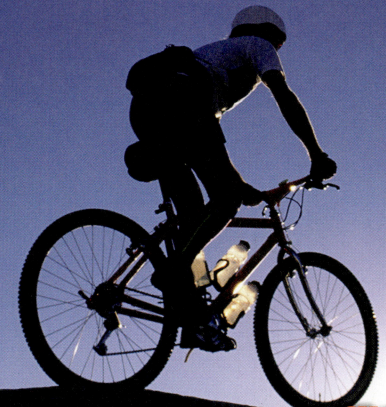

## Objectives

After reading this chapter, you should be able to:

- Describe the benefits of changing to a healthier lifestyle.
- Describe the Stages of Change model used in changing to a healthy lifestyle.
- Design a personal contract for changing a health-related behavior.

**It is not the strongest of the species that
    survives,
Nor the most intelligent,
But the ones most responsive to change.**

—Charles Darwin

## Focus on Lifestyle

It is important to take a healthy look at your lifestyle. More than half of the leading causes of death in this country are preventable.

Actual causes of death reflect lifestyle and behavioral factors, such as smoking and physical inactivity, that contribute to this nation's leading killers, including heart disease, cancer, and stroke Figure 1.1 . By changing these unhealthy behaviors people can improve their health and reduce their risk of disease.

Many individuals do not worry about their health until they lose it. Many have unsuccessfully tried various diets and a succession of exercise programs. This chapter offers methods, if used, that will enable you to develop a healthier lifestyle by changing a health-related behavior.

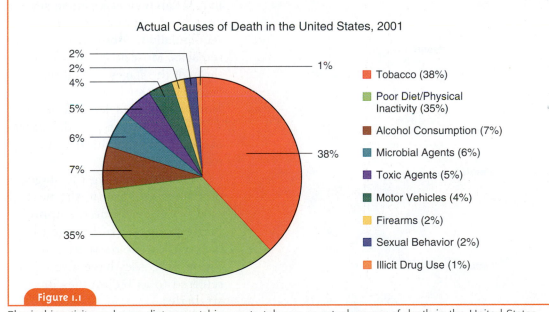

**Figure 1.1**

Physical inactivity and poor diet are catching up to tobacco as actual causes of death in the United States. (*Source:* Modified from http://www.cdc.gov/nccdphp/factsheets/death_causes2000_access.htm.)

## Changing Behavior

It is never very easy to change, and for some individuals, it is extremely difficult. Why do some people find it so difficult to adhere to a healthy lifestyle while others find it easier? One answer involves the short-term pleasure of inappropriate behavior and the delayed nature of its negative health consequences. Some prefer dealing with life by playing the odds that they will not contract a problem like heart disease or cancer.

Research reveals that good educational programs can increase knowledge and foster positive attitudes. However, these factors have not been found to reliably influence long-term behavior change toward healthier lifestyles. While mastery of accurate information is necessary, it may not sufficiently empower most people to allow them to control their behavior. Conversely, the ability to use self-management techniques often helps individuals make lifestyle changes.

Prochaska and colleagues developed the Transtheoretical Model of Change, better known as the Stages of Change model, which can help us to change a problem behavior (Prochaska, Norcross, and DiClemente 1994). This model says that people move through a series of stages of change (some call it a readiness to change). Its authors describe behavior change as a process, not an event. Change does not happen overnight—it could take weeks, months, or even years.

In adopting healthy behaviors (e.g., regular physical activity) or eliminating unhealthy ones (e.g., eating saturated fat), people progress through five stages related to their readiness to change. At each stage, different intervention strategies help them progress to the next stage. The five distinct stages are:

1. Precontemplation
2. Contemplation
3. Preparation
4. Action
5. Maintenance

Progression through the stages of change is cyclical rather than linear. Rarely does a person successfully go through the stages sequentially without encountering setbacks. Most people will recycle through the stages several times before being successful (Prochaska, Norcross, and DiClemente 1994). **Figure 1.2** represents the stages of change in a graphical cyclic manner.

After identifying the stage of change you are in, the next step is to determine the appropriate processes of change to be used for the particular stage. These processes have also been referred to as techniques or strategies.

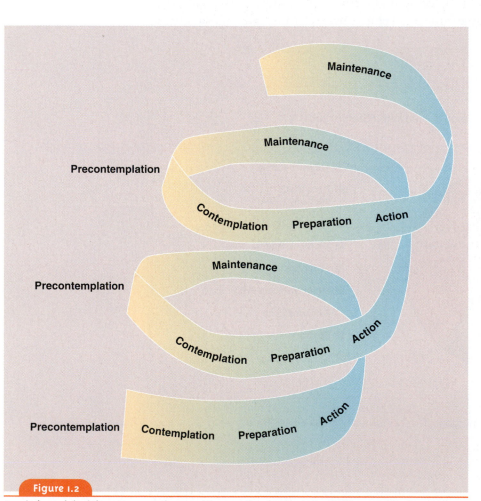

**Figure 1.2**

A spiral model of the stages of change. (*Source:* Prochaska J. O., DiClemente C. O., and Norcross J. C. In search of how people change: Applications to addictive behaviors. *American Psychologist* 1992; 47:1102–1114. Copyright ©1992 by the American Psychological Association. Reprinted by permission.)

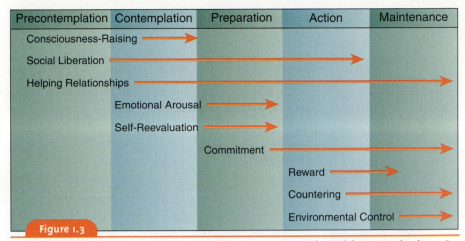

Figure 1.3 matches the processes of changes and the stages of change.

Refer to Table 1.1 for the major processes of change. These are activities and experiences that individuals engage in when they attempt to change a behavior.

The key to successful change is to determine what stage you are in, and then to decide what processes (strategies) to use. There is no set time frame for each stage; you may spend more time in one stage than another. Change is a process that is unique to the individual and situation.

Figure 1.3

Select appropriate processes to promote change. (*Source:* Adapted from Prochaska J. O., Norcross J. C., and DiClemente C. O. *Changing for Good.* New York: Quill, 2002. www.changecompanies.net/change_model.htm.)

## Table 1.1 Processes That Promote Change

| Processes of Change | Stages of Change | Examples of Techniques |
|---|---|---|
| **Consciousness-raising:** increased awareness | Precontemplation Contemplation | Read news stories or a book; watch a TV program; talk with a friend or doctor |
| **Social liberation:** societal support for the healthy behavior change | Precontemplation Contemplation Preparation Action | Availability of a health club; restaurants offering low-fat/low-carb foods |
| **Helping relationships:** support system of family, friends, and co-workers | All five stages | Discuss your plans with others; join with another who is working on the behavior |
| **Emotional arousal:** emotional experience related to the unhealthy behavior | Contemplation Preparation | Personal testimony of someone who has solved a similar behavioral problem; seeing someone suffering the harmful consequences of his or her unhealthy behavior |
| **Self-reevaluation:** understanding that your behavior is how you are known | Contemplation Preparation | See yourself as fit |
| **Commitment:** making a firm commitment to change and believing that it can be done | Preparation Action Maintenance | Make a New Year's resolution; tell others about your intentions |
| **Reward:** increasing the rewards for positive behavioral change and decreasing the rewards for unhealthy behavior | Action Maintenance | Reward the behavior change (e.g., buying new clothes, movie ticket) |
| **Countering:** substituting healthy behavior for an unhealthy behavior | Action Maintenance | Take a walk instead of watching TV |
| **Environmental control:** avoiding triggers or using cues | Action Maintenance | Avoid dessert parties; leave encouraging messages on a calendar or stuck to the mirror or refrigerator |

*Source:* Adapted from Prochaska J. O., Redding C. A., and Evers K. The Transtheoretical Model and Stages of Change, in *Health Behavior and Health Education: Theory, Research, and Practice*, Glanz K., Lewis F. M., and Rimer B. K. (eds.), San Francisco: Jossey-Bass, 1996.

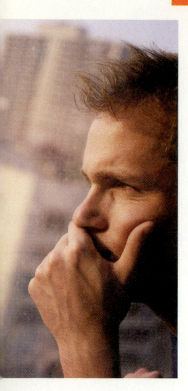

In addition to the stages and processes, the Stages of Change model features several other unique insights:

### Weighing Pros and Cons

At each stage, a person weighs the pros and cons of adopting a new behavior. To help people move toward change, it is necessary to make the pros outweigh the cons. This is especially true in the precontemplation and contemplation stages.

### Temptation

Change is difficult and a combination of cravings, emotional stress, and social situations can lead a person back to old habits. Not only is this possible, but it should also be expected. Should you slip or have a setback, do not think of this as a failure, but learn from it. What caused this setback? Now that you have learned this, avoid it next time! Remember: Change is a cycle that can move both forward and backward. Either way, the process continues!

# Stage 1: Precontemplation

Precontemplation is the stage in which you are not ready to make a change in your life in the foreseeable future. Many individuals in this stage do not believe they have a problem and have often constructed defenses that aid in the denial of the problem. Many of us know that it is important to make healthy choices, but in a world full of temptations and unhealthy alternatives it is often difficult to find the strength to make those changes in our lives.

### Difficulty Living a Healthy Lifestyle

People often find it difficult to adhere to a healthy lifestyle of self-control because of:
- Firmly established habits
- Immediate gratification—people often want instant results or pleasure
- Delayed negative health consequences of an unhealthy lifestyle—it may take years or even decades before the effects are seen; "it won't happen to me" belief in which it is assumed that poor health happens to others but not me; prefer dealing with life by taking risks or playing the odds that they will not contract a disease or get injured
- Too much scientific information, which sometimes overwhelms or confuses
- Fear of failure—often based on past failed attempts
- Feeling a loss of control over one's life
- Too many choices from which to pick for type of exercise, food, and weight control

# Stage 2: Contemplation

The contemplation stage occurs when you are aware that a problem exists and are seriously thinking about overcoming it, but have not yet made a commitment to take action. This is a time of reflection. Finding the reasons to change, the motivation to reach a goal, and the strength to make a plan work requires a lot of soul-searching. This stage can take a good amount of time and should not be rushed. As important as it is to make a healthy change in your life, take the time to find what truly motivates you and your behavior. This stage is the key to a successful course of action.

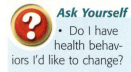

**Ask Yourself**
- Do I have health behaviors I'd like to change?
- Do I participate in activities that do not promote health?
- Do I practice behaviors passed down through my family?

**The Inside Track**

**Failure and Change**

American society does not accept failure. In fact, those who fail are seen as "bad" or "inadequate." You must change your outlook on failure when it comes to behavior. There's an old saying: "without failure, there is no learning." It may take many tries, and many failures, before you find an approach that works. You must simply keep trying!

# What Helps Change a Lifestyle?

Factors that influence an individual to change may include:

- Increasing knowledge—this can influence one's behavior, but often may not be enough to influence people to change. The maxim "Why do we do what we do, when we know what we know?" illustrates that knowledge often is insufficient to affect behavior.

- Motivation, having a reason—a person may want to change to avoid sickness, to look and feel better, to live longer, or because of pressure from a spouse, child, or friend.

- Readiness—motivation is required, but may involve physical capabilities as well. Another maxim—"You can lead a horse to water, but you can't make it drink"— may reflect a lack of motivation or perhaps the physical inability to act for a variety reasons.

- Landmark events—resolutions to change often occur at the start of a new year, during a personal health crisis, on a birthday, upon the birth of a child, or the death of someone close to you.

- Self-management techniques—the ability to employ them helps individuals to make lifestyle changes.

## Motivation

Motivation is what drives us to make changes. No matter how big or how small the change may be, we must be inspired to make choices. Finding what inspires or motivates you is an essential step in making a successful adjustment in your lifestyle.

Motivations for change could include:

- Improving self-image and/or self-esteem
- Being a role model for someone else
- Improving relationships with family and peers
- Reducing stress
- Reducing risk of disease

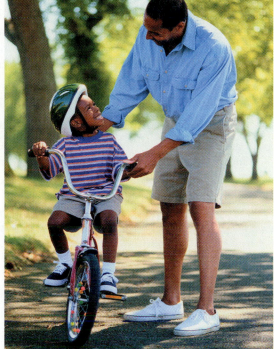

## Locus of Control

Life involves many struggles for control. Sometimes external factors can control aspects of your life for a moment. At other times the power is in your hands. The key to change is locating what controls a certain behavior. A locus of control is the figurative place where a person locates the source of responsibility in his or her life. It can be external or internal.

**An external locus of control could be:**

- Believing others' actions determine your actions
- Environmental factors—weather, location, and so on
- Another person or social group
- Blaming outside influences for your behavior

**An internal locus of control might be:**

- Self-expectations
- Internal thoughts ("I can do this")
- How open one is to change

To create a successful change in your life, you must be the one who takes the responsibility for your actions. Individuals with an internal locus of control are more likely to see their behavior as something they can adapt or change. If you believe it is within your abilities, you may experience greater success!

# Stage 3: Preparation

The preparation phase combines intention and behavior. Here you will monitor your behavior, analyze and identify patterns in your activity, and then set a goal. The most important concept in this stage is honesty. It is easy to try and make your behavior fit a certain pattern or profile. Sometimes the truth isn't what we want to see, but it is imperative to set realistic goals and to achieve real changes. When in the preparation stage, individuals are intending to take action within the next 30 days.

## Self-Monitoring

Self-monitoring means observing and recording one's own behavior. This process is necessary to:

- Make you aware of the size and seriousness of a problem
- Provide a benchmark to compare your original behavior (the point at which you began to try to change) with your later behavior

Behaviors need recording as they occur, not days later. Self-monitoring devices to measure the frequency of a behavior include:

- A health notebook, journal, or diary to record the occurrence of a behavior
- Counters to collect data (e.g., pedometers, golf counters)
- Graph paper (horizontal axis represents time—usually days—and vertical axis represents the amount of the behavior to be changed—body weight, exercise, number of hours of sleep) **Table 1.2**

**Ask Yourself**

- Why do I want to make this change?
- For whom am I changing? If we choose to change for our own well-being instead of trying to garner the attention of others, we are more likely to maintain the progress.

| Table 1.2 | Self-Managed Behavior Change Graph |
|---|---|

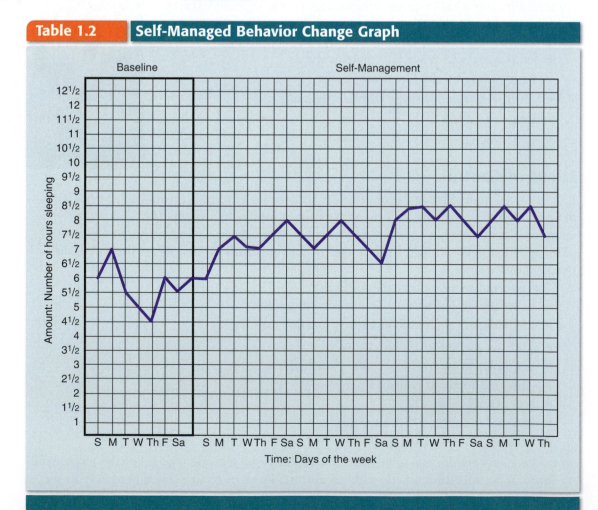

## Analysis

Once you have gathered your data, sit back and review your record. You are looking for patterns or clues about why and how you engage in the unhealthy behavior you wish to change. You should look at the following:

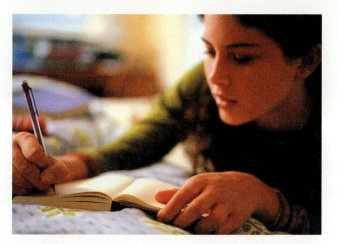

- **Time.** When during the day or week do you find yourself resorting to the activity? Is it linked with another activity (e.g., smoking after a meal or with a beer)?

- **Place.** Is there a specific place that you tend to be during the activity (e.g., making unhealthy diet choices on the way to class)?

- **Reason.** Can you link the behavior with a mood or an event that might trigger it (e.g., indulging in comfort food before an exam)?

Sometimes these aspects may not be immediately clear. Take a few days to look over your log. Remember that you are analyzing your behavior, not you as an individual. Keep a positive outlook—this behavior may be less than perfect, but you are making strides to change it, and that is more than the majority can say!

## Goal Setting

At this point, you have determined the where, when, and why for your behavior in question. The next step is to set a goal. Don't rush through this step. You may think that the goal is obvious, but certain factors must be taken into consideration for this goal to be effective. It must be:

- **Realistic.** While it is good to aim high, watch out for making your goal a bit too ambitious. If you set an unrealistic goal, you will become frustrated along the way and lose your motivation quickly. Aim for a moderate expectation—one that will challenge you but is within your ability. Remember that you can always set a higher goal once you reach this one.

- **Quantitative.** Many times people set goals that are very abstract (i.e., wanting to lose weight). That is a fine ambition, but it is not an effective goal. You want your goal to be quantitative so that you can track your progress. A more effective goal would be to lose 10 pounds, or to stretch for 30 minutes three times a week. Try to define your goal in some type of measurable unit: minutes, pounds, number of servings, percentages, quantities, and so on.

- **Broken down in steps.** If you start out thinking that you are aiming toward this one big goal from the beginning, you will find that it is easy to get discouraged during the first few weeks. You need to choose a goal that can be broken down into smaller intermediate steps—mini goals—along the way. For example, if the goal is to stop drinking soda, perhaps the mini goals could be to cut back to three sodas per day, then two, then one, and so on. Make sure your mini goals are quantitative.

- **Tracked on a timeline.** Having the ambition to live a healthy lifestyle is different than trying to achieve your goal. The ambition can be carried with you for as long as you want. The goal, however, must have an end date. By using a timeline it is easier to keep your progress on track. The end date is not the end of the healthy behavior. After you have completed your goal within the time frame you chose, be sure to continue practicing the healthy habits until they stick!

- **Important to you.** If you do not feel that this goal is important or worthwhile, it will not be a success. It does not matter how many people tell you that your goal is great, you have to believe in it yourself. If you don't, go back and revise the goal until it fits with your expectations and your motivation.

Having a plan and a contract will help further your success as you begin to reach toward your goal. See a personal contract in Figure 1.4.

**The Inside Track**

**Graduated Regimen Implementation**

Starting a new behavior or stopping a behavior all at once is difficult.

Graduated programs can shape desired behaviors. Example: slowly start exercising.

## The Plan

The plan is where you break your goal down into manageable steps. Your plan should include:

- What you will need. Do you need a newly stocked cabinet with healthier food? Do you need a gym membership? What equipment will you need for each of your steps?
- What is your timeline? When will you start this plan? When is your ending date for your goal?
- The steps you will take. Your goal should be broken down into smaller mini goals, each with its own timeline.

PERSONAL CONTRACT

Start Date: ______________________ Finish Date: ______________________

The Goal: ______________________________________________

Motivation (benefits): ______________________________________________

Identify your current stage of change: ______________________________

Match your current stage of change and other stages you anticipate progressing through with the appropriate processes of change (see Figure 1.3):

______________________ ______________________

______________________ ______________________

What specific techniques will you use for each of the processes identified above (see Table 1.1)?

| Processes | Specific techniques |
|---|---|
| | |
| | |
| | |
| | |
| | |

Stage of change on the finish date:

| Mini goals | Date | Reward |
|---|---|---|
| | | |
| | | |
| | | |

I, ______________, agree to work toward a healthier lifestyle and in doing so shall comply with the terms and dates of this contract.

Signature: ______________________ Date: ______________________

Witness: ______________________ Date: ______________________

Figure 1.4

A personal contract to bind yourself to your chosen course of action.

## Tipping Point

### Contracting with Others

- Contracting with another person makes the contract a public commitment.
- This person should have a meaningful relationship with you—a roommate, friend, parent, or relative, for example.
- Have this person review your contract and sign it as a witness to your new commitment.
- A commitment to friends and family is less likely to be broken than just a personal commitment.

## The Contract

Write a contract binding yourself to the chosen course of action. Your contract should include:

- **Start date** Write the date that you will begin your plan.
- **Finish date** Write the date when you will have completed your goal.
- **The goal** Be specific and concise.
- **Motivation (benefits)** Determine what is in it for you.
- **Identify your current stage of change.**
- **Identify the processes (strategies) of change** Use Figure 1.3 for each possible stage of change.
- **For each process of change to be used, identify a specific technique.** See Table 1.1.
- **Identify the stage of change when you finish.**
- **Mini goals with rewards** What are the intervals along the way that will indicate you are making progress?
- **Your signature** Sign your name as a sign of your commitment to your plan.
- **Witness signature** Have a close friend or family member sign your contract as well.

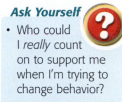

**Ask Yourself**
- Who could I *really* count on to support me when I'm trying to change behavior?
- What challenges will I face when I try to change?

# Stage 4: Action

The action stage is where you begin to move toward a healthier behavior. You have your motivation, your internal locus of control, and your goal. You are ready to make this change! Action involves the most observable behavioral changes and requires considerable commitments of time and energy.

## Tipping Point

### Rewards

- Self-contracting means you establish and administer your own rewards.
- Rewards are meant as motivation to keep the momentum going until you reach your goal.
- Rewards should be given immediately and frequently but in moderate amounts.
- Tailor your rewards to your individual taste—make sure they are desirable enough to motivate you.
- The reward should not be associated with the negative behavior you are trying to change. For example, if you are trying to lose weight, don't make your reward a brownie.

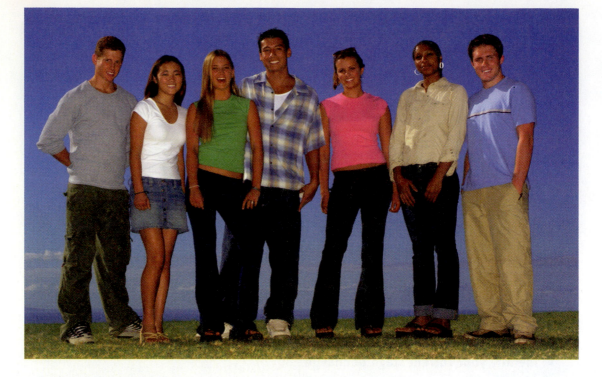

Sometimes the action phase can dwindle down, leaving the success of your plan vulnerable to barriers.

The five main barriers to successful change are:

- Social impact
- Stress
- Postponing
- Justification
- Denying responsibility

## Social Impact

There can be both positive and negative social impacts on your plan to change a behavior.

Positive social impacts may be in the form of:

- Structured support groups
- Cheerleading by friends and family
- Role models—people around you to whom you look up to and admire

Negative social impacts may include:

- Feeling like the odd one out
- Peer pressure
- Attending functions that tempt you to break your contract

Let those around you know that you are trying to change this specific behavior. They may be able to offer tips and suggestions to help you along. More importantly, if you explain your goals to them, they are more likely to respect your decision and less likely to pressure you into relapsing into old behavior patterns.

## Stress

One of the biggest barriers to changing lifestyle behaviors is stress. Stress can occur anywhere in our daily lives and without the correct management techniques it can lead you away from your goal. Eating comfort food, drinking, and engaging in other reckless behavior are common ways that many people deal with stress—none of which are effective or

## Tipping Point

### Dealing with Negative Social Impact
- Realize that this is your individual goal. Not everyone around you will have the same intentions as you.
- Stay committed to your goal. Review your contract before you go out to remind yourself how important this change is to you.
- Try and choose healthy alternatives whenever possible.
- Be a role model to others. By sticking with your plan and committing yourself to a healthier lifestyle, you may motivate others to do the same!
- Have a friend who wants you to push the limits of your goal? Assign that person as your personal coach or cheerleader. By making him or her feel like a responsible party in your plan, that individual may very well take on a role of support rather than peer pressure!

healthy. Learning effective coping techniques can not only make it easier for you to stay on track with your plan of action, but will also help you to create a better sense of wellness overall. You will cover stress and its impact on your health more completely in Chapter 8.

When life throws curve balls at you, try these helpful tips to calm down and get back on track:

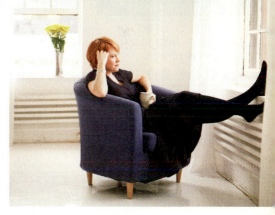

- Close your eyes and count to 10. Take deep breaths between each number.
- Have a CD on hand with calming music. Put it on and focus on the music for 5 minutes.
- Keep a journal. Record how you feel; sometimes just getting your thoughts on paper can help release tension.
- Go for a short brisk walk. The change of scenery and fresh air can renew your mood.
- Stop, stretch your muscles, and breathe deeply.

## Postponement

After that initial surge of motivation in the beginning of the action phase, it can get difficult to muster the energy to continue to make the healthy choices. Many times the steps to reaching your goal get pushed aside or postponed until a later point in time. It is best to stop the procrastination as soon as you feel yourself slipping into that mindset.

When you realize that you are postponing a step in your plan:
- Stop and identify out loud that you are procrastinating.
- Try to pin down why you are avoiding that particular step. For example, is cold weather causing you to avoid going to the gym? Or is that healthy dish too time-consuming to make?
- Once you have identified why you are postponing a particular step, try to revise that step to fit better with your life. For example, buy a few exercise videos for working out at home when the weather is bad. Or, find simpler recipes that still offer the same nutritional value.

## Justification

Many times when we procrastinate we justify or rationalize our actions. We make excuses for why we have not completed the task. It is important to catch yourself if you find that you are justifying not meeting your goal or one of your steps. Your plan may quickly

### What's the word. . .

**stress** The physical and emotional tension that comes from situations the body perceives as threatening.

**procrastination** Pushing a task to a later point in time.

**rationalization** Making excuses for not carrying out a task.

---

## Tipping Point

### Avoiding Procrastination

- Mark your calendar, daily planner, or appointment book.
- Leave messages on the refrigerator, bulletin board, or wall calendar; next to the bed; or on the bathroom mirror.
- Set your alarm, enter your goal in your computer, or have a friend call you.

---

become a slippery slope where nothing is accomplished, but everything is rationalized. When you feel yourself making excuses:

- Say your excuse out loud and listen—is it credible?
- Write down those times when you push your task off and explain why you did so. If you find yourself falling off course with your goal, these logs will provide a good resource describing when and why you aren't meeting each step.
- Understand that there will be times when you can't complete a step that second. Make sure that you are justifying the valid procrastinations, not the ones made out of low motivation.

### Denying Responsibility

*What's the word...*

**blaming** Placing the responsibility of an unmet goal on someone else.

Along with justification can come **blaming**. Blaming occurs when you displace the responsibility for missing a step or not completing a goal onto someone else (external locus of control). Because of *him/her/them* or what *they* did, the goal was not met. This is an easy trap to fall into as it is convenient and gives the appearance that you are not at fault. You are the victim. No matter how good blaming looks on paper, it will not help you reach your goal. You will still be left with an unfinished plan. It is important to accept responsibility for your own actions.

## Stage 5: Maintenance

After at least 6 months in the action stage, the person may move into the fifth stage: maintenance. This phase is when you keep up the new healthier habits that have replaced the old habits. Change is maintained more easily now. There may be an initial excitement

## Reflect ›››› Reinforce ›››› Reinvigorate

### Knowledge Check

*Answers in Appendix D*

1. What is the first stage of change?

   A. Preparation
   B. Precontemplation
   C. Action

2. An effective plan for changing a behavior should have:

   A. The steps to be taken
   B. How long it will last
   C. List of items needed
   D. All of the above

associated with making a change in which your motivation and commitment will both be high and the outlook toward your goal is positive.

Many of the activities used in the maintenance phase are the same as you'll use if you are in the action phase, just with small adaptations. For instance:

- **Rewards** You still need to set reward dates; however, they are more distant and the rewards should become smaller as the behavior becomes more natural.
- **Environmental control** Once the first set of influences is overcome, new ones can be established.

## Issues to Face in Maintenance

### Relapse

Relapse can occur at any stage of the change process. It can be triggered by many things: an extra stressful day or week, an unexpected event, low levels of motivation. If you find yourself relapsing along the way, try to identify a reason. Are you losing motivation? Is your plan unrealistic? Do you not have the right equipment or facilities?

This is a process; nothing is set in stone. You have the freedom to go back and revise your goal at any time. Don't be afraid to reevaluate your plan. If something is not working for you, find alternatives that will still help you change the behavior. Most importantly: Do not give up! A relapse is normal—it doesn't mean that you will never complete your goals. It is a minor setback that can be overcome.

### Acceptance

Acceptance is the finish line. The old unhealthy behavior has been fully replaced at this point. Not only have you completed your goal, but you have also integrated healthy habits into your daily routine. Be aware that this stage may not come quickly. Achieving your goal and dealing with relapses may take a long while, but your healthy new lifestyle is definitely worth it.

# Conclusion

Lifestyle change is a process that involves many steps and a lot of persistence. It is possible to have multiple changes taking place at once. The chapters in this text provide a wealth of information on many different aspects of healthy living. By incorporating each topic into your daily life, you will be working toward a more rounded sense of wellness.

3. Which factors influence a person to change?
   A. Obtaining more knowledge
   B. The ability to use self-management skills
   C. Having a reason
   D. All of the above

For each of the following, identify which stage of change the person is in, two strategies that may move the person to the next stage, one significant barrier the person may face, and a method to overcome that barrier.

4. Experiencing an episode or time frame when current behavior goes back to previously discontinued behavior is called:

   A. Maintenance

   B. Relapse

   C. Action

   D. Acceptance

5. When an individual makes excuses for not taking action on an issue, he or she is said to be:

   A. In denial

   B. Preparing

   C. Procrastinating

   D. In action

6. Lateisha has researched the benefits of becoming active. She has developed a scheme to move forward and is scheduled to begin taking steps in 2 weeks. What stage is Lateisha in?

   A. Contemplation

   B. Preparation

   C. Action

   D. Maintenance

7. The individual behavior responsible for more deaths than any other behavior is:

   A. Alcohol consumption

   B. Use of illegal drugs

   C. Irresponsible sexual behavior

   D. Tobacco use

8. The strategy that substitutes a healthy behavior for an unhealthy one is called:

   A. Reinforcement

   B. Self-evaluation

   C. Countering

   D. Emotional arousal

## Modern Modifications

The chapters in this text illustrate a wide variety of the important aspects of a healthy lifestyle. In each chapter there will be a section in which you will be given a chance to:

- Take a moment to look at your lifestyle in the terms of the topic discussed. What would you like to change in that area of your life?

- Go through and pick one of the suggestions provided. These suggestions are meant to be easily absorbed into your daily routine and offer immediate opportunities for change.

- Congratulate yourself. You are one step closer to a happier healthier lifestyle. Even small changes can make a big difference!

## Critical Thinking

1. Angela had been involved in ballet for many years, and she now wants to begin dancing again. She knows she lacks the flexibility to do so, but is willing to work on it—she just isn't sure how.

2. Max has been smoking since he was 12 (he is now 22). He looks forward to that first drag in the morning and is unconcerned with all the "hype" about cancer. Everyone in his family smokes and no one has ever gotten cancer!

## Going Above and Beyond

### Websites

MedlinePlus: Exercise and Physical Fitness
*http://www.nlm.nih.gov/medlineplus/exercisephysicalfitness.html*

Physician and Sports Medicine
*http://www.physsportsmed.com*

*Morbidity and Mortality Weekly Report*
*http://www.cdc.mmwr.gov*

Transtheoretical Model
*www.uri.edu/research/cprc/transtheoretical.htm*

### References and Suggested Readings

Marcus B., et al. Assessing motivational readiness and decision-making for exercise. *Health Psychology* 1992; 22:257–261.

Prochaska J. O. Strong and weak principles for progressing from precontemplation to action on the basis of twelve problem behaviors. *Health Psychology* 1994; 13:47–51.

Prochaska J. O. and Markus B. H. The Transtheoretical Model: Applications to Exercise, in *Advances in Exercise Adherence*, Dishman R. K. (ed.), Champaign, IL: Human Kinetics, 1994.

Prochaska J. O., Norcross J. C., and DiClemente C. O. *Changing for Good.* New York: HarperCollins Publishers, 1994. Reprinted by Quill, 2002.

Prochaska J. O. and Velicer W. F. The transtheoretical model of health behavior change. *American Journal of Health Promotion* 1997; 12:38–48.

U.S. DHHS. *Healthy People 2010.* Washington, DC: DHHS, 2000.

———. *Physical Activity and Health: A Report of the Surgeon General.* Atlanta, GA: DHHS, 1996.

Zimmerman G. L., et al. A "Stages of Change" approach to helping patients change behavior. *American Family Physician*, March 1, 2000: American Academy of Family Physicians.

# Preparing for Physical Activity and Exercise

## Objectives

After reading this chapter, you should be able to:

- Identify the health-related concerns of inactivity.
- Identify the health benefits of physical activity.
- Choose activities using the Physical Activity Pyramid.
- Describe the principles behind a successful workout.

# Recent Trends of Inactivity and Health-Related Concerns

Daily activity may affect health more than any other factor—more than physical environment, even more than genetics. Diseases and disabilities need not be inevitable consequences of the aging process.

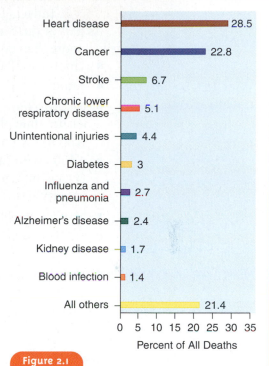

## The Dangers of Inactivity

Millions of Americans suffer from chronic illnesses that can be prevented or improved through regular physical activity. Inactivity can contribute to or exacerbate each of the following conditions that relate to the leading causes of death Figure 2.1:

- Coronary heart disease
- Heart attacks
- Diabetes
- Colon cancer
- Bone fractures
- High blood pressure
- Obesity

The risk for developing each of these disorders is decreased with as little as 30 minutes of activity per day.

# Components of Physical Fitness

It is easy to become confused regarding the terms of physical activity and exercise. In this context, physical activity is any activity that engages the body, while exercise is considered a series of coordinated movements specifically intended to increase physical performance. Both physical activity and exercise are essential when creating a balanced workout.

## Physical Activity

Physical activity includes any activity that gets you up and moving throughout the day. These activities could include grocery shopping, mowing the lawn, taking the dog for a walk, or shoveling a driveway. While they may not be specifically intended to increase your muscular or cardiovascular endurance, daily physical activities are just as important as structured exercise.

## Exercise

Four different elements of exercise provide the basis of a balanced workout program. These components are made up of structured activities aimed at increasing specific elements of fitness. The Centers for Disease Control and Prevention (CDC) defines these "components of physical fitness" as:

- **Cardiorespiratory endurance:** "the ability of the body's circulatory and respiratory systems to supply fuel during sustained physical activity."

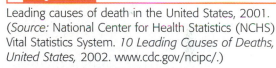

**Figure 2.1**

Leading causes of death in the United States, 2001. (*Source:* National Center for Health Statistics (NCHS) Vital Statistics System. *10 Leading Causes of Deaths, United States,* 2002. www.cdc.gov/ncipc/.)

Figure 2.1 (bar chart — Percent of All Deaths):
- Heart disease: 28.5
- Cancer: 22.8
- Stroke: 6.7
- Chronic lower respiratory disease: 5.1
- Unintentional injuries: 4.4
- Diabetes: 3
- Influenza and pneumonia: 2.7
- Alzheimer's disease: 2.4
- Kidney disease: 1.7
- Blood infection: 1.4
- All others: 21.4

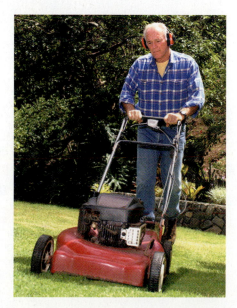

- **Muscle strength and endurance:** "the ability of the muscle to exert force during an activity . . . and . . . the ability of the muscle to continue to perform without fatigue."
- **Flexibility:** "the range of motion around a joint."
- **Body composition:** "the relative amount of muscle, fat, bone, and other vital parts of the body."

## Who Is Active?

Fewer than 50% of adults achieve the recommended amount of regular physical activity **Figure 2.2**. In fact, 16% of all adults are not active at all (NCCDPHP 2001).

As part of the National Health Survey, the National Center for Health Statistics interviewed more than 68,000 adults age 18 and older and found the following:

- Three out of 10 adults were physically active on a regular basis.
- Young white males were most likely to exercise.
- Nearly 8 out of 10 adults with graduate-level degrees engaged in some form of leisure-time physical activity, or twice as many as people having less than a high school diploma.
- Adults with incomes of at least four times the poverty level were twice as likely to engage in regular leisure-time physical activity as adults with incomes below the poverty line.
- Married men and women were most likely to be physically active.
- Single adults who had never been married were most likely to engage in strengthening activities such as weight lifting.
- Widowed adults were less likely than married adults to engage in physical activities.

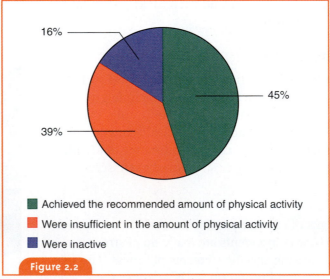

16%

45%

39%

■ Achieved the recommended amount of physical activity
■ Were insufficient in the amount of physical activity
■ Were inactive

**Figure 2.2**

Physical activity statistics in the United States, 2001. (*Source: National Center for Chronic Disease Prevention and Health Promotion (NCCDPHP). U.S. Physical Activity Statistics: 2001 state summary data,* 2001.)

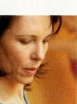

- Approximately 67% of adults living in the western United States were physically active compared to 56% of those living in the South.
- Adults living in the suburbs were more likely to be physically active than those in urban or rural areas.
- Nearly half of young adults aged 12–21 are not vigorously active on a regular basis.

# Benefits of Physical Activity

Deciding to become physically active brings many benefits. A common misconception, however, is that increasing your activity level helps only your physical health. This couldn't be more wrong. The benefits of physical activity involve all aspects of wellness, which combine to create an improved sense of well-being.

According to the National Center for Chronic Disease Prevention and Health Promotion (NCCDPHP), regularly participating in moderate to vigorous intensity physical activity "reduces feelings of depression and anxiety, promotes psychological well-being and reduces feelings of stress," as well as "lowering risk of developing coronary heart disease, stroke, non-insulin-dependent (type 2) diabetes mellitus, high blood pressure, and colon cancer by 30–50 percent." **Figure 2.3** gives more information on the effects of being physically active.

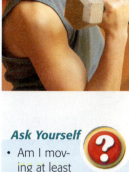

**Ask Yourself**
- Am I moving at least 30 minutes every day?

As you can see, being active not only improves the physical domain of your personal wellness, but also has a direct influence on your emotional health and may positively influence your social and environmental dimensions. Specific benefits include increases in self-esteem, risk reduction for many diseases, strong bones, promotion of a healthy weight, reduction in feelings of stress, provision of time for personal reflection, an increase in outdoor time, and provision of quality time with family and/or friends.

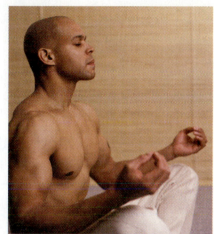

Exercise is a great way to relieve stress. It reduces muscle tension; stimulates regular, deep breathing; increases blood levels of endorphins; and creates an opportunity to free the mind from worries. The next time you exercise, see if you can become aware of these four stages of stress relief through exercise.

**Stage 1: Paying Attention**

At the beginning of an exercise session, focus your mind on the activity and allow any thoughts that arise to pass out of your mind. When you notice them, simply say to yourself, "Oh, I have a thought," and bring yourself back to focusing on your activity.

**Stage 2: Interested Attention**

After a period of concentrating and letting go, you no longer have to concentrate on eliminating distractions, and you sense a flowing with the activity.

**Stage 3: Absorbed Attention**

Absorption with the activity is so great that it is very difficult for you to be distracted by what is going on around you. You may experience altered perceptions of space and time, and your mind may move through thoughts and images without your direction. The experience can be dreamlike, except that you are entirely awake and attentive.

**Stage 4: Merging**

You are no longer aware of any separation between you and what you are doing. The experience of union is complete: physical, mental, and spiritual. You attain a complete loss of self-consciousness, and even though you may be working your body very hard, mentally and spiritually you feel very calm.

**Figure 2.3**

Stages of exercise-induced relaxed concentration. (*Source:* Edlin G., et al. *Health and Wellness,* 7th ed. Sudbury, MA: Jones and Bartlett, 2002:142.)

**2**

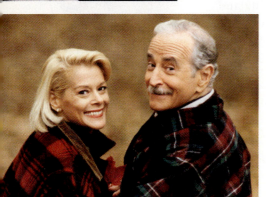

# Before Starting

## Check Your Health Status

Moderate physical activity, like walking the dog, gardening, or working around the house, is not dangerous for most people, and no medical clearance is needed.

Complete the Physical Activity Readiness Questionnaire (PAR-Q) (Lab 2-1). If you answered "yes" to any of the checklist items, discuss your answers with a physician *before* having your fitness assessed or starting a fitness program.

The American Heart Association suggests that you see a doctor before exercising if:

- You have a heart condition
- You take medicine for your heart and/or blood pressure
- You get pains in your chest, left side of your neck, or your left shoulder or arm when you exercise
- Your chest has been hurting for about a month
  - You tend to get dizzy, lose consciousness, and fall
  - Mild exertion leaves you breathless
  - You have bone or joint problems that a doctor told you could be worsened by exercise
  - You have an overweight or obesity problem
  - You have a medical condition, such as insulin-dependent diabetes, that requires special attention in an exercise program
  - You are middle-aged or older (40 years for men; 50 years for women)

## Gather the Basics

### What Do I Need to Begin?

- Loose, comfortable clothes
- Walking or cross-training shoes—preferably in good condition
- Hat and sunscreen, if you plan to be outdoors
- Bottle of water
- A safe place to walk
- Time—will vary depending on the speed and distance you walk and an adequate amount of time to warm up and cool down

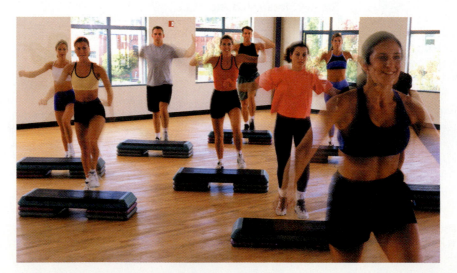

# Components of Physical Fitness and the Physical Activity Pyramid

The Physical Activity Pyramid  Figure 2.4  promotes a balanced "diet" of weekly physical activity. It suggests a healthy dose of daily physical activity combined with certain amounts of the four components of exercise.

Each component of physical fitness has its place in the pyramid. At the base is general *physical activity*. These activities simply get you moving. *Cardiorespiratory endurance* is the next level. These activities will probably make you sweat, raise your heartbeat, and keep it there for a minimum of 20 minutes. On the third level, you find *muscular strength and endurance* activity as well as *flexibility* activities. All four categories will be covered in much greater depth in their own chapters later in the text.

At the top of the pyramid is sedentary activity. Sedentary activities do not involve movement and in greater amounts have a negative impact on personal health status.

The pyramid follows the Frequency, Intensity, Time, and Type (FITT) guidelines:

- **Frequency** of the activity: The number of times an exercise or group of exercises is performed within a certain time frame. Usually this is measured in sessions per week. How frequently you perform a certain exercise depends on the intensity of the exercise.

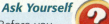

**Ask Yourself**

Before you begin your activity, ask yourself the following questions:

- Am I adequately rested to be physically active?
- Am I hydrated (about 2 cups water 2–3 hours before activity; 1 cup just before)?
- Did I warm up (light activity for 5–10 minutes)?
- Did I stretch the major muscle groups?

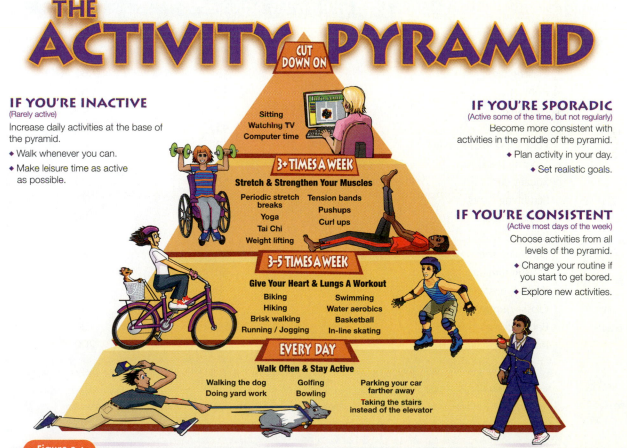

**Figure 2.4**

The exercise and physical activity pyramid. (*Source:* The Activity Pyramid © 2003 Park Nicollet Health Innovations, Minneapolis, MN, 1-888-637-2675. Reprinted with permission.)

- **Intensity** of the activity: The amount of energy exerted while performing an exercise.
- **Time** or duration of the activity: The measurement of how long an exercise or group of exercises takes to complete.
- **Type** of activity: The classification of exercise. Daily activity, cardiorespiratory endurance, muscle strength, and flexibility are all different types of activities.

## Cumulative Moderate Activity

It can be difficult to set aside large blocks of time each day for exercise when you are first beginning a fitness regimen. The great news about daily physical activity (Level 1 on the pyramid) is that you can accumulate a moderate amount of activity throughout the week. A moderate amount of physical activity is roughly equivalent to physical activity that uses approximately 150 calories of energy per day, or 1000 calories per week. This can be achieved in a variety of ways. **Table 2.1** illustrates the number of calories burned per minute for a variety of daily activities. If you have only a couple of short intervals of time to work out each week, you would choose a more intense exercise. If you have large frequent blocks of time, less vigorous exercise may be more appropriate.

For every physical activity or exercise session be sure to **warm up** before and **cool down** after. Skipping over or rushing through these two phases of an activity can be dangerous.

| **Table 2.1** | **Calories Used by Everyday Activities*** | |
| --- | --- | --- |
| | **Calories Used in 10 Minutes†** | |
| **Activities** | **Women** | **Men** |
| Walking fast | 45 | 60 |
| Painting | 45 | 60 |
| Weeding | 45 | 60 |
| Washing a car | 45 | 60 |
| Playing tag with a child | 50 | 67 |
| Mowing the lawn | 55 | 73 |
| Square dancing | 55 | 73 |
| Scrubbing floors | 55 | 73 |
| Hiking off-trail | 60 | 80 |
| Biking to work | 60 | 80 |
| Shoveling snow | 60 | 80 |
| Moving furniture | 60 | 80 |
| Walking upstairs | 70 | 93 |
| Cross-country skiing | 80 | 106 |
| Backpacking | 80 | 106 |
| Running upstairs | 150 | 200 |

*Use an average of 200 calories per day by doing these activities and decrease your risk of disease and live longer, without ever going near a gym or treadmill.

†Figures are for a 132-pound woman and a 176-pound man. All values are approximate and will vary from person to person.

*Source:* Edlin G., and Golanty E. *Health and Wellness,* 8th ed. Sudbury, MA: Jones and Bartlett, 2004:133.

**What's the word...**

**frequency** How often; the number of times an exercise or group of exercises is performed within a certain time frame.

**intensity** How hard; the amount of energy exerted while performing an exercise.

**time** How long; the duration of an exercise or group of exercises.

**type** The classification of exercise.

**The Inside Track**

**Intensity levels**

**Light-intensity:** You should be able to sing while doing the activity.

**Moderate-intensity:** You should be able to carry on a conversation comfortably while engaging in the activity.

**Vigorous-intensity:** You become winded or too out of breath to carry on a conversation.

## The Warm-up

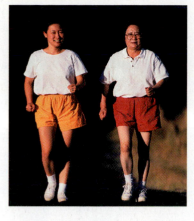

- Takes 5 to 10 minutes of low-intensity movement, such as walking, before stretching inactive muscles.
- Prepares your body for physical activity by gradually increasing muscle temperature and metabolism.
- Increases blood flow and oxygen delivery to the muscles, protects tendons, and lengthens short, tight muscles.
- Gives the body a chance to redirect blood to active muscles.
- Gives the heart time to adapt to increased demands.
- Ends with stretching the major joints with some range-of-motion movements.

## The Cool-down

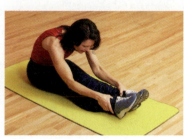

- Takes 5 to 10 minutes using the same muscles just exercised at a reduced pace.
- Consists of light, general movements and stretching or ending your chosen physical activity gradually.
- Helps to avoid the pooling of blood in the muscles and to remove metabolic end-products such as lactic acid and carbon dioxide.
- Determines how you feel several hours after your activity, as it can reduce muscle soreness, cramps, and stiffness.
- Ending with stretching also improves flexibility. Some experts feel it is best done at the end of the cool-down rather than while warming up.

### What's the word...

**warm-up** The 5–10 minutes of low-intensity movement at the beginning of a workout that prepares the body for activity by increasing muscle temperature and metabolism.

**cool-down** The 5–10 minutes at the end of a workout involving light movement and stretching.

**overload** Placing a greater-than-normal amount of stress (within reason) on the body to make it function at a higher capacity.

**specificity** The type of physical changes you desire in your body relates directly to the type of exercise you choose.

**progression** The gradual increase of the level and intensity of exercise.

**reversibility** The principle that states that the results of physical fitness are not permanent.

# The Principles of a Successful Workout

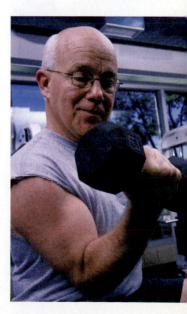

Physical fitness is dependent on many different factors. The following principles should be taken into account when designing an exercise program:

**Overload.** For an exercise to have an effect on the body, some level of stress must be placed on it. Overload refers to placing a greater-than-normal amount of stress (within reason) on the body in an attempt to make it function at a higher capacity, thereby increasing endurance and/or strength.

**Specificity.** The type of physical changes you desire in your body relates directly to the type of exercise you choose.

**Progression.** By gradually increasing the frequency, intensity, and time of exercise, the body is able to gain improvement in strength and endurance.

**Reversibility.** The results of physical fitness are not permanent. If you become inactive for an extended period of time, you may lose a good portion of strength and endurance that you have built up. It is important to maintain your fitness level with regular activity.

**Consistency.**　The only way to keep in shape is to participate in physical activities on a frequent and regular basis. Sporadic bouts of exercise will not result in increased fitness levels.

**Individual differences.**　We all differ in the maximum level of fitness we can and want to achieve. What works for one person may not work as well for another.

**Safety.**　Train, don't strain. Safety involves being aware of all aspects of your exercise routine. From learning the correct way to use a machine to knowing the limits of your body, there are numerous things that you should pay attention to in order to keep your body safe and healthy while you exercise.

**Rest.**　Your body needs rest to recover from strenuous workouts. Back-to-back high-intensity workouts merely break down muscles and never give them a chance to grow stronger.

## Tipping Point

### Tips for Workouts

- Hard-workout days should be followed by easy-workout days or rest.
- Alternate between lifting weights and aerobic exercise from day to day.
- High-energy days should be your harder-workout days.
- On low-energy days simply rest or perform a light workout.
- Most of all: Listen to your body!

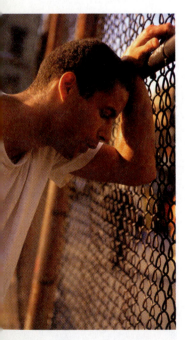

## Stay Motivated

Selecting an exercise that is right for you is just the first step in a successful exercise program. Making the necessary adjustments in your life to accommodate this new lifestyle change can be difficult. Procrastination, social pressures, stress, and busy schedules can hinder progress. Here are proven strategies to help motivate you to start exercising and to stay with it:

- Develop an exercise habit. Keep at it, knowing the more consistent you are in the beginning, the more fixed your new activity will become.
- Reserve a time slot each day for working out, and don't let anything interfere.
- Don't let others lead you astray. Inform everyone of your exercise time and that you would appreciate them respecting your choice.
- Seek support from friends and family, and believe that you can succeed.
- Be patient with yourself. Some days you will be more motivated or have more time than other days. A brief period of not exercising is not a disaster.
- Plan ahead and follow your plan. Decide when, where, how often, and with whom you will work out. Be prepared to exercise.
- Team up. Exercising with others can motivate you when you'd rather not exercise. But it can have a down side. A less motivated or less optimistic partner, for example, can drain you.
- Set realistic exercise goals. Set goals that you not only know you can achieve, but that are specific, not vague.

- Keep an exercise record. Place an exercise log on your refrigerator, in your bedroom, or in your office and record each session.
- Have fun. Customize your approach to make exercise more enjoyable. For instance, read, watch television, or listen to your favorite music while pedaling a stationary cycle.
- Add variety. Select activities that you enjoy. Cross-training helps.
- Affirm your efforts out loud each morning.
- Listen to your body. Your body may need a break at times.
- Complement exercise. In addition to exercising, be sure to eat a low-fat, balanced diet, sleep well, and avoid unhealthy influences like smoking and high stress.

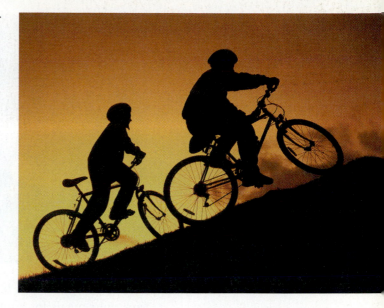

## For Exercise Drop-outs: How to Get Started Again

More than half the people who enroll in supervised exercise programs drop out within the first 6 months. So chances are, if you start exercising, at some point you are going to stop. Despite your best intentions, vacations, illnesses, and work responsibilities may wreak havoc on your regimen. How can you keep little breaks in your exercise program from meaning that you will never again break a sweat?

- Stop beating yourself up. Remind yourself that it is just a temporary suspension of your program. Look upon every relapse as a learning experience.
- Reevaluate your goals. Are you going to plan to stay on a 2-hour-a-day program 365 days a year for 10 years? If so, you're setting yourself up to fail. Instead, set realistic goals that include more activity some days and less on others.
- Get going. Perform some kind of physical activity today.
- Continually plan. If you are planning a trip or your workload picks up, think of strategies for incorporating short periods of physical activity into your day, which may prevent relapse.
- Most people find themselves starting over again at some point in time after dropping out of an exercise program. It is difficult to determine the long-term impact of a start-stop-start-stop pattern of exercise on health, although there may be a cumulative beneficial effect.

## Stay Safe

Physical activity comes with safety risks. Learning how to protect your body from injury and illness can make your fitness program that much more enjoyable. Here are some general guidelines for staying safe while staying active:

- Do not exercise if you have a cold or flu, and never exercise if you have a fever, chest pain, or breathing problem.
- Drink plenty of water. Do not wait until you are thirsty to drink water. You should be drinking 7–10 ounces of water for every 10–20 minutes of activity (Pfeiffer and Mangus 2004).

**What's the word. . .**

**exercise log** A record of your activity that includes the type, duration, and intensity of each exercise each day.

**cross-training** Combining the components of fitness in a workout program, instead of focusing on only one area.

**2**

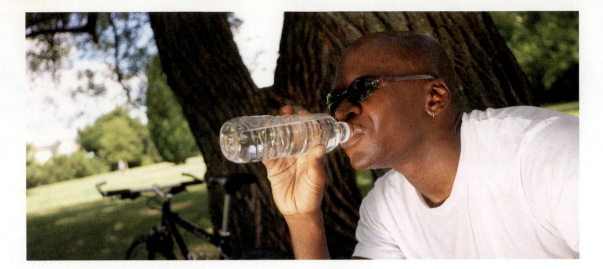

- Do not exercise if you have not had enough sleep, are fasting, or have just eaten. Save your meals for after exercise, and wait at least 2 hours after a heavy meal before exercising.
- Factors that can negatively affect your ability to handle extreme temperatures include not dressing appropriately for conditions, inadequate nutrition, dehydration, alcohol consumption, certain medications, and health conditions such as diabetes and heart disease.
- Wear the proper clothing, shoes, and equipment to prevent injuries.

## Be the Best and Expect the Best

Physical activity is essential to healthy living. It can ward off disease, relieve stress, and help increase self-esteem. By subscribing to a balanced diet of exercise and accumulating a moderate amount of daily physical activity, you are well on your way to a life of wellness. The following chapters in this book are designed to give you a gradual learning experience in fitness. The upcoming material will answer your questions, help you increase your understanding of physical activity, and encourage you to achieve a healthy lifestyle.

### Tipping Point

**Dress properly by following the guidelines below:**
- Wear clothing specific to the activity.
- Clothes should be comfortable and allow you to move freely.
- Cotton or cotton/polyester blend is recommended to allow for sweat evaporation.
- **Do not** wear clothing that restricts sweat evaporation. Sweating is how the body regulates its internal temperature.
- Wear additional clothing in layers to warm up or cool down as needed.
- The best protection against wind and rain is an outer layer that allows heat loss and sweat evaporation (e.g., Gortex).
- Women should consider wearing an exercise bra, and men, sports underwear (e.g., compression shorts or jockstrap).
- Protective equipment is needed for some activities (e.g., helmets for bikers and in-line skating).

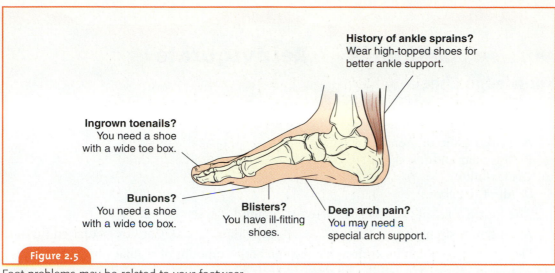

**History of ankle sprains?**
Wear high-topped shoes for better ankle support.

**Ingrown toenails?**
You need a shoe with a wide toe box.

**Bunions?**
You need a shoe with a wide toe box.

**Blisters?**
You have ill-fitting shoes.

**Deep arch pain?**
You may need a special arch support.

**Figure 2.5**

Foot problems may be related to your footwear.

## Tipping Point

The American Orthopedic Foot and Ankle Society makes several recommendations for selecting a good fitting shoe ( **Figure 2.5** and **Figure 2.6** ):

- Have both feet measured when they are at their largest: at the end of the day or after a run, walk, game, or practice.
- Wear your workout socks.
- Try on the shoes, because sizes vary by manufacturer.
- Make sure both shoes fit.
- Ensure that the shoe provides at least one thumb's width of space from the longest toe to the end of the toe box.

A variety of athletic shoes exist: running/jogging, walking, tennis, court, and cross-training. Properly sized socks help prevent blisters, ingrown toenails, and absorb perspiration.

Athletic shoes should have:

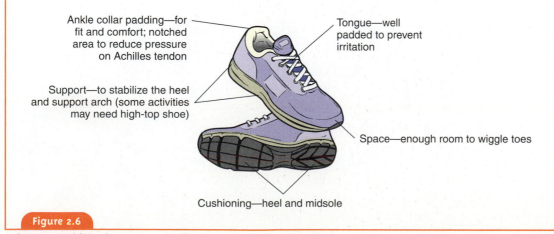

Ankle collar padding—for fit and comfort; notched area to reduce pressure on Achilles tendon

Tongue—well padded to prevent irritation

Support—to stabilize the heel and support arch (some activities may need high-top shoe)

Space—enough room to wiggle toes

Cushioning—heel and midsole

**Figure 2.6**

Select your athletic footwear carefully.

### The Inside Track

If you start to notice pain in your feet, ankles, legs, or knees even though you haven't changed your exercise routine, worn-out shoes may be a factor. Place your old shoes on a table or other flat surface and look at them from the back. If they lean inward or outward or show signs of excessive wear, such as badly worn edges of the sole, it's probably time for a new pair.

## Reflect >>>> Reinforce >>>> Reinvigorate

### Knowledge Check

*Answers in Appendix D*

1. The component(s) of physical fitness include:

   A. Cardiorespiratory endurance
   B. Muscular endurance
   C. Flexibility
   D. All of the above

2. The fourth level of the Physical Activity Pyramid is reserved for:

   A. Muscular strength       B. Rest       C. Stretching       D. Cardiovascular endurance

3. Less than _____ of adults achieve the recommended amount of regular physical activity.

   A. 16%       B. 27%       C. 39%       D. 50%

4. Mike has started going to the gym with his roommate. While lifting weights, Mike notices that his roommate can lift 30 pounds more than Mike can. Mike should not get discouraged because this disparity is due to:

   A. Individual differences
   B. Overload
   C. Consistency

5. Jim is on the track team. He used to stretch first thing when he went to practice, but recently his coach told the team that they should be stretching after their warm-ups. The coach changed the workout order because:

   A. The team was too impatient to stretch before their warm-up
   B. Stretching is safer when the muscles are warmer
   C. Stretching is not an important aspect of a workout

6. Amelia needs to buy a new pair of shoes for exercising. She has a history of ankle sprains. She should find shoes that offer:

   A. A wider toe box
   B. Special arch support
   C. A high-topped style that offers more ankle support

7. Deciding to pursue leg extensions to work directly on the quad muscles in the legs is an example of:

   A. Progression
   B. Specificity
   C. Overload
   D. Consistency

8. Joanie used to work out all the time, and she was pleased with her body. Now she is rarely active; she has gained weight and feels sluggish. The change in Joanie reflects what principle of fitness?
   A. Reversibility
   B. Progression
   C. Overload
   D. Safety

9. What is the acronym used to remember the dimensions of designing a workout?
   A. SPLAT
   B. BUFF
   C. WORK
   D. FITT

10. Which of the following is not a general rule related to clothing for exercise?
   A. Wear cotton or cotton blends to absorb sweat effectively.
   B. Clothing should allow you to move freely.
   C. Wear protective gear when necessary.
   D. All are general rules for exercise.

## Modern Modifications

Try these suggestions when you find yourself becoming sedentary:

- Take breaks from long periods of sitting. Get up and stretch every 15 minutes. Walk across the room a few times.
- While watching television do a couple of simple exercises. Try sets of crunches, leg lifts, or modified push-ups during the commercials.
- While sitting in class or at a computer for an extended period of time, sit only on the front 6 inches of the seat, keeping your back straight. Correct posture will naturally engage your abs and other muscle groups as you sit.
- Do not use the remote. Get up to change the channels or turn the power on/off.

## Critical Thinking

1. Leroy is a predominantly sedentary person but has decided to begin physical activity in 2 weeks. What stage is Leroy in? Based on the Physical Activity Pyramid, what activities should be in Leroy's plan for the first week?

2. Consider the activities you do around your house in the evening. Identify five moderate-level activities you could integrate into your evening routine.

## Going Above and Beyond

### Websites

American Alliance for Health, Physical Education, Recreation, and Dance
*http://www.aahperd.org*

American College of Sports Medicine
*http://www.acsm.org*

American Council on Exercise
*http://www.acefitness.org*

American Heart Association
*http://www.justmove.org*

Canada's Physical Activity Guide
*http://www.hc-sc.gc.ca/hppb/paguide*

CDC Physical Activity Information
*http://www.cdc.gov/nccdphp/phyactiv.htm*

Health A to Z
*http://www.healthatoz.com*

Medicine and Science in Sports and Exercise
*http://www.acsm-msse.org*

MedlinePlus: Exercise and Physical Fitness
*http://www.nlm.nih.gov/medlineplus/exercisephysicalfintess.html*

Physician and Sports Medicine
*http://www.physsportsmed.com*

## References and Suggested Readings

American College of Sports Medicine. *ACSM's Guidelines for Exercise Testing and Prescription,* Baltimore, MD: Lippincott Williams and Wilkins, 2000.

Balady G. J. Survival of the fittest—More evidence. *New England Journal of Medicine* 2002; 346:852–854.

Blair S. N., et al. Is physical activity or physical fitness more important in defining health benefits? *Medicine and Science in Sports and Exercise* 2001; 33(suppl 6):S379–S399.

Edlin G., et al. *Health and Wellness,* 7th ed. Sudbury, MA: Jones and Bartlett, 2002:142.

National Center for Chronic Disease Prevention and Health Promotion (NCCDPHP). *Components of Physical Fitness.* 2003. www.cdc.gov/nccdphp/dnpa/physical/components/index.htm [June 21, 2004].

NCCDPHP. *U.S. Physical Activity Statistics: 2001 State Summary Data.* 2001. http://apps.nccd.cdc.gov/PASurveillance/StateSumResultV.asp [June 18, 2004].

———. *Why Should I Be Active?* 2004. www.cdc.gov/nccdphp/dnpa/physical/importance/why.htm [June 18, 2004].

National Center for Health Statistics (NCHS) Vital Statistics System. *10 Leading Causes of Deaths, United States.* 2001. www.cdc.gov/ncipc/ [June 18, 2004].

Pescatello L. S. Exercising for health: The merits of lifestyle physical activity. *Western Journal of Medicine* 2001; 174:114–118.

Pfeiffer R. and Mangus B. *Concepts of Athletic Training,* 4th ed. Sudbury, MA: Jones and Bartlett, 2004:265.

U.S. DHHS. *Healthy People 2010.* The Healthy People 2010 Database, April 2004 Edition. http://wonder.cdc.gov/scripts/broker.exe [June 18, 2004].

———. *Physical Activity and Health: A Report of the Surgeon General.* Atlanta, GA: DHHS, 1996.

## CHAPTER 3

# Improving Cardiorespiratory Endurance

## Objectives

After reading this chapter, you should be able to:

- Differentiate between *aerobic* and *anaerobic* activities.
- Describe the benefits of cardiorespiratory exercises.
- Measure and assess your cardiorespiratory endurance.
- Design an appropriate cardiorespiratory exercise program.

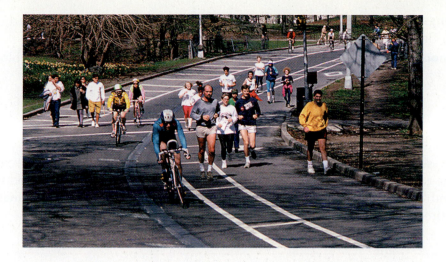

# The Doorway to Cardiorespiratory Activity

From a health standpoint, cardiorespiratory endurance activity is about as close as you can get to an elixir for physical health and well-being. It can help you lose weight, ease stress, boost your immune system, and reduce the risk of certain diseases.

There are a few *buzz words* that are basically synonymous with cardiorespiratory activity:

- Cardiovascular activity
- Cardiopulmonary activity
- Aerobic exercise

Merriam-Webster's dictionary defines *aerobic* as "occurring only in the presence of oxygen." When linked with exercise, *aerobic* refers to any activity that increases oxygen intake and heart rate.

When you exercise aerobically:

- You repeatedly contract large muscle groups, such as your legs and arms.
- You increase your breathing and your heart rate.

Examples of aerobic exercises include:

- Walking (brisk pace)
- Jogging/running
- Bicycling: road or mountain
- In-line skating or rollerblading
- Swimming
- Cross-country skiing
- Treadmill
- Stationary bicycle
- Stair climber
- Rowing machine
- Aerobic dancing

To understand how you benefit from these kinds of activities, you must first have a basic understanding of how the cardiorespiratory system works.

# Basic Physiology

The cardiorespiratory system consists of the following components:

- **Heart:** a muscle required to continuously deliver oxygen-rich blood to all the organs of the body

**3**

- **Lungs:** organs that provide the body with oxygen and rid the body of carbon dioxide through respiration
- **Blood vessels:** a system of arteries, veins, and capillaries that transport blood to and from the heart

# Cardiovascular Processes

The processes of respiration and circulation (pulmonary and systemic) are all connected within the cardiovascular system. Working together, the heart, lungs, and blood vessels deliver and transport oxygen to the body without stopping. **Figure 3.1** outlines this intricate process in eight basic stages.

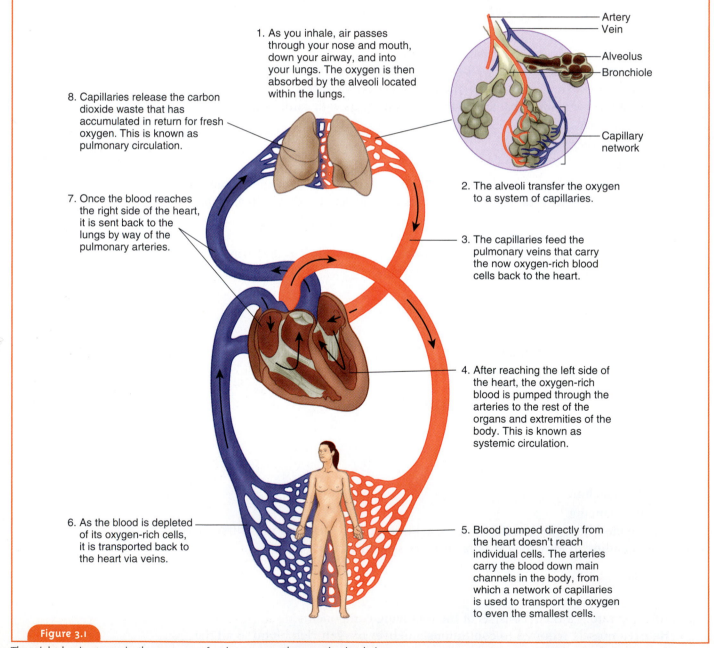

1. As you inhale, air passes through your nose and mouth, down your airway, and into your lungs. The oxygen is then absorbed by the alveoli located within the lungs.

Artery
Vein
Alveolus
Bronchiole
Capillary network

8. Capillaries release the carbon dioxide waste that has accumulated in return for fresh oxygen. This is known as pulmonary circulation.

2. The alveoli transfer the oxygen to a system of capillaries.

7. Once the blood reaches the right side of the heart, it is sent back to the lungs by way of the pulmonary arteries.

3. The capillaries feed the pulmonary veins that carry the now oxygen-rich blood cells back to the heart.

4. After reaching the left side of the heart, the oxygen-rich blood is pumped through the arteries to the rest of the organs and extremities of the body. This is known as systemic circulation.

6. As the blood is depleted of its oxygen-rich cells, it is transported back to the heart via veins.

5. Blood pumped directly from the heart doesn't reach individual cells. The arteries carry the blood down main channels in the body, from which a network of capillaries is used to transport the oxygen to even the smallest cells.

**Figure 3.1**

The eight basic stages in the process of pulmonary and systemic circulation.

The ability of the body to deliver oxygen to and from the heart is critical. The more active you are, the more efficient your pulmonary and circulatory systems become. The less active you are, the weaker your heart muscle will be. Being sedentary and out of shape may have a more detrimental effect on your health than other well-known risk factors such as smoking, high blood pressure, and heart disease (Myers et al. 2002).

The basic idea underlying cardiorespiratory or aerobic training is to place greater demands on the heart than what is required during rest. By regularly overloading the heart in this fashion, it will become stronger. This results in the heart pumping more blood and delivering more oxygen to the body per heartbeat, creating a lower resting heart rate. See Lab 3-1 to determine your current resting heart rate.

# Benefits of Cardiorespiratory Endurance Exercise

Regular endurance exercise can benefit the body in many healthy ways. Following are the short- and long-term benefits achieved by exercising regularly, using the cardiorespiratory system.

## Short-Term Benefits

Many people start a physical activity program because of its long-term benefits; however, it is the short-term benefits that keep them motivated to continue the habit.

### Relaxes and Revitalizes
Physical activity reduces mental and muscular tension and increases concentration and energy levels. Regular aerobic exercise releases endorphins.

### Increases Stamina
Exercise may cause fatigue immediately after the activity. Over the long term, though, it will increase stamina and reduce fatigue.

### Offers a Break from Daily Routine and Stress
Planned or unplanned physical activity can be enjoyable and provide a release from day-to-day stress and boredom.

### Helps You Feel Good About Yourself
Physical activity can improve your self-esteem and self-confidence, and enhance your general sense of well-being.

## Long-Term Benefits

### Decreases Risk of Heart Disease
The American Heart Association (AHA) has identified physical *inactivity* as a risk factor for cardiovascular diseases—primarily heart attacks and strokes, which are the leading causes of death in the United States (AHA 1995).

### Decreases Risk of Cancer
Physical activity lowers the risk of colon and breast cancer. Other types of cancers may also be less likely to occur in active people.

### Lowers Blood Pressure
High blood pressure increases the risk of heart disease, stroke, and kidney disease. Inactive people are more likely to develop high blood pressure than those who are active. Aerobic exercise can reduce the risks of high blood pressure.

**The Inside Track**

Before menopause, women have less cardiovascular disease than men do. After menopause, women's risk is closer to men's.

**What's the word. . .**

endorphins Proteins produced in your brain that serve as your body's natural painkiller. Endorphins also reduce stress, depression, and anxiety.

**The Inside Track**

Women's bone density is typically greatest in their mid-20s to mid-30s, but then declines slowly until menopause, which becomes a time of rapid bone loss. Physical activity performed during younger years will help women maintain good bone mass at menopause. Even physical activity begun later in life or during menopause will help slow the loss of bone.

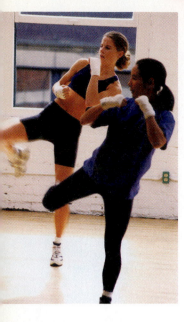

## Lowers Body Fat

**Obesity** is a risk factor for heart disease and a culprit in other diseases as well. Aerobic exercise preferentially burns fat, resulting in a decrease in total body fat.

## Improves Muscular Health

Aerobic exercise stimulates the growth of blood vessels and capillaries in the muscles, providing for more efficient oxygen delivery to the muscles and helping to remove irritating metabolic waste products such as lactic acid. This can reduce pain in those who have fibromyalgia and chronic low-back pain.

## Reduces Number of Sick Days

Many studies report that people who exercise regularly are less susceptible to minor viral illnesses, such as colds or flu, because of an improved immune system.

## Decreases Chance of Premature Death

In 1986, results from the Harvard Alumni Health Study published in the *New England Journal of Medicine* for the first time linked exercise with increased life spans. Since then, additional research has supported this finding.

## Decreases Cholesterol and Triglyceride Levels

High blood cholesterol and triglyceride levels increase the risk of heart disease. Regular exercise raises the level of *good* cholesterol, or high-density lipoprotein (HDL), which may help clear blood vessels and lower the level of *bad* cholesterol, or low-density lipoprotein (LDL). HDLs and LDLs are discussed further in Chapter 6.

## Decreases Risk of Diabetes

Physical activity lowers the risk of type 2 diabetes. Because it helps increase the ability of insulin to regulate blood sugar, it can decrease the need for drugs in those who already have **type 2 diabetes** (AHA 2004b).

## Decreases Risk of Osteoporosis

Gradual bone loss that may lead to fractures can be delayed by regular exercise. Exercise also is known to promote bone formation.

## Decreases Arthritis Symptoms

Regular exercise helps keep joints flexible and helps build muscle to support the joints.

---

**What's the word. . .**

**obesity** Excessive amounts of body fat.

**type 2 diabetes** A disease that involves the inability to produce an adequate amount of insulin.

---

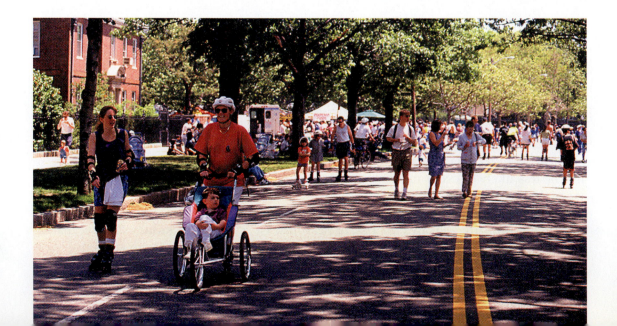

## Assessing Cardiorespiratory Fitness/Endurance

Cardiorespiratory fitness or endurance is largely determined by habitual physical activity. As defined earlier in the chapter, aerobic, or cardiorespiratory, exercise involves oxygen. When you assess your cardiorespiratory endurance, you are actually measuring how efficiently your system is using oxygen.

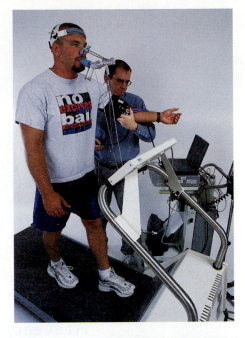

### Maximal Oxygen Uptake

Determining maximal oxygen uptake ($VO_{2max}$):
- Is the best measure of cardiorespiratory fitness
- Reveals how much oxygen is delivered to body tissues
- Requires an exercise physiology laboratory with trained personnel to analyze a person's oxygen intake

Maximal tests can be substituted with submaximal tests, which are a comparable way to score the $VO_{2max}$. They are less expensive, require little to no equipment, and are, therefore, more practical.

### Submaximal Tests

Submaximal tests can give a fairly good estimate of $VO_{2max}$:
- Monitoring your heart rate is necessary for these tests.
- Large numbers of people can be tested at one time.
- The tests require little equipment.
- Test results can be affected by a person's motivation and pacing ability.

The following tests are commonly used to judge cardiorespiratory endurance. The instructions for each are provided in the corresponding lab:
- *Rockport Fitness Walking Test (Lab 3-2, Activity 1)*
- *YMCA Step Test (Lab 3-2, Activity 3)*
- *1.5-Mile Run/Walk Test (Lab 3-2, Activity 2)*

Please complete the PAR-Q, Lab 2-1, before taking any of these tests.

> **What's the word...**
>
> **maximal oxygen uptake ($VO_{2max}$)** How efficiently the cardiorespiratory system uses oxygen.

## Designing a Cardiorespiratory Endurance Exercise Program

Every person has individual needs. Your exercise program should consist of physical activities that are right for your body and your endurance level, and that make you feel good, both mentally and physically. As you proceed with your program, make sure that you:
- Warm up and cool down
- Follow the FITT (Frequency, Intensity, Time, Type) guidelines
- Progress safely

### Warm-up

Begin each exercise session with a warm-up.
- Usually the warm-up involves the same activity as the workout, but at a low intensity.
- You can also simply swing your arms from side to side for a couple of minutes or walk around at a steady pace.

> **The Inside Track**
>
> A common mistake is stretching before muscles are warmed up. Not only is it difficult to stretch cold muscles, but there are risks to exercising heavily on muscles that are not warm, especially as you get older.

**3**

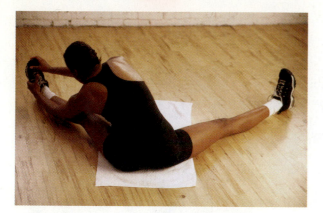

- After 5 to 10 minutes, stretch the primary muscles used in the warm-up before proceeding to the cardiorespiratory endurance exercise. A thorough list of stretching and flexibility exercises is provided in Chapter 4.

## Cool-down

End each exercise session with a cool-down.
- The cool-down should last 5 to 10 minutes and be done at a low intensity.
- Allow your heart rate, breathing, and circulation to return to normal.
- Stretch the primary muscles used.

## FITT Guidelines

After the warm-up, the FITT guidelines are an easy way to remember the essential facts for a good and effective aerobic exercise **Table 3.1**.

## Frequency

The American College of Sports Medicine (2000) recommends exercising 3 to 5 days each week within the target heart rate zone for cardiorespiratory fitness. More frequent exercising provides few additional benefits and may increase the likelihood of injury. Significant fitness loss occurs within 2 weeks of becoming inactive.

## Intensity

There are several ways to monitor exercise intensity. Five popular methods include:
- Maximum heart rate method
- Heart rate reserve method using the Karvonen formula
- Rate of perceived exertion method
- Calories burned
- Talk-test method

**The Inside Track**

Those who are considered obese should avoid vigorous-intensity workouts and should consult a doctor before beginning an exercise regimen.

| Table 3.1 | Aerobic FITT Guidelines | |
|---|---|---|
| Frequency | Start with 3 days per week and work up to 5 days per week. Exercising aerobically more than 5 days per week can lead to injury and is not necessary for promoting health. | |
| Intensity | Based on maximum heart rate:<br>70% to 85% | Based on heart rate reserve:<br>60% to 80% |
| Time | 20 to 60 minutes, within your target heart rate zone | |
| Type | Choose an aerobic activity that:<br>    Increases breathing, elevates heart rate, and maintains that heart rate level for an extended period<br>    Uses repetitive, rhythmic, large-muscle movements performed continuously over an extended time<br>Start-and-stop sports such as tennis, racquetball, and basketball are also aerobic, if skill levels allow for continuous play and are intense enough to raise heart rate to target levels. | |

*Source:* Adapted from American College of Sports Medicine.

Both the maximum heart rate and heart rate reserve methods are heart rate–based measurements. They work by measuring increases in heart rate. These methods provide a quick and easy way to gauge the intensity of your workout. However, an increase in heart rate is not the training stimulus; heart rate increase is merely indicative of the oxygen consumption required during the exercise.

## Maximum Heart Rate Method

According to the American College of Sports Medicine (ACSM), you should exercise using 70% to 85% of your maximum heart rate. To calculate your maximum heart rate, refer to Lab 3-1. To find your target heart rate zone, multiply your maximum heart rate (MHR) by 70% (low end of the range) and 85% (high end of the range):

Maximum HR _____ × 70% = _____ Low End of Target Zone
Maximum HR _____ × 85% = _____ High End of Target Zone

Take your pulse during your workout to determine whether the intensity of the exercise has increased your heart rate to the target zone.

## Calculating Heart Rate Reserve Using the Karvonen Formula

For this method you will need to calculate both your resting and maximum heart rates. Begin by finding your maximum heart rate, then subtract your resting heart rate from that number:

Maximum HR _____ − Resting HR _____ = _____ Heart Rate Reserve (HRR)

The ACSM recommends a target range of 60% to 80%. So, multiply the new value by 60% (low end of the range) and 80% (high end of the range).

HRR _____ × 60% = _____ New Value + Resting HR = _____ Low End of Target Zone BPM
HRR _____ × 80% = _____ New Value + Resting HR = _____ High End of Target Zone BPM

*What's the word...*

**target heart rate zone** A range of heart rates used to maintain optimal effects during aerobic exercise.

**pulse** The surge of blood that can be felt on certain points on the body each time the heart pumps blood into the arteries.

**rate of perceived exertion (RPE)** A person's own perception of the intensity of his or her exercise.

## Rate of Perceived Exertion

A person's own perception of the intensity of his or her exercise can often be as accurate as the heart rate in gauging exercise intensity. The Borg scale shown in **Figure 3.2** lets you determine your rate of perceived exertion (RPE). This scale consists of numerical ratings for physical exercise followed by their associated descriptive ratings (Borg 1982). Measurements are based on a 20-point scale. Six is no exertion and 20 is maximum exertion. To judge perceived exertion:

- Estimate how difficult it feels to do the exercise.
- Do not be concerned with any one single factor such as shortness of breath or work intensity.
- Concentrate on the total inner feeling of exertion.
- Multiplying the rating of perceived exertion by 10 roughly approximates the heart rate during exercise. These numbers were chosen because when multiplied by 10, they roughly equal the resting and maximum heart rate values of 60 and 200 beats per minute, respectively.

  For example, Mary Susan perceives she is exerting a 14 while dancing in her Scottish dance class. She multiplies that number by 10. This estimates that Mary Susan's heart rate for this kind of exercise is at or around 140.

- Once accustomed to a particular exercise, you will be able to estimate your heart rate based on your RPE. Most people should work out at a perceived exertion rate between 12 and 15.

**3**

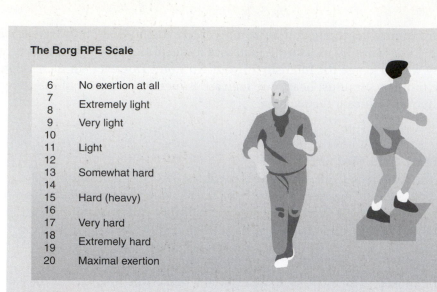

**The Borg RPE Scale**

| | |
|---|---|
| 6 | No exertion at all |
| 7 | |
| 8 | Extremely light |
| 9 | Very light |
| 10 | |
| 11 | Light |
| 12 | |
| 13 | Somewhat hard |
| 14 | |
| 15 | Hard (heavy) |
| 16 | |
| 17 | Very hard |
| 18 | |
| 19 | Extremely hard |
| 20 | Maximal exertion |

**Figure 3.2**

The Borg RPE Scale. Rating of perceived exertion (RPE) can be used to monitor your response to physical activity. (*Source:* For correct usage of the scale, see the instruction and administration given by Borg G. *Borg's Perceived Exertion and Pain Scales.* Champaign, IL: Human Kinetics, 1998; or the folder published by Borg on the RPE scale or the CR10 scale, Borg Perception, Furuholmen 1027, 762 91 Rimbo, Sweden.)

### Calories: Not Just Used for Dieting

Calories per hour is the amount of energy that an exerciser expends when maintaining the same exercise intensity for an hour. This value is calculated by most exercise machines and pedometers.

It is possible, of course, to calculate the number of calories you would burn by participating in a variety of activities. The basic formula is to multiply your weight (in pounds) by the number of minutes in the activity by a caloric expenditure figure. Caloric expenditures for several common activities are found in **Table 3.2**.

For example, if you weighed 120 pounds, and you bicycled at a moderate pace for 30 minutes, you would take $120 \times 30 \times 0.05$. The result indicates you burned 180 calories during that activity.

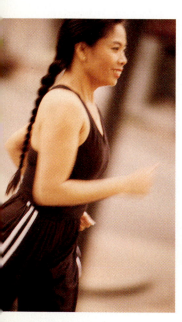

### Talk-Test Method

The talk-test method of measuring intensity is simple. A person who is active at a light-intensity level should be able to talk while doing the activity. One who is active at a moderate-intensity level should be able to carry on a conversation comfortably while engaging in the activity. If a person becomes winded or too out of breath to carry on a conversation, the activity can be considered vigorous.

### Determining the Appropriate Intensity for Your Workout

Now that you have calculated your target zone, determining the intensity level at which you should exercise is quite simple. The ACSM says that exercising at 70% to 85% MHR or 60% to 80% HRR for 20 to 30 minutes, excluding the time spent warming up and cooling down, enables most individuals to achieve good health, fitness, and weight man-

| Table 3.2 | Caloric Expenditures |
|-----------|----------------------|

| Activity | Calories per Minute per Pound | Calories per Hour per 150 Pounds | Activity | Calories per Minute per Pound | Calories per Hour per 150 Pounds |
|----------|-------------------------------|----------------------------------|----------|-------------------------------|----------------------------------|
| Archery | 0.034 | 305 | Rowing<br>  Light (2.5 mph)<br>  Vigorous | <br>0.036<br>0.118 | <br>325<br>1062 |
| Badminton<br>  Moderate<br>  Vigorous | <br>0.039<br>0.065 | <br>350<br>585 | Running<br>  6 mph (10-min mile)<br>  10 mph (6-min mile)<br>  12 mph (5-min mile) | <br>0.079<br>0.1<br>0.13 | <br>710<br>900<br>1170 |
| Basketball<br>  Moderate | <br>0.047 | <br>423 | Soccer | 0.06 | 540 |
| Baseball | 0.031 | 279 | Swimming<br>  25 yd/min<br>  50 yd/min | <br>0.058<br>0.071 | <br>520<br>640 |
| Bicycling<br>  Slow (5 mph)<br>  Moderate (10 mph)<br>  Fast (15 mph) | <br>0.025<br>0.05<br>0.072 | <br>225<br>450<br>550 | Table tennis | 0.025 | 225 |
| Dancing<br>  Moderate<br>  Fast | <br>0.045<br>0.064 | <br>405<br>575 | Tennis<br>  Moderate<br>  Vigorous | <br>0.046<br>0.06 | <br>415<br>540 |
| Fishing | 0.018 | 165 | Volleyball<br>  Moderate<br>  Vigorous | <br>0.036<br>0.065 | <br>325<br>585 |
| Gardening | 0.024 | 220 | Walking<br>  2 mph<br>  3 mph<br>  4 mph<br>  5 mph | <br>0.022<br>0.03<br>0.039<br>0.064 | <br>200<br>270<br>350<br>576 |
| Golf | 0.029 | 260 | | | |
| Hill climbing | 0.06 | 540 | | | |
| Jogging (4.5 mph) | 0.063 | 565 | Wrestling | 0.091 | 820 |
| Karate | 0.087 | 785 | | | |

agement goals. Your individual level of fitness will ultimately determine where you fall within this range.

When starting an exercise program, aim at the lowest value of your target zone during the first few weeks. Gradually build up to the higher values of your target zone—this may take at least 1 month or up to 6 months or more. The ACSM recommends that healthy adults gradually advance or progress in a cardiorespiratory exercise program to avoid muscle aches, pain, and discouragement.

You should always be able to catch your breath and speak comfortably while exercising. Feeling effort or maybe even slight discomfort is normal during some exercise. You should, however, never sense pain. Always warm up slowly and cool down gradually.

| Table 3.3 | Comparing Intensity of Physical Activity | | |
|---|---|---|---|
| **Intensity** | **Heart Rate Reserve (HRR) %** | **Maximal Heart Rate (MHR) %** | **Rating of Perceived Exertion (RPE)** |
| Very light | <25 | <30 | <9 |
| Light | 25–44 | 30–49 | 9–10 |
| Moderate | 45–59 | 50–69 | 11–12 |
| Hard | 60–84 | 80–89 | 13–16 |
| Very hard | >85 | >90 | >16 |
| Maximal | 100 | 100+ | 20 |

*Source:* Adapted from Public Health Service. *Surgeon General's Report on Physical Activity and Health.* Washington, DC: U.S. Government Printing Office, 1996.

## The Correlation Between Frequency and Intensity

Exercise classified as moderate or Level 1 in the Physical Activity Pyramid is recommended on a daily basis. If your goal is to:

- Maintain or improve general fitness—exercise at a moderate to hard intensity
- Maintain or increase performance-related fitness—occasionally exercise at a hard to very hard intensity

Exercise intensities of very hard to maximal should be performed only by individuals in excellent aerobic condition. Exercise in this range cannot be sustained for long time periods and is primarily performed to develop the anaerobic energy system and improve performance in activities such as sprinting. **Table 3.3** describes the relationships between exercise intensity and HRR, MHR, and RPE.

## Time or Duration of Exercise

A cardiorespiratory endurance session should vary from 20 to 60 minutes (single session or several sessions of 10 or more minutes each) to gain significant aerobic and fat-burning benefits. This does not include the warm-up and cool-down phases of your program. All beginners, especially those who are out of shape, should take a very conservative approach and train at relatively low intensities for 10 to 25 minutes. As you get into better shape, you can gradually increase the amount of time you exercise.

Gradually increase the duration of exercise before you increase the intensity. For example, when beginning a brisk walking program, be more concerned with increasing the number of minutes of the exercise session before you increase how fast you walk or add a hilly terrain.

## Type of Aerobic Activities

To choose the best exercises for you, consider the following:

- Choose exercise that involves several muscle groups and that is weight bearing. This will require the greatest amount of energy and oxygen to perform.
- Choose the exercises that you enjoy the most.
- Alleviate boredom and decrease your risk for injuries by cross-training or alternating the types of exercise you perform.

**Table 3.4** provides a few choices of indoor and outdoor aerobic activities, and the pros and cons of why you may or may not choose one of these activities for your exercise.

| Table 3.4 | Types of Indoor and Outdoor Aerobic Activity | |
|---|---|---|
| **Activity** | **Pros** | **Cons** |
| **Walking** | • Most popular of all activities<br>• No age limit—a lifetime activity<br>• Convenient<br>• Easily incorporated into lifestyle<br>• Little skill involved<br>• No cost<br>• Fewer injuries than jogging or running<br>• You can take in seasonal changes or walk through city streets and people watch<br>• This is a weight-bearing exercise<br>• Uses most major lower-body muscle groups | • Not active enough for some<br>• Takes three times longer to get the same aerobic benefit as from running<br>• Injuries can occur, such as shin splints and blisters |
| **Jogging/running** | • Convenient<br>• High levels of cardiorespiratory fitness benefits in short time periods<br>• Few skills needed<br>• Impact on hard surface builds stronger bones and offers protection against osteoporosis<br>• Euphoric feeling or "runner's high"<br>• In bad weather, you can run on an indoor track, if one is available<br>• Low cost—just need a good pair of running shoes<br>• Because it is often done outdoors, you get to view nature and a change of scenery | • Frequent, chronic injuries from impact to muscles, tendons, ligaments, and bones<br>• Injuries such as shin splints and stress fractures due to:<br>  • Improper warm-up<br>  • Excessive distances<br>  • Impact of feet and legs on ground<br>  • Wearing inadequate shoes<br>• Dangerous when done on roads with traffic<br>• Poor outdoor conditions (i.e., snow, pollution) may prohibit |
| **Bicycling: road or mountain** | • No age limit—a lifetime activity<br>• Fewer injuries than running because there is less impact on legs and feet<br>• Because it is done outdoors, you get to view nature and a change of scenery | • May be difficult to locate a safe place to ride<br>• Injuries include painful knees, feet, back, and saddle soreness<br>• Cost for the bike and other gear such as helmet, gloves, water bottle, sunscreen, and glasses |

*continues*

## Table 3.4 — Types of Indoor and Outdoor Aerobic Activity, *continued*

| Activity | Pros | Cons |
|---|---|---|
| **In-line skating or rollerblading** | • Lots of fun—curving, turning, gliding, sprinting, and spinning<br>• Change of scenery<br>• Works thighs, hips, and buttocks muscles | • There is a learning curve, which could make the beginning stages a bit dangerous<br>• May be difficult to locate a safe place to skate<br>• Some people have difficulty stopping<br>• Injuries may result from collisions, falling, and blisters<br>• Requires skill and balance<br>• Coasting loses the aerobic effects<br>• Costs for skates, helmet, wrist guards, knee guards, elbow guards, and gloves |
| **Swimming** | • Fewer injuries because there is no impact on legs and feet<br>• Good for people who are:<br>  • Injured and want to keep exercising<br>  • Pregnant<br>  • Overweight<br>• Works every part of the body, with an emphasis on the upper body<br>• Refreshing<br>• No age limit—lifetime activity | • You must locate a swimming pool and an available lane for swimming laps<br>• Requires skill<br>• Repetitive arm motions can result in pain and inflammation, leading to tendonitis and bursitis<br>• Swimming laps can be repetitive and seem boring<br>• Not a social activity<br>• Since this exercise doesn't involve impact, it does not help build bone density<br>• Risk of infections in the ears, eyes, and sinuses |
| **Cross-country skiing** | • Involves both lower and upper body, including most major muscle groups when poles are used<br>• Rigorous workout obtained when at higher altitudes, in cold weather, and from added weight of clothing<br>• Scenery changes<br>• Low impact | • Exposure to cold conditions can lead to frost-nip, frostbite, or hypothermia<br>• Requires accessibility to snow<br>• Skiing downhill decreases the aerobic effect |

| Table 3.4 | Types of Indoor and Outdoor Aerobic Activity, *continued* | |
|---|---|---|
| **Activity** | **Pros** | **Cons** |
| **Treadmill** | • Easily accessible no matter what the weather conditions<br>• Good for beginners, many levels<br>• Easy to use<br>• Easier on joints than walking or jogging on asphalt and concrete surfaces<br>• Can watch TV while exercising<br>• Some machines have various personal high-tech computer programs that monitor heart rate | • Can get monotonous<br>• Can stumble and slide off<br>• Expensive to own; may require health club membership |
| **Stationary bicycle** | • Great thigh workout<br>• Gives knees a rest<br>• Can read or watch TV while exercising<br>• Easy to use | • With stationary bikes you have added convenience, but lose the ability to ride outdoors<br>• Expensive to own; may require health club membership |

*continues*

| Table 3.4 | Types of Indoor and Outdoor Aerobic Activity, *continued* | |
|---|---|---|
| **Activity** | **Pros** | **Cons** |
| **Rowing machine** | • Total body workout using most major muscle groups<br>• Can watch TV while exercising<br>• Will prepare you for outdoor rowing or paddling on a canoe or kayak | • Can strain back if not performed correctly<br>• Repetitive motion can become boring<br>• Requires coordination |
| **Aerobic dancing** | • Enjoyable<br>• Can be done with a class or individually at home with a video or a televised class<br>• Camaraderie can develop within a group of people working out together<br>• Low injury rates<br>• Different styles and variations of classes may be classified as below:<br>  - High impact—more jumping and faster movement<br>  - Low impact—less jumping and slower movement<br>  - Aquatic—done in the water<br>  - Step aerobics using a 6- to 12-inch step—increase impact and weight-bearing movement<br>  - Kick boxing—uses movements of kick boxing for added variety and strength<br>  - Circuit—uses weights and aerobics to work out upper body as well as to increase aerobic endurance | • Possible injuries could occur, such as shin splints, tendonitis, muscle strain, back strain, and stress fracture<br>• Cost of class or travel time to a gym |

## Progression

There is a tendency when first beginning a fitness regimen for people to do too much too quickly. Keep in mind that just because you don't meet your goal the first day, it doesn't mean that you won't get there eventually. Slow and consistent improvement is the safe way to train.

If you have been sedentary, begin by taking a brisk walk or by bouncing on an exercise ball for 5 to 10 minutes. Gradually increase the duration of the activity by 10% per week until you can perform 20 to 60 minutes continuously. Your training intensity during these exercise sessions should be between 70% and 85% of the maximum heart rate.

Reference Table 3.5 for the ACSM's recommendations on how to progress in a cardiorespiratory exercise program.

| Table 3.5 | Progression for Cardiorespiratory Exercise | | | |
|-----------|-------------|----------------------|-------------------|----------------|
| **Program Stage** | **Week Number** | **Frequency (days/week)** | **Intensity (% HRR)** | **Time (minutes)** |
| Initial Stage | 1 | 3 | 40–50 | 15–20 |
| | 2 | 3–4 | 40–50 | 20–25 |
| | 3 | 3–4 | 50–60 | 20–25 |
| | 4 | 3–4 | 50–60 | 25–30 |
| Improvement stage | 5–7 | 3–4 | 60–70 | 25–30 |
| | 8–10 | 3–4 | 60–70 | 30–35 |
| | 11–13 | 3–4 | 65–75 | 30–35 |
| | 14–16 | 3–5 | 65–75 | 30–35 |
| | 17–20 | 3–5 | 70–85 | 35–40 |
| | 21–24 | 3–5 | 70–85 | 35–40 |
| Maintenance stage | 24+ | 3–5 | 70–85 | 30–45 |

*Source:* Adapted from American College of Sports Medicine. *ACSM's Guidelines for Exercise Testing and Prescription.* Philadelphia: Lippincott Williams and Wilkins, 2000.

## Rules for Progression

1. Increase only one FITT component at a time. It is best to increase duration first.
2. Increase your exercise workout by no more than 10% per week. Increasing too fast will lead to injury.
3. Stop exercising and seek immediate health care if you experience any of the following:
   - Tightness in your chest
   - Severe shortness of breath
   - Chest pain or pain in your arms or jaw, often on the left side
   - Heart palpitations
   - Dizziness, faintness, or feeling sick to your stomach

## Overtraining

Overtraining occurs when an individual does not give the body sufficient time to recover between workouts. Some signs that you may be suffering from excessive training are:

- General aches and pains that do not seem to subside
- Leg, muscle, and joint soreness or injury
- Insomnia
- Inability to relax or irritability
- A sense of feeling drained of energy
- Decreased workout performance
- Dehydration
- Greater sickness (e.g., colds, sore throat, other minor ills)

If you begin to recognize these symptoms, the best option is to stop your routine and allow your system to recover. The body can heal only during rest, and it is important to listen to your body when it tells you to slow down! You may want to visit a physician to rule out any significant ailment. Once you have given yourself time to recover, you should be able to return to a reasonable level of activity (use the Physical Activity Pyramid as your guide).

# Conclusion

Aerobic activity can increase your overall wellness by boosting your immune system, easing stress, improving your self-image, and reducing the risk of certain diseases. When you exercise, you strengthen your heart, making it pump oxygen-rich blood to the rest of the

## Reflect ›››› Reinforce ›››› Reinvigorate

### Knowledge Check

*Answers in Appendix D*

1. Circulation between the heart and lungs is called:

   A. Pulmonary circulation
   B. Systemic circulation
   C. Cardiovascular circulation

2. What does aerobic mean?

   A. Exercising with a pain in your chest
   B. Exercising using oxygen
   C. Exercising for more than 60 minutes

3. The body's natural painkiller that is produced in the brain is:

   A. Histamine
   B. Endorphins
   C. Oxygen

4. Gary is 18 years old and would like to improve his cardiorespiratory health. What should be his first step toward putting together an effective exercise program?

   A. Take a submaximal test to find his current cardiorespiratory fitness level
   B. Begin running 2 miles per week
   C. Bike for 40 minutes per day and gradually add in other activities

5. Marcia is 23 years old and has been told that stretching is an important component of cardiorespiratory training. When is the best time for Marcia to stretch?

   A. First thing when she gets to the gym
   B. 50 minutes after exercising, when her muscles have cooled down
   C. After she warms up for 5 to 10 minutes but before she starts her routine

6. Sylvia is 20 years old, walks 15 minutes per day, and would like to increase her level of activity. What is the safest way for Sylvia to progress with her cardiorespiratory training?

   A. Jog for the 15 minutes instead of walking
   B. Increase the duration of her walks by 10% each week until she feels comfortable walking for 60 minutes continuously
   C. Try running a mile once a week in addition to her daily walks

7. What is the recommended frequency for aerobic endurance workouts?

   A. Once each week
   B. 3–5 times each week
   C. Daily

8. How many calories will a 180-pound person burn hill-climbing for 45 minutes?

   A. About 400
   B. About 500
   C. About 700

body more efficiently. Submaximal tests assess how efficiently the cardiorespiratory system uses oxygen.

When designing your fitness program, make sure to follow the FITT guidelines. Always warm up and cool down, and progress slowly. Choose activities that are appropriate for your fitness level, patience, interests, and schedule. Most importantly, have fun!

9. James is in the middle of his aerobic routine. He can still speak with his partner, but occasionally he must stop talking to catch his breath. At what intensity level is James most likely working?
   A. Light
   B. Moderate
   C. Hard
10. Aerobic workouts should last for how long each session?
   A. 10 to 20 minutes
   B. 20 to 60 minutes
   C. 60 to 90 minutes

## Modern Modifications

Try a couple of these suggestions to add a little more heart-friendly activity to your daily routine:

- Park at the farthest spot in the parking lot and walk briskly or jog to the door.
- Take the stairs—avoid the escalator and elevator as much as possible.
- Turn up the stereo and dance. Cut loose for a couple of minutes when your favorite song comes on the radio.
- When shopping, walk the length of the mall between entering stores.
- Put away the leaf-blower and snow-blower—pick up a rake or shovel instead.
- After you take the dog for a walk, stay outside and play with the dog for an extra 30 minutes.
- Join an intramural team. It's great exercise, you meet new people, and it is a fun way to spend a couple of hours!

## Critical Thinking

1. Now that you have a basic understanding of cardiorespiratory endurance, consider the role that it plays in your life. At what stage of change are you regarding cardiorespiratory endurance? What would an appropriate target zone be for you to begin a new routine? After reviewing the variety of activities in Table 3.4, which three are most appropriate for you? Why? What strategies can you employ to counter the "cons" of the activities you've chosen?

**3**

## Going Above and Beyond

### Websites

American Academy of Orthopedic Surgeons
*http://orthinfo.asos.org*

American Heart Association
*http://www.americanheart.org* or *http://www.justmove.org*

Cooper Institute for Aerobics Research
*http://www.cooperinst.org*

MedlinePlus: Exercise and Physical Fitness
*http://www.nlm.nih.gov/medlineplus/exercisephysicalfitness.html*

Physician and Sports Medicine
*http://www.physsportmed.com*

Runner's World Online
*http://www.runnersworld.com*

Shape Up America! Fitness Center
*http://shapeup.org/fitness*

Walking
*http://walking.miningco.com*

## References and Suggested Readings

American College of Sports Medicine (ACSM). ACSM position stand: The recommended quantity and quality of exercise for developing and maintaining cardiorespiratory, muscular fitness and flexibility in healthy adults. *Medicine and Science in Sports and Exercise* 1998; 30:975–991.

———. *ACSM's Guidelines for Exercise Testing and Prescription.* Philadelphia: Lippincott Williams and Wilkins, 2000.

American Heart Association (AHA). A statement on exercise: Benefits and recommendations for physical activity programs for all Americans. *Circulation* 1995; 91:580.

———. Cholesterol. 2004a. *http://www.americanheart.org* [June 14, 2004].

———. Diabetes mellitus. 2004b. *http://www.americanheart.org* [June 14, 2004].

———. Resting heart rate. 2004c. *http://www.americanheart.org* [June 14, 2004].

———. Target heart rate. 2004d. *http://www.americanheart.org* [June 14, 2004].

Blair S. N. and Jackson A. S. Physical fitness and activity as separate heart disease risk factors: A meta-analysis. *Medicine and Science in Sports and Exercise* 2001; 33:762–764.

Borg G. A. Psychophysical basis of perceived exertion. *Medicine and Science in Sports and Exercise* 1982; 14:377.

Carroll J. F. and Kyser C. K. Exercise training in obesity lowers blood pressure independent of weight change. *Medicine and Science in Sports and Exercise* 2002; 34:596–601.

Cooper K. H. *The Aerobics Program for Well-Being.* Toronto: Bantam Books, 1982.

Erikssen G. Physical fitness and changes in mortality: The survival of the fittest. *Sports Medicine* 2001; 31:571–576.

Fletcher G., et al. American Heart Association: Statement on exercise. *Circulation* 1992; 86:726.

Merriam-Webster Dictionary. "Aerobic" and "obesity." 2004. *http://www.merriam-webster.com* [June 14, 2004].

Myers J., et al. Exercise capacity and mortality among men referred for exercise testing. *New England Journal of Medicine* 2002; 346:793–801.

Public Health Service. *Surgeon General's Report on Physical Activity and Health.* Washington, DC: U.S. Government Printing Office, 1996.

UC Davis Health System. The Well-Connected Report—Exercise. March 2000. *http://wellness.ucdavis.edu/wellconnected/exercise29.html* [June 14, 2004].

## CHAPTER 4

# Increasing Flexibility

## Objectives

After reading this chapter, you should be able to:

- Define flexibility and describe the benefits of increased flexibility.
- Explain the factors influencing flexibility.
- Assess flexibility.
- Explain the difference between ballistic, static, dynamic, and proprioceptive neuromuscular facilitation (PNF) stretching.
- Describe various types of stretching exercises.
- Implement stretching into an exercise program.
- Explain how low-back pain can be prevented.
- Describe which exercises can help prevent back pain.
- List the ways to improve your posture.

# What Are the Benefits of Flexibility?

Flexibility offers the following benefits:

- Increases joint movement (mobility)
- Improves circulation, bringing nutrients to keep tissues healthy and transporting wastes out of the tissues
- Improves performance in some activities
- Improves posture and personal appearance
- Is valuable during the cool-down phase of a workout
- Prevents low-back problems
- Improves coordination and balance, which helps maintain an independent and active lifestyle in the elderly
- Helps reduce excess stress by lowering anxiety and boosting feelings of self-confidence

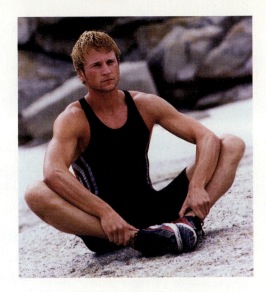

# What Determines Flexibility?

- Flexibility is an important part of physical fitness, but it is often overlooked during workouts.
- Flexibility is achieved by stretching. Stress causes muscles to contract and tighten. Stretching helps muscles relax, relieving pain from muscular stress.
- There are two kinds of stretching: static and dynamic.

## Factors That Influence Flexibility

- *Muscle temperature.* Warm muscles stretch more easily than cold muscles.
- *Physical activity.* Sedentary individuals are less flexible; active individuals tend to maintain or even increase flexibility.
- *Injury.* Injury can limit range of motion, but a good rehabilitation program can help regain all or part of a joint's flexibility.
- *Body composition.* Most muscular individuals have good flexibility because they have trained their muscles through a full range of motion. Overly bulky muscles may limit movement (known as being "muscle bound"), but this is rare. Fat can also limit movement and flexibility.
- *Age.* As a person ages, flexibility declines due more to inactivity than to the aging process itself. Flexibility can be maintained by doing stretching activities regularly.
- *Disease.* Diseases such as arthritis can make it uncomfortable or even painful to move joints. Arthritic individuals can improve their joint mobility through exercise.

**What's the word. . .**

**flexibility** Ability to move a joint smoothly through a full range of motion.

**stretching** Primary method of improving flexibility.

**static or passive stretching** Muscle is stretched naturally without force being applied.

**dynamic or active stretching** Muscle is taken beyond its normal range of motion with help from a partner.

# Assessing Flexibility

You cannot determine flexibility with one test because the flexibility of one joint does not affect flexibility in other joints.

**4**

## Precautions

Take the following precautions when testing your flexibility:

1. Warm up before doing a test.
2. Stop the test if pain occurs.
3. Do not perform fast, jerky movements.
4. If any of the following criteria apply, seek medical advice before performing a test:
   a. Presently suffering from acute back pain
   b. Currently receiving treatment for back pain
   c. Ever had a surgical operation on your back
   d. Health-care professional told you never to exercise your back

## Sit-and-Reach Test

**Step 1:** Sit on the floor with your legs straight, knees together, and toes pointing toward the ceiling.

**Step 2:** Place one hand over the other. Place the tips of your two middle fingers on top of each other.

**Step 3:** Slowly stretch forward without bouncing or jerking. Stop when you feel tightness or discomfort in your back or legs.

**Step 4:** Repeat the test three more times. Record your score by using **Table 4.1**. Record your scores as follows:

First attempt:    ____ points

Second attempt:    ____ points

Third attempt:    ____ points

Total points =    ____ divided by 3 = ____ **your score**

Score your results by averaging your three attempts.

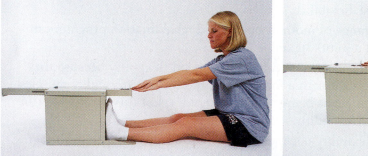
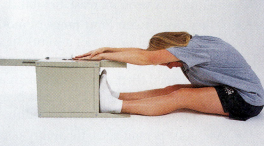

| Table 4.1 | Scoring Results for the Sit-and-Reach Test | |
|---|---|
| **If you reached . . .** | **You get . . .** |
| More than 2 inches past your toes | 1 point—excellent |
| To your toes and up to 2 inches past | 2 points—good |
| Up to 4 inches from your toes | 3 points—fair |
| More than 4 inches from your toes | 4 points—poor |

*Source:* Imrie D. and Barbuto L. *Back Power.* Toronto: Stoddart, 1988.

| Table 4.2 | Scoring Results for the Shoulder Flexibility Test | |
|---|---|---|
| **If . . .** | **Your flexibility is . . .** | |
| You can clasp your hands together | Very good. | |
| Your fingertips almost touch | Good, but needs work. | |
| You are not within an inch of touching your fingertips together | Poor; needs a lot of work. | |

*Source:* Imrie D. and Barbuto L. *Back Power.* Toronto: Stoddart, 1988.

## Shoulder Flexibility Test

**Step 1:** Bring your right hand over your shoulder and down between your shoulder blades.

**Step 2:** Bring your left hand around the small of your back and up between your shoulder blades.

**Step 3:** Try to touch the fingertips of both hands behind your back.

**Step 4:** Have someone measure the distance between your fingertips.

**Step 5:** Do the test the other way: left hand over your head and down between your shoulder blades, right hand reaching behind your back up to your shoulder blades.

**Step 6:** Try to touch the fingertips of both hands behind your back.

**Step 7:** Have someone measure the distance between your fingertips.

Score your results using Table 4.2.

## Other Flexibility Tests

There are many other tests that can be used to assess your flexibility. See Lab 4-1, Activity 3 for additional flexibility assessments.

# Maintain Your Flexibility

- The adage "use it or lose it" applies especially to flexibility.
- Stretch all the major muscle groups in the body (arms, shoulders, chest, back, legs).
- Do not stretch swollen joints.
- Stretch the muscle group slowly, until slight discomfort is felt (not pain).
- Do not hold your breath—breathe normally.
- Do not bounce at the end of a stretch.
- Hold the stretch for at least 10 to 30 seconds.
- Repeat the stretch four times.
- A workout to stretch all of the major joints will last 10 to 15 minutes.
- Do all at once or piecemeal throughout the day.
- Stretch at least 2 to 3 days per week; every day is okay.

**Ask Yourself**
- Am I doing some light activity before I attempt to stretch out?

**What's the word. . .**
**stretch reflex** An involuntary muscle contraction against a quick stretch.

**The Inside Track**

**Physiology of Stretching**

Areas within your muscles and tendons protect them from overstretching or tearing during a quick stretch by creating a **stretch reflex**. For example, someone tapping your leg just below the kneecap quickly stretches the quadriceps muscle. This makes your thigh contract and kick out your lower leg. The quicker the stretch, the stronger the reflex.

The protective action of tendons causes a stretched muscle attached to the tendon to relax, and signals its opposing muscle to contract. This protects the stretched muscle and tendon from tearing.

By stretching slowly during exercise, you avoid contracting the muscle you are trying to stretch. As a stretch is held, your muscles and tendons adapt to the new length.

**4**

## Informal Stretching

Stretching can be done virtually anywhere. When you need a quick break, you want a short stress reliever (during a test, for instance), or you sense discomfort in a muscle group during the day, use stretching as a means to relieve the pain. In addition, these activities can be fun if you choose to do them with a friend, while listening to music or television, or during your own time. Here is an example of a routine you can do anywhere, anytime:

- Clasp your hands together and stretch out in front of you.
- In the same position, stretch your hands over your head.
- Lean right.
- Lean left.
- Clasp your hands behind your back and open up your chest area.
- Stretch your wrists by bending your wrists back, then down, then in a circle.
- Lift your shoulders up to your ears, then down and back. Do that five times.
- Take your right hand and put it on your left shoulder. With your left hand, gently push your right elbow, pushing your right hand past your shoulder and stretching the back of your right arm.
- Stretch your left arm in the same manner.

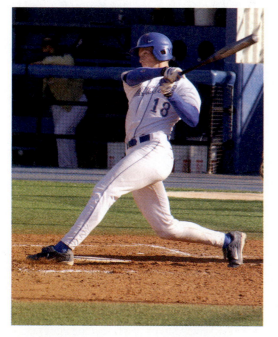

- Put your hands flat on your desk, palms down, and push your chair out, stretching your back.
- Feel free to add more stretches for a variety and to avoid boredom! Remember, SIT UP STRAIGHT! Good posture starts now!

## Stretching as Part of the Exercise Routine

Stretching, of course, also needs to play a role in your exercise routine. Muscles that are ill prepared for activity can easily be injured, and stretching assists you in staying healthy and being able to participate in exercise activity.

Don't stretch to warm up. Rather, warm up so that you have a more productive and successful stretch. Be sure to do 5 to 10 minutes of light activity to increase the blood flow to your muscles before completing your preparatory stretch.

Not all activities emphasize the same muscle groups. While you should stretch all major muscle groups to some degree, a review of **Table 4.3** will indicate the major muscle groups that require specific attention for a variety of activities.

### Tipping Point

**Rewards**

- Avoid **ballistic stretching**—for example, bending forcefully to touch your toes with your knees straight and bouncing while you reach. Ballistic stretching may do more harm than good, because the muscles may shorten reflexively. This type of stretching is not recommended for most people. However, some athletes believe that controlled ballistic stretching can better prepare a muscle for sustained activity, especially one requiring a burst of speed.

| Table 4.3 | Sport-Specific Recommendations for Stretching | | | | | | | | |
|---|---|---|---|---|---|---|---|---|---|
| | **Running** | **Golf** | **Tennis** | **Volleyball** | **Basketball** | **Aerobics** | **Soccer** | **Martial Arts** | **Swimming** |
| Neck | | | X | X | | | X | | X |
| Shoulder roll | | | X | | | X | | X | |
| Back scratch | X | X | X | X | | | X | X | |
| Rack | | X | | | | | X | | X |
| Reach up | | X | X | | | X | | | X |
| Arm circles | X | | | | | | | | X |
| Arm across chest | | | X | X | X | X | X | X | |
| Wall press | | X | X | | X | | | X | X |
| Hamstring | X | | X | X | X | X | X | X | |
| Modified hurdler | | X | | X | | | X | | |
| Knee to chest | X | | X | X | X | X | X | X | |
| Calf | X | | X | X | X | X | X | X | |
| Butterfly | X | | X | X | X | X | X | X | |
| Heel to buttock | X | X | X | X | X | X | X | X | |
| Lunge | X | | X | | X | X | X | X | X |
| Skater lunge | | X | | | | | | X | |
| Curl up | | X | | X | | | | | |
| Elbow to knee | X | X | X | | X | | | X | |

As stated earlier, the best stretching occurs when the muscles are already warm. As such, the cool-down stretch is very important. You will gain the most flexibility by incorporating stretches of all major muscle groups after your exercise routine is complete.

# Types of Stretching

Stretching techniques include static stretches, ballistic stretches, and PNF (proprioceptive neuromuscular facilitation).

## Static Stretching

Static stretching is the most practical type of stretching. It is effective, causes less pain, and is usually easier to do.

Perform a static stretch by:
1. Slowly and gently stretch the muscle to the point of discomfort and hold that position for 10 to 30 seconds.
2. Slightly back off and, while holding this position, relax.
3. Take a deep breath and exhale.
4. Slowly and gently stretch again to the point of discomfort (this point should be beyond the first step).

See ( Table 4.4 ) for proper stretching exercises and ( Table 4.5 ) for potentially harmful exercises that should be avoided.

## Ballistic Stretching

Ballistic stretching uses bouncing, repetitive movements to force a stretch past the normal range of motion.

**4**

## Table 4.4 | Proper Form for Stretching Exercises

### Neck

Ear to shoulder          Chin to chest          Look right and left

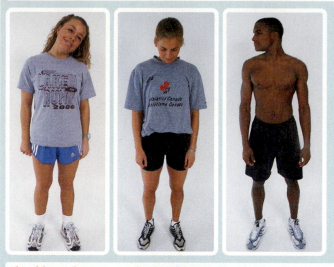

### Shoulders, chest, upper back, and abdominals

Shoulder roll          Back scratch          Handcuff stretch          Rack

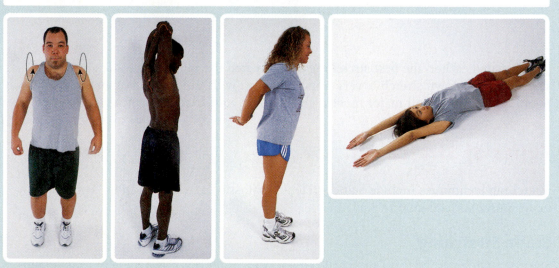

Reach up          Slow arm circles                    Arm across chest          Wall press

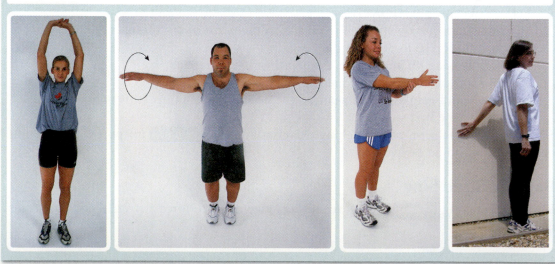

## Hamstrings, groin, and lower back

Supine hamstring stretch                Modified hurdler

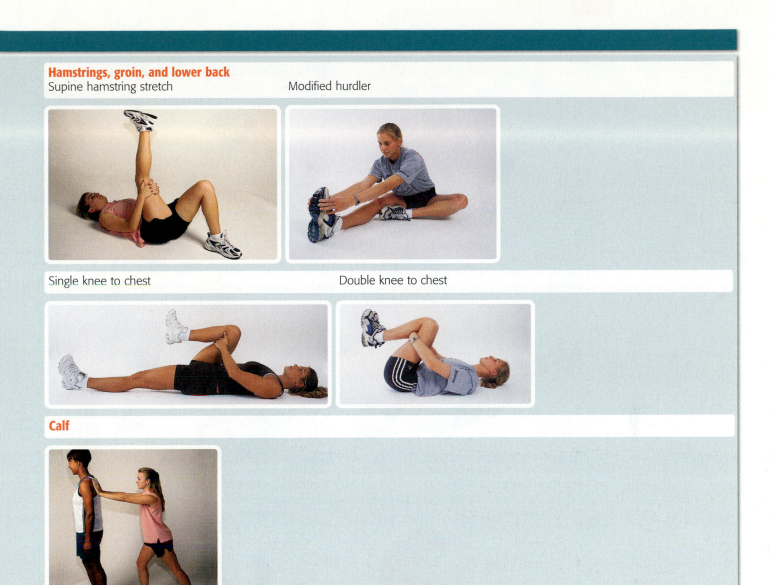

Single knee to chest                    Double knee to chest

## Calf

## Quads, inner thigh, and hips

Butterfly

Standing heel-to-buttock
(do not perform without your
health-care provider's advice if you
have knee pain or knee surgery)

Standing lunge          Side (skater) lunge

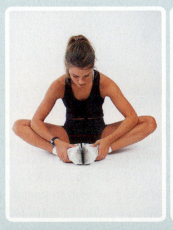
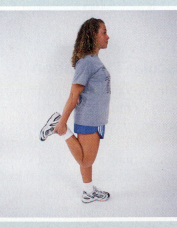
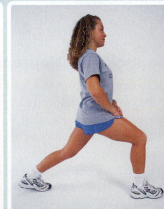

**4**

## Table 4.5 | Potentially Harmful Exercises to Avoid

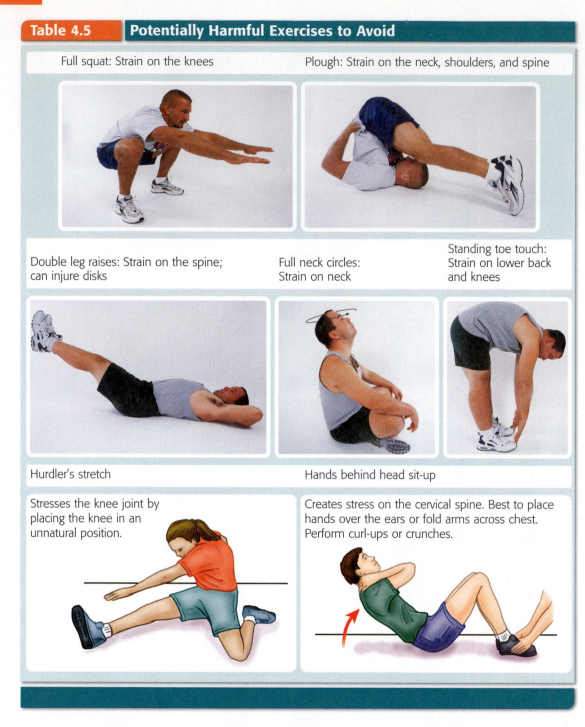

Full squat: Strain on the knees

Plough: Strain on the neck, shoulders, and spine

Double leg raises: Strain on the spine; can injure disks

Full neck circles: Strain on neck

Standing toe touch: Strain on lower back and knees

Hurdler's stretch

Hands behind head sit-up

Stresses the knee joint by placing the knee in an unnatural position.

Creates stress on the cervical spine. Best to place hands over the ears or fold arms across chest. Perform curl-ups or crunches.

## Proprioceptive Neuromuscular Facilitation

Proprioceptive neuromuscular facilitation involves tightening a muscle as hard as you can right before you stretch it. The theory behind PNF is that the act of tightening or squeezing exhausts the muscle so that it becomes relaxed and more receptive to the stretch.

PNF may be the most effective type of stretching (static stretching is almost as good), but it usually requires a partner, takes more time, and can cause more muscle soreness. There are several PNF techniques. An example of one method of performing a PNF stretch follows:

- Do a near-maximum 6-second isometric contraction of the muscle you wish to stretch.
- Immediately relax the muscle for 2 seconds, then have a partner push the muscle into a static stretch for 10 to 15 seconds.

# Back Fitness

More than 80% of North Americans suffer back pain in their lifetime. Low-back pain, both acute and chronic, centers on the muscles supporting the spine. Age and physical condition are the major factors associated with low-back pain, along with the trauma of lifting something in the wrong way or injuring yourself in an activity or sport. Being overweight, poor posture, stress, and occupation (e.g., computer programmers and truck drivers) may contribute to the pain. There is also recent research indicating a link between smoking and lower-back pain.

## Preventing Low-Back Pain

To prevent low-back pain:
- Exercise regularly to improve the strength of your back and abdominal muscles.
- Maintain correct posture in sitting and standing, especially while studying and working on a computer.
- Warm up before engaging in physical activity.
- Keep the spine straight up and down when lifting an object. **Do not** bend over. Use the muscles of your legs and hips to lift.

## Exercises for the Lower Back

The following exercises will help to stretch and strengthen your lower back:
- Curl-up

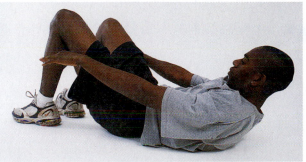

- Knee to chest

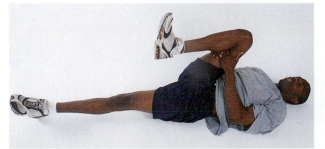

- Elbow-to-knee stretch

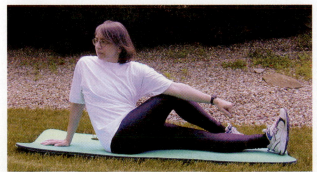

**4**

■ Cat and camel

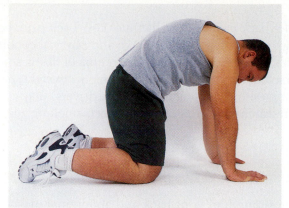

■ Lunge stretch

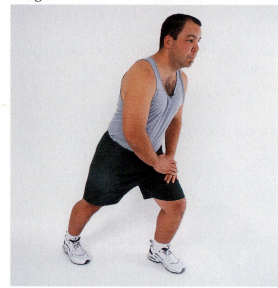

■ Modified chest lift

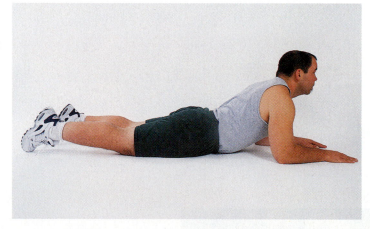

## What Is Poor Body Posture?

You can evaluate your posture by standing in front of a three-panel mirror, of the kind often found in fitting rooms. See Figure 4.1 for guidance on good and poor posture.

# Why Have Good Posture?

- Good posture makes your bones align properly.
- This bone alignment allows for muscles, joints, and ligaments to work properly.
- Internal organs are in the right position and can work more effectively (allows for deep breathing and proper digestion).
- Good posture lessens the risk of lower-back pain.
- Good posture can project the body image that you are strong and proud.

# Signs of Poor Posture

- Head aligned in front of center of gravity (can cause headaches, dizziness, and neck, shoulder, and arm pain)
- Too much outward curve in upper back (can shorten breath by squeezing lung area; can cause neck, shoulder, and arm pain)
- Too much inward curve in lower back (can cause low-back pain, painful menstruation)
- Abdomen sticks out too far (can cause **lordosis**, low-back pain, painful menstruation)
- Knees extend backward too much (can cause knee injury and lordosis) **Figure 4.2**

# Ways to Improve Your Posture

- **Sit correctly:** Distribute weight evenly on both hips, bend knees at a right angle, legs should not be crossed and feet should be flat on the floor, keep back straight and shoulders back
- **Stand correctly:** Hold head up with chin in, ears should be in line with shoulders, shoulders should be back, chest forward, knees straight, stomach tucked in
- **Lift correctly:** Keep back straight and bend at knees and hips, keep feet in wide stance, lift object using leg muscles, moving in a steady motion
- **Lie in bed correctly:** Lie on your side with your hips and knees slightly bent; put a flat pillow between your knees **Figure 4.3**

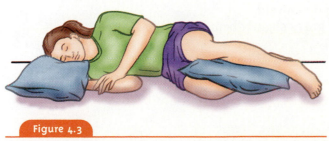

**Figure 4.3**

To improve your posture, sleep on your side with your hips and knees slightly bent.

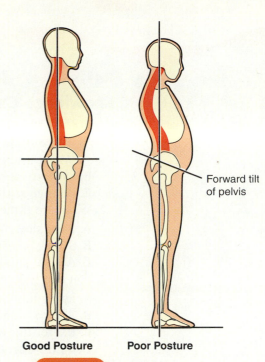

**Good Posture**    **Poor Posture**

Forward tilt of pelvis

**Figure 4.1**

Good posture depends on the pelvic tilt and abdominal muscles. Only when the pelvis is level is it at its strongest.

> **What's the word. . .**
> **lordosis**
> Excessive pelvic tilt.

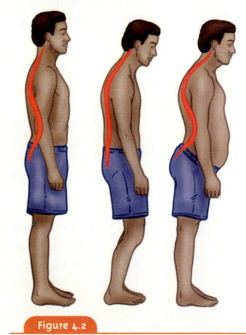

**Figure 4.2**

Left to right: good posture (pelvic tilt); poor posture (lordotic back, pelvis tilted too far forward; pelvis tilted too far back)

## Reflect ›››› Reinforce ›››› Reinvigorate

### Knowledge Check

*Answers in Appendix D*

1. In assessing your flexibility, you should:
   
   A. Warm up before you do a stretch test
   B. Do fast moves to get your muscles warm
   C. Bounce at the end of each movement

2. What are three basic types of stretching?
   
   A. Fast, slow, ballistic
   B. Static, ballistic, PNF
   C. Active, passive, quick

3. You can help prevent low-back pain by:
   
   A. Lying flat on your back while sleeping
   B. Always standing with your legs at least 2 feet apart
   C. Exercising your back and abdominal muscles regularly

After standing around waiting for a delayed gun, you bolt from the starting line of a 5K, feeling fit and ready to have a great race. As you sizzle through the first half-mile, you marvel at how fast you are running and how easy the pace feels to you. Suddenly, agonizing pain stabs you, and you are forced to hobble to a complete stop. You realize that you have torn your hamstrings so badly that you probably won't run at anything faster than a very slow jogging pace for at least 6 to 8 weeks.

4. Can stretching before exercising help prevent muscle injuries?
   
   A. Yes
   B. No

5. Which is the safest type of stretching for most people?
   
   A. Ballistic
   B. Static
   C. Proprioceptive neuromuscular facilitation (PNF)

Craig, as a dentist, bends over patients daily for long hours. When he was younger, he experienced no back problems. However, in middle age, he has experienced severe back pain.

6. Does flexibility decrease as a person ages?
   
   A. Yes
   B. No

7. Could having a "pot belly" affect Craig's flexibility?
   
   A. Yes
   B. No

8. The best sleeping position for your posture is:
   
   A. On your back, with your face and toes pointed toward the ceiling
   B. On your stomach, facing downward
   C. On your side, with your knees slightly bent

9. How long should you hold each stretch during your exercise routine?
   A. 5–10 seconds
   B. 10–30 seconds
   C. 30–45 seconds
10. When first starting your exercise routine, how often should you perform stretching exercises?
    A. Rarely, as injury may occur
    B. Only on days where aerobic activity is performed
    C. Daily, to improve flexibility

## Modern Modifications

Think about the activities you do and the postures you assume each day. Are there ways you can improve your flexibility and posture just by changing the way you do these activities? When you are sitting or standing, are you:

- Arching your back?
- Rounding your shoulders?
- Letting your head slump forward?

When you are lying down, are you:

- Tilting your pelvis down?
- Arching your back?

While lying on your back, you should have just enough room between the small of your back and the floor to slide a computer mouse under there. You know your posture is bad if your back is touching the floor (squishing the mouse) or arching (the mouse could do jumping jacks).

Consciously change what you do during each activity or posture. For instance:

- While sitting, keep your back straight, lean slightly forward, and use a footrest to keep your knees higher than your hips.
- While standing, use a footrest to raise one leg to help you keep your back straight.
- When lifting, bend at the knees, **not** at the waist, lift slowly, and push with your legs. Don't twist.
- Do one different stretching exercise each morning, at noon, and each evening before going to bed.

## Critical Thinking

1. Consider your current level of activity. What role does flexibility and stretching play in your workouts? Identify three to five ways you can improve your flexibility based on the suggestions in the chapter.
2. What rationalizations do you believe you might hear from someone who does not practice stretching as a portion of his or her routine? What are the risks the individual may be taking by avoiding this piece of the routine?

**4**

## Going Above and Beyond

### Websites

American Academy of Orthopaedic Surgeons
*http://orthoinfo.aaos.org*

Georgia State University: Flexibility
*http://www.gsu.edu/~wwwfit/flexibility.html*

MedlinePlus
*http://www.nlm.nih.gov/medlineplus*

National Institute on Aging
*http://www.n.a.nih.gov/exercisebook*

Physician and Sports Medicine
*http://physsportsmed.com*

## References and Suggested Readings

Canham-Chervak M., et al. Does stretching before exercise prevent lower-limb injury? *Clinical Journal of Sport Medicine* 2000; 10:216.

Gleim G. W. and McHugh M. P. Flexibility and its effect on sports injury and performance. *Sports Medicine* 1997; 24:289–299.

Hodges P. and Jull G. Does strengthening the abdominal muscles prevent low back pain? *Journal of Rheumatology* 2000; 27:2286–2288.

Knudson D. Stretching: From science to practice. *Journal of Physical Education, Recreation and Dance* 1998; 69:38–42.

———. Stretching during warm-up: Do we have enough evidence? *Journal of Physical Education, Recreation and Dance* 2000; 70:271–277.

Patel A. T. and Ogle A. A. Diagnosis and management of acute low back pain. *American Family Physician* 2000; 61:1779–1786.

Shrier I. Stretching before exercise: An evidence based approach. *British Journal of Sports Medicine* 2000; 34:324–325.

Shrier I. and Gossal K. Myths and truths of stretching. *Physician and Sports Medicine* 2000; 28:57–63.

## CHAPTER 5

# Increasing Muscular Strength and Endurance

## *Objectives*

After reading this chapter, you should be able to:

- Explain the difference between muscular strength and muscular endurance, and identify how training differs for each.
- Describe the changes that take place in your body as a result of muscle training.
- Explain the differences in muscle fibers and their functions.
- Assess muscular strength and endurance.
- Describe effective individual muscle-training exercises.
- Design an effective muscle-training program.

## Muscular Endurance

Muscular endurance describes how long or how many times (number of repetitions) you can lift and lower a given weight. It can be assessed by determining the number of repetitions of a particular exercise that can be performed.

For most people, developing muscular endurance is more important than muscular strength. Muscular endurance is usually more important in carrying out everyday activities.

## Muscular Strength

As you lift and lower a weight, your muscle must generate enough force to move that weight. Muscular strength can be assessed by determining the amount of weight that can be lifted in one repetition of an exercise. Strength can be developed by increasing the amount of weight that can be lifted in an exercise after a lower weight can be lifted 10–12 times easily.

## What Are the Benefits of Muscular Strength and Endurance?

Muscular endurance and muscular strength are important components of physical fitness. Your ability to perform physical tasks can be enhanced by strength and endurance training. The benefits of strength and endurance training are that you will:

- Improve at physical work, sports, and recreation
- Look better and feel better about yourself
- Maintain a healthy body weight
- Better manage stress and anxiety
- Help prevent osteoporosis (brittle-bone disease)
- Have good posture and avoid back and neck pain
- Digest food better (and possibly lower your risk of colon cancer)
- Experience fewer injuries and have better balance

## How Does Weight Training Change Body Composition and Metabolism?

Exercising the muscles changes the ratio of fat to muscle fiber and speeds up weight loss. The more muscle, the higher the metabolic rate and the more calories your body will burn on its own. It will be easier to keep your weight where you want it by eating right and exercising.

Exercising also slows degeneration of muscle and nerves with age. It keeps the bones strong, helping you to avoid osteoporosis. Being stronger when you are older keeps you from falling down as easily. Falls are the number one cause of injury for seniors!

Weight training keeps more of your motor nerves connected to the muscles they control. And you are better able to make quick and powerful moves.

## Gender Differences for Weight Training

Men are, on average, larger and stronger than women, because they have more muscle mass. But women have about the same strength in the lower body and only a small percentage less in the upper body. Why? Men have more androgens (hormones that cause facial hair, deep voice, and other sex-linked characteristics). Also, male muscles tend to activate faster, adding to muscle power.

<aside>
**What's the word...**

**muscular endurance**
The ability of muscles to apply force repeatedly.

**muscular strength**
The force muscles can exert against resistance.
</aside>

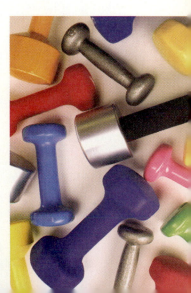

## What's the word...

**hypertrophy** Increase in bulk or size by thickening of muscle fibers.

**atrophy** Progressive loss (wasting) of muscle mass.

**isometric** Muscle contraction without movement at the joint.

## The Inside Track

### Will Weight Training Give Women Bulky Muscles?

Women do not develop large muscle mass as a result of weight training because they lack the male hormones in the quantity necessary for significant hypertrophy to occur.

The principal advantages of weight training for women are (1) greater strength as they age, (2) better bone density, and (3) easier maintenance of desired weight without fat.

# What Are the Different Types of Muscle Fiber?

Muscles consist of many muscle fibers. Larger muscle fibers mean a larger and stronger muscle (hypertrophy). When muscle fiber size diminishes it is called atrophy. Two types of muscle fibers exist according to their contraction speed and energy source:

- *Fast-twitch fibers* contract quickly and forcefully, but fatigue more rapidly than slow-twitch fibers. They rely on anaerobic energy metabolism.
- *Slow-twitch fibers* do not contract as rapidly or strongly as fast-twitch fibers. They are fatigue resistant and rely on aerobic energy metabolism.

Endurance activities (i.e., jogging) use slow-twitch fibers; power and strength activities (i.e., sprinting) use fast-twitch fibers. Weight training can increase the size and strength of both fiber types.

Everyone has both types of muscle fiber. Your genetics determine the proportion of each type of fiber in your body.

# Assessing Your Muscular Strength and Endurance

Muscular fitness is determined by assessing muscular strength and endurance.

- Muscular strength: Because muscular strength is specific to the muscle group, the testing of one group of muscles does not provide accurate information about the strength of other muscle groups. For a comprehensive assessment, strength testing must involve several major muscle groups. Standard tests use free weights. The heaviest weight you can lift only one time through the full range of motion for a specific muscle group is considered your maximum strength for that muscle group.
- Muscular endurance: Muscular endurance is specific to each muscle group. Few tests of muscular endurance have been developed. The YMCA developed a bench-press test for muscular endurance, using a standard weight. (Using the bench press to test strength is preferred by some experts. It is not a fair test for smaller, lighter individuals, however.) See Lab 5-1, Activity 1 for complete instructions on how to perform this assessment.

Also see Labs 5-2 and 5-3 for assessing muscular strength and endurance.

# Modes of Exercise

## Isometric (Static) Exercises

Isometric (static) exercise contracts muscle without changing muscle length (does not involve muscle movement) **Figure 5.1** .

- Do these exercises against an immovable object (e.g., a wall) to provide resistance.
- You can use isometric exercises to strengthen muscles after an injury or surgery.

### Advantages

- Require no or little equipment or expense
- Low risk of muscle soreness
- Can be done in a small space
- Rapid strength improvement

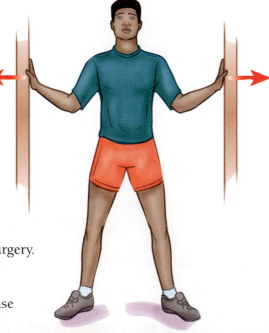

**Figure 5.1**

Isometric (static) exercise.

## Disadvantages

- Difficult to devise a full-body workout
- Not very motivating

## Isotonic Exercises

Isotonic (dynamic) exercise contracts muscle in a way that changes muscle length (involves muscle movement). Isotonic is the most popular type of exercise for increasing muscle strength. It can be performed with weight machines **Figure 5.2** , free weights, or your own body (i.e., push-ups). Two kinds of muscle contractions occur **Figure 5.3** :

- *Concentric contractions* occur when the muscle applies force as it shortens.
- *Eccentric contractions* occur when the muscle applies force as it lengthens.

For example, during an arm curl, the biceps muscle works concentrically as the weight is raised toward the shoulder, and eccentrically as the weight is lowered.

## Advantages

- Improve strength across entire range of motion
- Help improve joint flexibility
- More motivating

## Disadvantages

- Require more exercise equipment
- Higher risk of muscle soreness

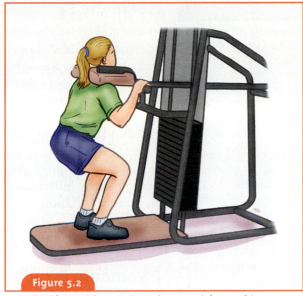

**Figure 5.2**

Isotonic (dynamic) exercise using a weight machine.

**What's the word. . .**

**isotonic** Muscle contraction where tension is constant while length increases.

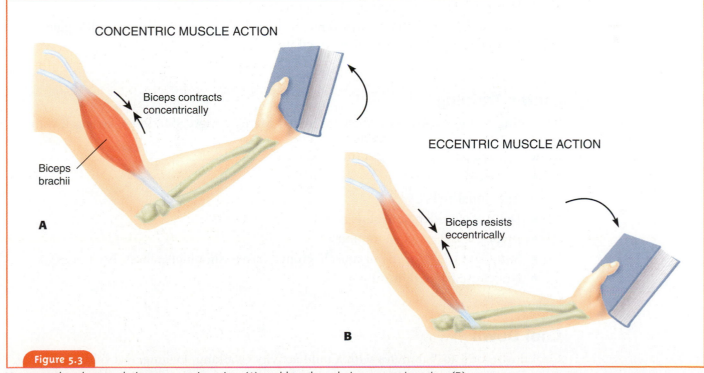

CONCENTRIC MUSCLE ACTION

Biceps contracts concentrically

Biceps brachii

A

ECCENTRIC MUSCLE ACTION

Biceps resists eccentrically

B

**Figure 5.3**

Your muscles shorten during concentric action (A) and lengthen during eccentric action (B).

**5**

## Isokinetic Exercises

**Isokinetic** exercise combines the advantages of both isometric and isotonic exercises. It uses special apparatus to provide a maximum resistance to the muscles, as in isometric exercise, but throughout the full range of motion, as in isotonic exercise. This equipment is often used by individuals who are in rehabilitation **Figure 5.4**.

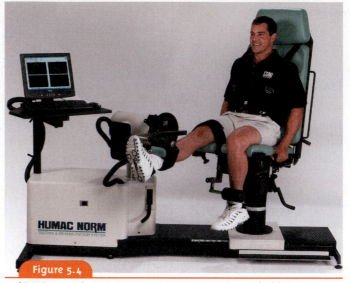

**Figure 5.4**

Isokinetic exercise apparatus. *Source:* Image provided by CSMI, www.csmisolutions.com. All rights reserved.

## Plyometric Exercises

**Plyometrics** involves doing abrupt, explosive movements, such as bounding on and off a box, or jumping off a platform and immediately leaping upward. It develops quick-twitch muscle fibers but risks incurring injury. Do plyometric exercises only after you have developed well-conditioned muscles.

# Getting Started with Weight Training

### Warm Up

Begin with a 5- to 10-minute warm-up. This will:
- Prepare the heart muscle and circulatory system
- Warm the muscles, making them more flexible

To warm up, use low-intensity exercises (biking, stair-climbing, treadmill/jogging). When you begin to sweat, you are warmed up.

### During Training

According to the American College of Sports Medicine (ACSM 1998), strength training should be:
- Progressive
- Rhythmic
- Individualized
- Done at a moderate to slow speed
- Involve a full range of motion
- Stimulate all of the major muscle groups (arms, shoulders, chest, back, legs)
- Not cause labored breathing

### Cool Down

Cool down for 2 to 5 minutes with a mild activity (walking, jogging, or cycling). Stretch *after* exercise—warm muscles stretch farther and are less likely to tear.

# Where Should You Exercise?

## At a Health Club/Gym: Advantages

- Availability of professional supervision and trainers
- Many exercise options, including aerobic options
- Social climate: meet new friends
- Influence of motivated exercisers

## At Home: Advantages

- Convenient: no concerns about appearance, travel time, parking, gym hours
- Private: avoids strangers, not intimidating if you feel weak and awkward
- No waiting in line; no noise from loud music and talking
- Cleaner: the germs on the bench and bars are yours
- Less expensive: no monthly payments for health club membership

# Fundamentals of Weight Training

- To get stronger, use few repetitions (6–8) with maximum weight. The number of repetitions performed without stopping to rest is called a set.
- To gain endurance, use many repetitions (12–15) with minimum weight.

If you train with weights on consecutive days, work the upper body one day and the lower body the next day.

Muscles need one day of rest between training sessions to recover and minimize injury.

## Training Frequency

The ACSM (1998) recommends specific training frequencies for various levels of ability:

*Beginning:* Train entire body 2 to 3 days per week.

*Intermediate:* Train entire body 2 to 3 days per week.

*Split workout:* Train each muscle group (upper and lower body) 1 to 2 days per week.

*Advanced:* Train 4 to 6 days per week.

*Elite bodybuilding:* Work out twice each day for 4 to 5 days per week—with appropriate steps taken to optimize muscle recovery and minimize risk of overtraining.

## Intensity

Intensity is the most critical part of resistance or weight training. It is the amount of weight used in each repetition.

## Progressive Overloading

The basis of strength training is progressive overloading. It increases the force your muscles can generate and helps you gain muscle strength without injury.

Progressive overloading strengthens individual muscle fibers and engages a larger proportion of available fibers in an activity. This makes you stronger.

If you can lift a certain weight for more than 12 reps with good form, you can increase the weight during your next training session.

> ### What's the word. . .
>
> **repetition (rep)** A single lifting and lowering of the weight.
>
> **set** Number of reps performed without stopping to rest.
>
> **progressive overloading** Increasing, from one session to another, the amount of weight you lift during a set.
>
> **repetition maximums (RM)** The maximum weight you can lift successfully once while using proper form.

## Tipping Point

### Determining Your Repetition Maximum

- Adjust the exercise intensity by knowing your repetition maximums (RM). Use free weights to determine your RM for each muscle group.

# Creating a Successful Training Program

Start a training routine consisting of one to two sets of 12 reps each for each major muscle group **Figure 5.5**. This takes about 30 minutes to perform. Do this routine two to three times per week.

- Change the exercises you perform for each muscle group every 4 to 8 weeks, even if you keep the same set and rep routine. Changing exercises will overload the muscles differently, increase your strength gains, and alleviate boredom.
- Gradually increase the weight you lift until you can lift it only 12 times with good form. If you can perform more reps easily, increase the weight.
- If you can't do 12 reps with good form, decrease the weight.
- Increase the weight by no more than 10% per week.
- See Lab 5-3 for tools for tracking your muscular training.

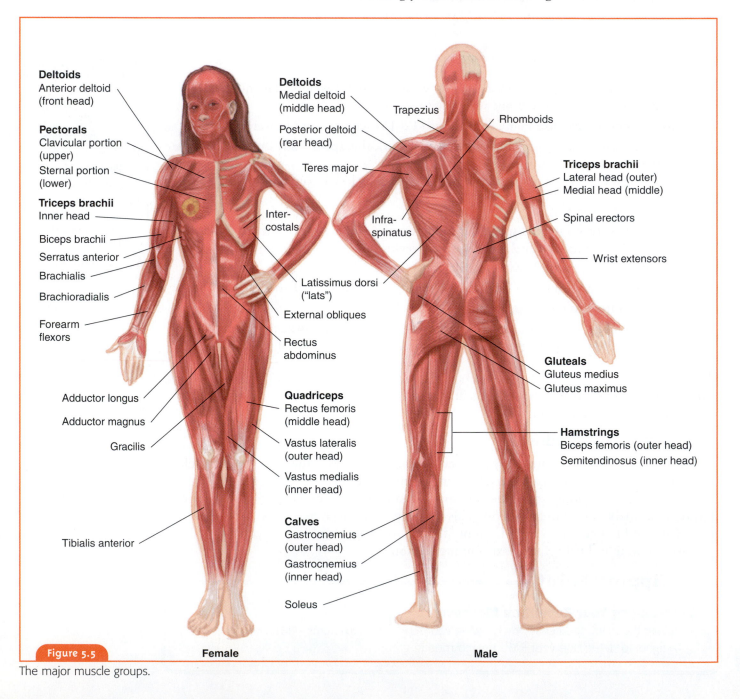

**Figure 5.5**

**Female**          **Male**

The major muscle groups.

## Exercise Guidelines

*For muscle strength:* Three to five sets, two to eight reps, with a weight that cannot be lifted more than eight times.

- Rest at least 120 seconds between sets.
- **Do not** perform maximum-weight lifts when strength training.

*For muscle endurance:* Two to three sets, 12 to 15 reps, with a weight that cannot be lifted more than 15 times.

- Rest 30 to 60 seconds between sets.

## Selecting Types of Exercise

Muscle balance refers to the strength ratio of opposing muscle groups across a common joint (e.g., the biceps and triceps muscle groups in the upper arm).

Perform exercises that target opposing muscle groups across joints. You will improve your joint function and reduce your risk of injury.

Select at least one exercise targeting each major muscle group.

## Exercise Sequence

The ACSM (1998) recommends the following order for exercises:

- Do large muscle group exercises before doing small muscle group exercises.
- Do multiple-joint exercises (e.g., squats) before doing single-joint exercises (e.g., leg curl). Why? Because single-joint exercises fatigue the smaller muscle groups needed to perform multiple-joint exercises.

An example of a multiple-joint exercise is the bench press, because your upper and lower arms move at the shoulder and elbow joints.

An example of a single-joint exercise is a biceps curl, because only your lower arm moves at the elbow.

To determine which exercises are multiple-joint exercises, watch and feel how many joints move while you perform the exercise.

Lower-back and abdominal exercises should be done at the end of your workout because these muscles are used during other exercises for balance and posture. If they are fatigued before doing other exercises, you may not be able to do those exercises properly.

Use Lab 5-3 to help you design your workout and to record your progress.

> **What's the word. . .**
>
> **multiple-joint exercise**
> An exercise in which two or more joints move together.

## Weight-Machine Training Safety

- Keep away from moving weight stacks.
- Stay away from moving parts of the machine that could pinch your skin.
- Do not lift in an awkward position.
- Beware of broken bolts, frayed cables, broken chains, or loose cushions.
- Be alert to what is happening around you.
- Be aware of the advantages and disadvantages of using weight machines **Table 5.1** .

### The Inside Track
**What Kinds of Equipment Do You Need?**

- Standard workout clothing
- Supportive shoes
- Fitted lifting gloves (optional)
- Exercise machine or free weights

| Table 5.1 | Advantages and Disadvantages of Weight Machines |
|---|---|
| **Advantages** | **Disadvantages** |
| ■ Recommended for beginners<br>■ Convenient<br>■ Safe: weight cannot fall on you<br>■ Less clutter: no weights scattered around<br>■ No spotters needed<br>■ No lifter needed to balance bar<br>■ Offer variable resistance<br>■ Ensure correct lifting movements, which prevents cheating when tired<br>■ Easy to use: require less skill than free weights<br>■ Easy to move from one exercise to the next<br>■ Easier to adjust<br>■ Easier to isolate specific muscle groups<br>■ Back support (on most machines)<br>■ Some offer high-tech options like varying resistance during lifting motion | ■ Limited availability: may need to go to a club<br>■ Expensive<br>■ Require a lot of space<br>■ Do not allow natural movements<br>■ Most machines have only one exercise<br>■ Less motivation: only working against resistance on a machine |

## Weight Machines: Circuit Training

Circuit training combines aerobic and strength exercise.
- Each exercise station takes 30 to 45 seconds to do.
- Stations alternate between upper and lower body exercises.
- The circuit is repeated two or more times per session.
- Do a circuit-training workout three times each week for aerobic conditioning and moderate increases in strength.

## Using Free Weights (Barbells, Dumbbells)

Olympic-style barbells with a narrow center bar for gripping and wider ends for loading weights are the most common in gyms.
- The bar is 5 to 7 feet long and weighs 30 to 45 pounds.
- The bell plates used to load the bars come in pounds and kilograms. They range from 2.5 to 45 lb (1.25 to 20 kg).
- Know if your gym uses plates in pounds or kilograms: 10 lb is much heavier than 10 kg. Use adjustable collars to keep plates on the bar.
- Depending on the style of collar, a pair of bells can add 1 to 5 lb to your bar.
- Be aware of the advantages and disadvantages of using free weights   Table 5.2 .

| Table 5.2 | Advantages and Disadvantages of Free Weights |
| --- | --- |
| **Advantages** | **Disadvantages** |
| ■ Allow dynamic movements<br>■ Allow a greater variety of exercises<br>■ Widely available<br>■ Require minimal space<br>■ Strength transfers to daily activities<br>■ Inexpensive<br>■ Offer greater sense of accomplishment<br>■ Most serious bodybuilders and lifters use free weights | ■ Not as safe as exercise machines: weights can fall off the end of the bar or can pin or smash you when muscles tire<br>■ Balancing is required, which can be difficult and dangerous (e.g., weights overhead or while doing squats)<br>■ Require spotters for some exercises<br>■ Allow cheating by swinging for momentum when muscles tire<br>■ Require more time to change weights<br>■ Can cause blisters and calluses<br>■ Clutter creates hazard when weights are scattered |

## Proper Free-Weight Lifting Techniques

- Keep weights as close to your body as possible.
- Do most of the lifting with your legs.
- Keep your hips and buttocks tucked in.
- Keep your hands dry.
- Wear gloves to prevent calluses and blisters.
- Wrap your thumbs around the bar when gripping it.
- When picking up a weight from the ground, keep your back straight and your head level or up.
- Warm up before lifting.
- Use spotters and collars with free weights.
- Start slowly and progress gradually.
- Perform exercises smoothly and with good form.
- Lift or push the weight forcefully during the active phase of the lift and then lower it slowly with control.
- Perform all lifts through the full range of motion to reduce the chance of injury and soreness. Do not lock (fully straighten) your knees or elbows when involved in an exercise, as this practice stresses the joint.
- Exhale when exerting the greatest force, and inhale when moving the weight into position for the active phase of the lift.
- Rest between sets if you perform more than one set of each exercise.
- If you feel pain during an exercise, stop immediately. Continue only if the pain subsides, but reduce the amount of weight.
- Soreness the next day is normal when first starting to exercise or when increasing the amount of weight you lift.
- Cool down after a workout.

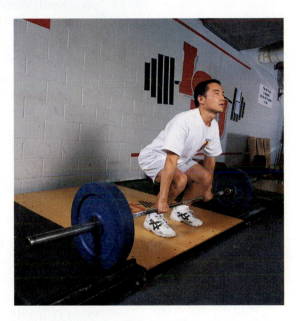

### What's the word. . .

**spotter** Another person who can help if the weight tilts or can help move a weight into position before or after a lift.

**collars** Devices used to secure weights to a barbell or dumbbell. Without collars the weights on one side of the bar will slip off.

**5**

## Improper Free-Weight Lifting Techniques

Do not do the following:

- Bend at the waist with legs straight
- Twist your body while lifting
- Jerk weights; lift smoothly and slowly
- Bounce weights against your body during an exercise
- Arch your back when lifting a weight
- Lift beyond the limits of your strength
- Hold your breath when lifting

## Training with Weights

These exercises may be done with free weights or with circuit-training machines.

### Bench Press

Muscles developed: pectoralis major, triceps, deltoids. See **Figure 5.6**.

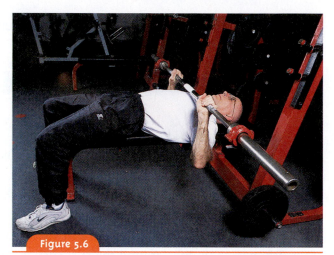

Figure 5.6

Bench press.

- Lie facing up on a bench, your feet flat on the floor, with your head, shoulders, and buttocks pressed down firmly.
- Grip the bar about shoulder width or slightly wider. Push the bar from a low point on your chest to a high point over your chin.
- Extend your arms, pause momentarily, then lower them slowly. Repeat.
- **Do not** arch your back or raise your buttocks during lifting.
- **Do not** bounce the bar off of your chest.

### Shoulder (Military) Press

Muscles developed: deltoids, triceps, trapezius. See **Figure 5.7**.

- Stand or sit with your feet shoulder-width apart. Keep your eyes straight ahead and your back straight. Place your hands shoulder-width apart. Push the bar overhead to arm's length, pause, then slowly lower it. Repeat.

### Biceps Curl

Muscles developed: biceps, brachialis. See **Figure 5.8**.

- Stand with your feet spread shoulder-width apart, palms facing out. In the starting position, the bar should rest against your thighs. Keep your elbows by your sides, bend your arms slowly to raise the weight up to your chest, pause, then slowly lower it. Repeat.

### Triceps Curl

Muscles developed: triceps. See **Figure 5.9**.

- Sit erect with your elbows and palms facing up, the bar resting behind your neck on your shoulders. Your hands should be shoulder-width apart. Slowly curl the weight overhead, pause, and slowly lower it. Repeat.

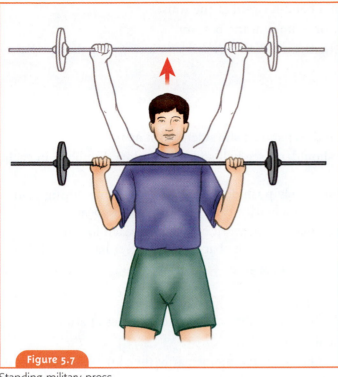

**Figure 5.7**

Standing military press.

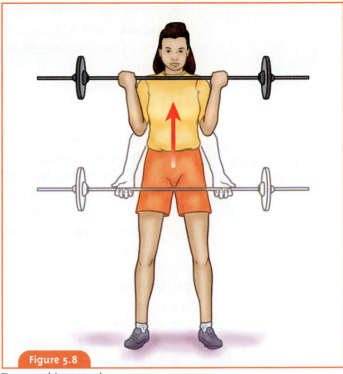

**Figure 5.8**

Two-arm biceps curl.

## Half Squat

Muscles developed: quadriceps, gluteus maximus, hamstrings, gastrocnemius. See **Figure 5.10**.

- Stand erect with the bar resting on your trapezius muscles (shoulder muscles), not your neck.
- Use an overhand grip, with your hands and feet spread shoulder-width part.
- Lower your weight by bending at the knees to a 90° angle (thighs parallel to floor), pause, and slowly return to an upright position. Repeat.

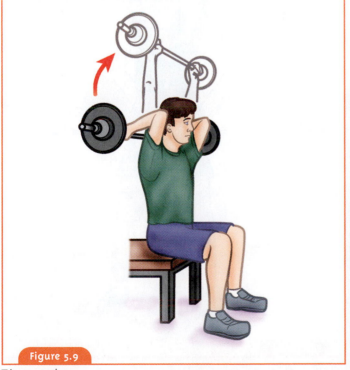

**Figure 5.9**

Triceps curl.

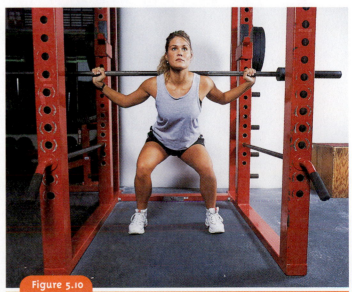

**Figure 5.10**

Half squat.

**5**

- Keep your back straight; do not bend forward at the waist.
- **Do not** squat beyond halfway or bounce at the bottom.
- Place a bench behind you so that you can sit down if you lose your balance. Use spotters.

### Heel Raise

Muscles developed: gastrocnemius, soleus. See Figure 5.11.

- Stand erect with your hands and feet spread shoulder-width apart.
- Hold the bar resting on your shoulders (see half squat) or hold a dumbbell in each hand. Use an overhand grip.
- With your feet flat on the floor, slowly push down on your toes while lifting your heels as high as possible, pause momentarily, then lower slowly. Repeat.
- You can also do this exercise by placing the front one third of each foot on the edge of a bottom stair or wood block, with the backs of your feet hanging off.

### Upright Rowing

Muscles developed: trapezius, deltoids, biceps. See Figure 5.12.

- In a standing position, grip the bar with palms down 4 to 8 inches apart.
- Keep your eyes straight ahead and chest high.
- Raise the bar until it reaches chin height, pause momentarily, then lower slowly. Repeat.
- Keep your weight close to the front of your body, and make sure that your elbows stay higher than your hands.

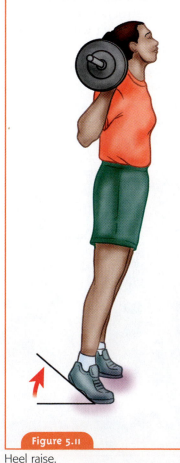

**Figure 5.11**

Heel raise.

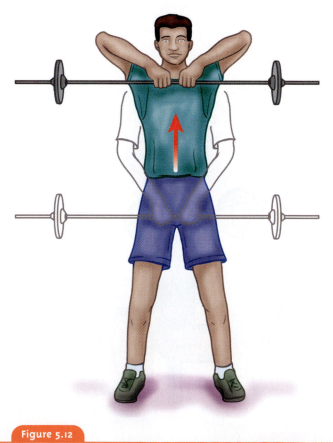

**Figure 5.12**

Upright rowing.

## Lunge

Muscles developed: thigh, gluteal. See Figure 5.13.

- Place the barbell behind your head or use a dumbbell in each hand.
- Keep the weight of the bar mainly on your trapezius muscles, not your neck.
- Your hands should be shoulder-width apart.
- Keep your head up and look forward, with your back straight.
- Slowly take a step forward and allow your leading leg to drop so that it is nearly parallel with floor. The lower part of your leg should be nearly vertical and your back should be kept upright.
- Pause momentarily, then take a stride with your other leg to return to a standing position.
- Repeat with your other leg.

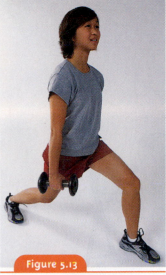

**Figure 5.13**

Lunge.

## Training without Weights

### Push-ups

Push-ups develop the triceps, deltoids, pectoralis major, abdominals, and erector spinae Figure 5.14.

- Keep your back as straight as possible. Flex your elbows. Lower your body until it almost touches the floor; pause momentarily, then raise yourself back up to the starting position and repeat.
- You can use a bench, chair, or stairway to support your hands, rather than the floor.
- Increase resistance by having someone push down on your way up.
- If you are unable to do push-ups as described, do modified push-ups by placing your lower body on your knees rather than on your feet Figure 5.15.

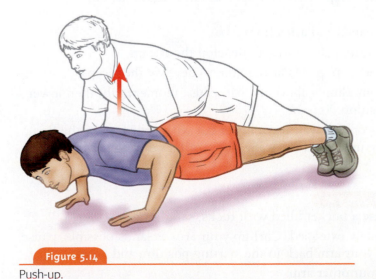

**Figure 5.14**

Push-up.

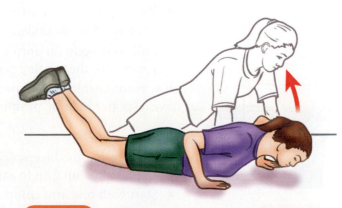

**Figure 5.15**

Modified push-up.

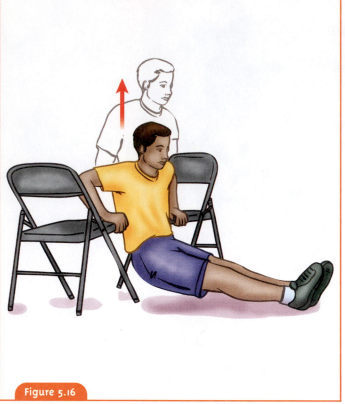

Figure 5.16

Modified dip.

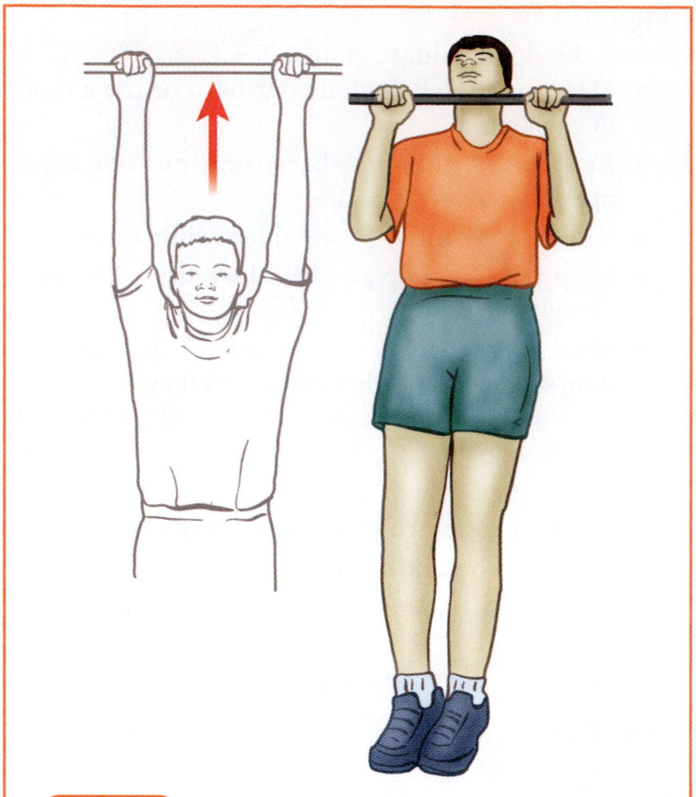

Figure 5.17

Pull-up or chin-up.

### Modified Dip

The modified dip develops the triceps, deltoids, and pectoralis major Figure 5.16 .

- Place your hands on opposite chairs or use parallel bars.
- With your knees slightly bent, dip down to at least a 90° angle at the elbow joint, pause momentarily, then raise yourself back up to the starting position. Repeat. Increase resistance by having someone push down on your way up.

### Pull-ups and Chin-ups

Pull-ups and chin-ups develop the biceps, triceps, trapezius, and latissimus dorsi
Figure 5.17 .

- Suspend yourself by your hands and arms from a bar.
- *Pull-ups:* Use an overhand grip, palms away, to develop the triceps.
- *Chin-ups:* Use an underhand grip, palms facing you, to develop the biceps.
- Pull your body up until your chin is above the bar, pause momentarily, then lower yourself to the starting position. Repeat.

If you are unable to do a pull-up this way, use a lower bar with your feet on the floor, or have a spotter help by pushing upward at the waist, hips, or legs during the exercise.

### Arm Curl

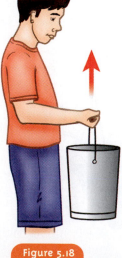

Figure 5.18

Arm curl.

Arm curls develop the biceps Figure 5.18 .

- Use a palms-up grip to raise a bucket filled with rocks, sand, or dirt.
- Start with one arm completely extended. Curl up your arm as far as possible, pause momentarily, then extend your arm back to the starting position and repeat.
- Repeat the exercise with your other arm.

### Curl-ups or Crunches

Curl-ups or crunches develop the abdominals and hip flexors **Figure 5.19**.

- Lie face up on the floor or an exercise pad, with your knees bent at a 90° angle and both feet flat on the floor.
- Fold your arms across your chest or place hands over your ears—do not lock your fingers behind your head.
- Slowly raise your upper torso into a curling motion until your shoulders have totally cleared the floor.
- Pause momentarily, then slowly return to starting position. Repeat.

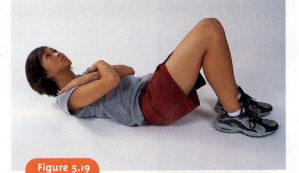

**Figure 5.19**
Curl-up.

### Twisting Curl-up

- Perform the crunch (preceding section), but as you raise your shoulders off the floor, twist your upper torso to bring your left shoulder toward your right knee.
- Slowly lower yourself back to the starting position.
- Repeat by doing each twist to an alternate side, or alternate sides from one rep to another.

### Lunges

These exercises are completed in the same fashion as lunges with weights, except that the hands are placed on the hips.

- Look straight ahead.
- From the "standing upright" position, step out and allow your leading leg to come almost parallel to the floor.
- Your back leg should come to a nearly vertical position.
- Pause, and return to the standing position.
- Repeat with your other leg.

### Step-up

This exercise requires a firm box, aerobic step, or step of a stairwell to complete.

- Position yourself facing the step.
- Step in an "up, up, down, down" cadence.
- Alternate the initial "step-up" leg.
- As your strength develops, you can increase the height of the step or quicken the pace of the cadence.

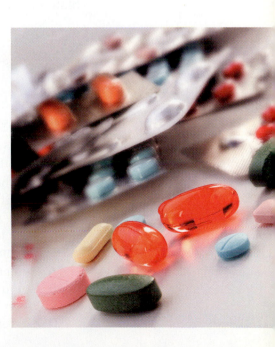

## Cautions About Supplements and Drugs

Many people take drugs and supplements to enhance the results of their weight training. This practice can be expensive and dangerous. The most common of these substances are anabolic steroids, synthetic derivatives of testosterone. Using this kind of drug helps bodybuilders develop abnormally large muscle mass—along with some undesirable secondary sexual characteristics.

Steroids increase protein synthesis, which promotes muscle growth and improves the ability of muscle to respond to training and recovery.

**5**

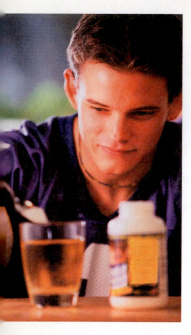

## Drugs with Undesirable Side Effects

- *Testosterone* has the same benefits and similar side effects as steroids.
- *Human growth hormone (HGH)* promotes muscle growth but can cause gigantism: abnormal enlargement of the joints, jaw, and skull.
- *Amphetamines* increase motor activity and delay fatigue but can cause chest pains, extreme confusion, aggressiveness, irritability, and hallucinations.
- *Creatine* is said to increase performance in brief, high-intensity exercises such as sprinting. Side effects include diarrhea, dehydration, and muscle cramping and tearing.
- *Caffeine* also increases motor activity and delays fatigue but can cause insomnia and abnormal heart rhythm.
- *Androstenedione dehydroepiandrosterone (andro-DHEA)* promotes muscle growth. It has similar side effects as steroids.
- *Erythropoietin (EPO)* increases red blood cells and the ability to transport oxygen to the muscles. A bad side effect is thickened blood, which can lead to strokes or heart problems.

Even though steroids have been used in the sports and athletic arenas for some time, their long-term effects are not completely understood. Well-known athletes from many sports such as track, football, and professional baseball have admitted to using such performance enhancers to improve the quality of their play. But the problem goes well beyond these individuals. Participants in cycling, bodybuilding, and even make-believe sports such as professional wrestling utilize performance-enhancing drugs.

The challenge in denouncing steroids is that deaths can only be circumstantially attributed to use. The "steroid" itself doesn't kill the user; rather death results from long term, high-level use. Lyle Alzado, a former professional football player, died from brain cancer he said was caused by more than 20 years of steroid use. As many as 10 professional wrestlers with a known history of heavy and consistent steroid use have died from complications directly related to the use of the drug in the last 5 years—either heart, liver, or emotional problems. It is estimated that more than 80 professional cyclists have died from drug use in the last 10 years. Countless reports of aggression, including some high-profile cases of suspected murder, are found in police blotters related to individuals known to have used performance-enhancing drugs.

## Reflect >>>> Reinforce >>>> Reinvigorate
### Knowledge Check
*Answers in Appendix D*

1. What is the measure of muscle strength?
   A. Number of repetitions in a set
   B. Length of muscle stretch
   C. Force against resistance
   D. Time taken to complete a workout
2. Which mode of exercise is most popular for increasing strength?
   A. Isometric
   B. Isotonic
   C. Plyometric
   D. Isokinetic

The numbers aren't staggering, but the relationship between steroid use and these problems becomes clearer all the time.

According to the professionals at Exercise Prescription (ExRx.com), this is what we know about performance-enhancing drugs:

- Because each person is unique, each responds differently to the use of steroids. However, people choose steroids based on what has worked for others—a dangerous proposition at best.
- The extent of the side effects experienced is affected by the type of enhancer used, dose, length of time and frequency of use, age at first use, and use of other drugs while on steroids.
- Most physical effects are reversible after the drug is discontinued for several months, with the notable exception of damage to the myocardium—the inner muscle of the heart.

Possible side effects in men include:
- Multiple changes in the risk factors for heart disease, including the previously noted changes in the myocardium, increased triglyceride levels, increased cholesterol levels, and hypertension
- Damage to the liver's ability to function properly
- Damage and/or changes to the reproductive system, including reduced sperm count and mobility, reduced testicle size, and gynecomastia (breast development)
- Reduced ability to fight disease
- For injected forms of steroids, increased risks for HIV/AIDS, hepatitis, and other blood-borne diseases

Possible side effects in women include:
- Menstrual abnormalities and changes in clitoris size
- Masculinization, including voice changes, breast shrinkage, baldness, body hair, and increased levels of testosterone
- Some irreversible effects

Both men and women have reported a fairly consistent pattern of emotional effects related to steroid use, although the relationship seems to reflect the type of steroid, not the amount taken. Most commonly reported are bouts of anger and violence, significant mood swings, depression, and changes in the perception of one's body.

3. Which of the following is an effect of muscle training on a person's body?
   A. Higher muscle-to-fat ratio
   B. Stronger bones
   C. Higher rate of metabolism
   D. All of the above
4. When the number of desired repetitions is accomplished during an exercise, it is the completion of one:
   A. Block
   B. Form
   C. Set
   D. Activity

5. Gradually increasing the weight one uses during a workout is called:
   - A. Repetition maximum
   - B. Progressive overload
   - C. Specificity
   - D. Muscular gain

6. Which of the following exercises is designed to help build muscles in the arm?
   - A. Curls
   - B. Squats
   - C. Deadlift
   - D. Extensions

7. Which of the following is an advantage of using machine weights?
   - A. They are available everywhere.
   - B. They are inexpensive.
   - C. They are easier for beginners to use.
   - D. They take up little space.

8. Which of the following would be a reason someone might choose *not* to use free weights?
   - A. Lack of variety in exercises
   - B. Limited availability
   - C. No spotters available
   - D. Too costly to purchase

9. A person who can help complete your lift if you cannot complete the exercise on your own is called a(n):
   - A. Spotter
   - B. Assistant
   - C. Grabber
   - D. Collar

10. Once an individual can lift a weight _____ times, it is recommended to increase the weight being used.
    - A. 6
    - B. 9
    - C. 12
    - D. 20

## Modern Modifications

Take a moment to look at your lifestyle in terms of strength training. Would you like to be stronger and more fit? Try these simple suggestions to get started:

- Do a set of push-ups (modified or regular, whichever you are comfortable with) first thing each morning. Only do 1 set of however many push-ups you can perform at the moment: 5, 10, 15, or whatever that number may be. Every week try adding 1 to 2 more push-ups to your routine.
- Do a wall squat while you are waiting for class or a meeting to start.
- Take a stress ball to work or class—improve your grip strength and your mood at the same time!
- Grab a can of soup and do some bicep curls while watching television.

## Critical Thinking

1. As Susan has gotten older, her upper arms have become flabby. She is very self-conscious when she raises an arm while wearing short sleeves. Describe the type of activities Susan can do to address her problem. Discuss specific types and forms of exercise as well as FITT principle descriptors. What may be the reason for her lack of firmness in the upper arms?

2. Phil wants to start a strength-training program. He has been told that exercise machines are better for beginners than free weights. Discuss the pros and cons of weight machines versus free weights. What would you suggest to Phil?

## Going Above and Beyond

### Websites

American College of Sports Medicine
*http://www.acsm.org*

Exercise Prescription
*http://www.exrx.net*

National Strength and Conditioning Association
*http://www.nsca-cc.org*

National Council of Strength and Fitness
*http://www.ncsf.org*

Physician and Sports Medicine
*http://www.physsportsmed.com*

### References

American College of Sports Medicine (ACSM). The recommended quantity and quality of exercise for developing and maintaining cardiorespiratory and muscular fitness and flexibility in healthy adults. *Medicine and Science in Sports and Exercise* 1998; 30:975–991.

Braill P. A., et al. Muscular strength and physical function. *Medicine and Science in Sports and Exercise* 2000; 32:412–416.

Ebben W. P. and Jensen R. L. Strength training for women. *Physician and Sports Medicine* 1998; 26:86.

Feigenbaum M. S. and Pollock M. L. Strength training: Rationale for current guidelines for adult fitness programs. *Physician and Sports Medicine* 1997; 25:44.

———. Prescription of resistance training for health and disease. *Medicine and Science in Sports and Exercise* 1999; 31:38–45.

Stamford B. Weight training basics. Part 1: Choosing the best options. *Physician and Sports Medicine* 1998; 26:115–116.

# Choosing a Nutritious Diet

# What Is a Healthy Diet?

Eating is one of life's greatest pleasures. Since there are many foods and many ways to build a healthy diet and lifestyle, there is plenty of room for choice.

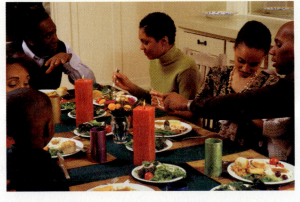

Eating is also a necessity. Nutrients must come from what you eat, because some nutrients cannot be made in the body at all, and others not in sufficient quantities.

The six classes of nutrients are proteins, fats, carbohydrates, vitamins, minerals, and water.

- Proteins, fats, carbohydrates, and water are macronutrients.
- Vitamins and minerals are micronutrients.

## Proteins

All the cells in your body are made up of proteins. Proteins vary in size, depending on how many amino acids are linked together. The proteins are made up of at least 20 different amino acids. Nine are called essential amino acids because the body cannot make them; they must be obtained from the diet. That is why you must eat protein—to take in the essential amino acids. Good sources of protein are fish, lean meat, poultry, milk, and beans.

### Complete and Incomplete Proteins

Eating protein made up of amino acids is necessary for good health. There are two types of proteins: *complete* and *incomplete*.

Complete proteins are found in animal products (e.g., meats, milk, fish, eggs).

Incomplete proteins generally have one amino acid in insufficient quantity (the limiting amino acid). Grains, legumes, and nuts are sources of incomplete proteins.

### How Much Protein Do You Need?

Many people eat high-protein foods because they think that proteins make them grow bigger and stronger.

- Each day adults need about 4 grams of protein for every 10 pounds of body weight (your ideal weight, that is). Athletes may need a bit more.
- You can estimate your protein intake by using food labels or by using the Food Guide Pyramid to get an ample amount of protein.

### What's the word. . .

**nutrients** Substances in food the body needs for normal function and good health.

**macronutrients** Nutrients needed by your body in relatively large amounts.

**micronutrients** Nutrients needed by your body in relatively small amounts.

**protein** Nutrient made up of amino acids that is needed for growth to build, repair, and maintain body tissues.

**essential amino acids** The nine protein amino acids that the body cannot make and, therefore, must come from foods you eat.

**complete protein** A protein that contains all the essential amino acids.

**incomplete protein** A protein lacking one or more of the essential amino acids.

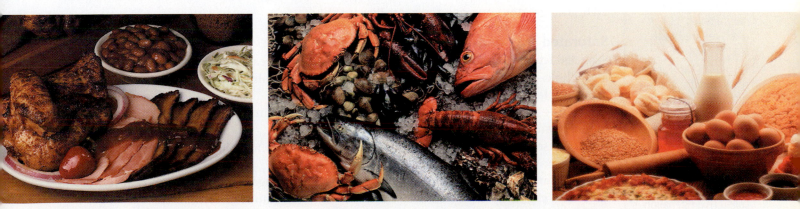

- Taking in a lot of protein increases your fluid needs, and may dehydrate you if you are not taking in enough fluids.
- Eating excessive amounts of protein for a long time requires lots of calcium since some of the calcium may be pulled from the bones. Excessive amounts may contribute to obesity, heart disease, and certain forms of cancer.
- Protein deficiency is the most common form of malnutrition in the world. It can manifest itself in two forms: kwashiorkor and marasmus. Kwashiorkor is the result of the body not receiving enough vitamins; it occurs mostly in children. Affected children tend to have swollen body tissues, particularly hands and feet, and bloated bellies. Marasmus results from lack of food. The chronic deficiency in protein results in severe **wasting** of body fat and muscles. People with marasmus have skeletal bodies (Insel, Turner, and Ross 2002).
- Although proteins provide energy, they are not the main source of energy for the body.

## Lipids (Fats, Oils)

**Lipids** (fats) may have a bad reputation, but not all fats are the same.

### Benefits of Fat Intake

Fats provide a major form of stored energy; they provide energy during exercise, in cold environments, and if starvation occurs. They:

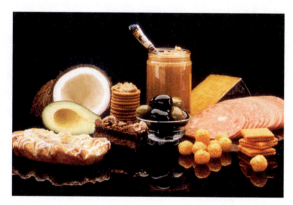

- Insulate your body
- Cushion internal organs
- Help carry other nutrients throughout your body
- Serve a structural role in making and repairing cells
- Satisfy hunger and add taste to many foods

### Cholesterol

**Cholesterol** is important in forming certain key hormones (e.g., testosterone and estrogen). The body makes cholesterol in the liver. Too much cholesterol in the blood is associated with an increased risk for heart disease. Deposits of cholesterol can build up inside the arteries, which may narrow an artery enough to slow or block blood flow.

Cholesterol is carried by **lipoproteins**. When you have your cholesterol checked, the results will show your total blood cholesterol level. If you fasted overnight before giving a blood sample, the test should also show separate counts for your **high-density lipoprotein (HDL)** and **low-density lipoprotein (LDL)**. In general, the higher your LDL and the lower your HDL, the greater your risk for heart disease.

### Saturated Fats and Trans Fats: The Bad Fats

**Saturated fats** are found primarily in animal foods (red meats, butter, poultry with skin, and whole-milk dairy products). Tropical oils such as palm and coconut are also high in saturated fat   **Table 6.1**  .

Taking in too much saturated fat can raise the amount of LDL cholesterol in your bloodstream, increasing your risk of heart disease.

Because saturated fat and cholesterol are not known to help prevent chronic diseases, they are not required in any diet.

**Trans fatty acids** are unsaturated fats converted (hydrogenated) to a form that has the same bad effects as saturated fats. Trans fats are often found in commercial baked goods, margarines, snack foods, processed foods, and fast foods.

---

### What's the word. . .

**wasting** Occurs when the diet lacks protein; the body breaks down body tissue (e.g., muscle) and uses it as a protein source.

**lipids** Fats or fatlike substances characterized by their insolubility in water or solubility in fat.

**cholesterol** Wax-like substance made by the body's liver and found in animal foods.

**lipoprotein** Allows cholesterol to dissolve in the blood and carries it through the bloodstream to all parts of the body; the two main types are high-density lipoprotein (HDL) and low-density lipoprotein (LDL).

**high-density lipoprotein (HDL)** Carries cholesterol from the blood back to the liver, which processes the cholesterol for elimination from the body. HDL is often referred to as *good* cholesterol.

**low-density lipoprotein (LDL)** Carries cholesterol from the liver to the rest of the body. When there is too much LDL cholesterol in the blood, it can be deposited on the walls of the coronary arteries. LDL is often referred to as *bad* cholesterol.

**saturated fat** Fat from meat, poultry, dairy products, and hardened vegetable fat.

**trans fatty acids** Fats produced by heating liquid vegetable oils in the presence of hydrogen. This process is called hydrogenation.

| Table 6.1 | Dietary Fats | |
|---|---|---|
| **Type of Fat** | **Main Sources** | **Effect on Blood Cholesterol Levels** |
| Monounsaturated | Olives; olive oil, canola oil, peanut oil; cashews, almonds, peanuts, and most other nuts | Lowers LDL; raises HDL |
| Polyunsaturated | Corn, soybean, safflower oil; fish | Lowers LDL; raises HDL |
| Saturated | Whole milk, butter, cheese, ice cream; red meat; chocolate; coconuts | Raises both LDL and HDL |
| Trans fatty acids | Most margarines; vegetable shortening; partially hydrogenated vegetable oil; deep-fried chips; many fast foods; most commercial baked goods | Raises LDL |

**What's the word...**

**unsaturated fat** Type of fat obtained from plant sources and fish; two types are monounsaturated and polyunsaturated.

**monounsaturated** High concentrations of unsaturated fat in canola, peanut, and olive oils.

**polyunsaturated** High concentrations of unsaturated fat in sunflower, corn, soybean oils, and fish.

**carbohydrate** Nutrient that is the body's main source of energy; consists of sugars and starches found in grains, vegetables, and fruits; two types are simple and complex.

**glucose** Simple sugar circulating in the blood.

**glycogen** Complex carbohydrates stored primarily in the skeletal muscles and liver. When energy is needed, glycogen is converted to glucose.

Food manufacturers hydrogenate foods to extend their shelf life. The more processed foods you eat, the greater your trans fat intake. Trans fatty acids are worse for cholesterol levels than saturated fats because they not only raise LDLs but also lower HDLs.

### Monounsaturated and Polyunsaturated Fatty Acids: The Good Fats

When unsaturated fats—monounsaturated and polyunsaturated—are eaten in place of carbohydrates, these good fats decrease LDL levels and increase HDL levels, and thus lower the risk of heart disease.

- Monounsaturated fatty acids are found in olive oil, canola, and peanut oils.
- Polyunsaturated fatty acids are found in fish, sunflower, corn, wheat, nuts, soybean, and vegetable oils. Fish (e.g., mackerel, salmon, sardines, swordfish) are sources of omega-3 fatty acids, which have the potential to lower heart disease risk. The American Heart Association recommends that everyone eat at least two servings of fish each week.

### High-Fat Diet and Your Health

A high-fat diet usually means saturated fat. It is associated with many diseases, including heart disease, cancer, obesity, and diabetes. However, a completely fat-free diet can be harmful, since certain fats are essential nutrients.

Limit the bad fats and replace them with good fats. Try to reduce your consumption of both trans and saturated fats as much as possible and replace them with polyunsaturated and monounsaturated fats.

## Carbohydrates

Carbohydrates are the main source of energy for your body. Your body breaks down most of them to a simple sugar, glucose, also called "blood sugar." Glucose is the most important source of energy for your body. It is stored in your liver and muscle as glycogen.

There are two types of carbohydrates: simple and complex.

- Examples of foods containing simple carbohydrates are table sugar, honey, fruit, milk, maple syrup, and molasses.
- Examples of foods containing complex carbohydrates are whole grains, fruits, vegetables, and legumes (peas and beans).

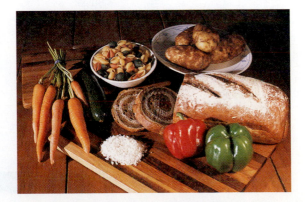

Complex carbohydrates consist of starch (digestible) and fiber (indigestible). For health reasons you should take in a sufficient amount of fiber every day.

### Glycemic Index and Glycemic Load

The glycemic index measures how different foods affect your blood sugar levels Table 6.2. For example, white bread and potatoes cause blood sugar to rise rapidly. Therefore, they are classified as having a high glycemic index. Apples and brown rice are

## Table 6.2 — Glycemic Index

| Cereals | GL | GI | Snacks | GL | GI | Pasta | GL | GI | Beans | GL | GI |
|---|---|---|---|---|---|---|---|---|---|---|---|
| All Bran | 9 | 51 | Chocolate bar | 12 | 46 | Cheese tortellini | 10 | 50 | Baked | 7 | 44 |
| Bran Buds + psyll | 6 | 45 | Corn chips | 17 | 72 | Fettucini | 15 | 32 | Black, boiled | 9 | 30 |
| Bran Flakes | 13 | 74 | Croissant | 17 | 67 | Linguini | 23 | 50 | Butter, boiled | 6 | 33 |
| Cheerios | 15 | 74 | Doughnut | 17 | 76 | Macaroni | 23 | 46 | Garbanzo, boiled | 11 | 34 |
| Corn Chex | 21 | 83 | Graham crackers | 14 | 74 | Spaghetti, 5 min. boiled | 16 | 33 | Kidney, boiled | 7 | 29 |
| Cornflakes | 21 | 83 | Jelly beans | 22 | 80 | Spaghetti, 15 min. boiled | 21 | 44 | Kidney, canned | 9 | 52 |
| Cream of Wheat | 17 | 66 | Life Savers | 21 | 70 | Spaghetti, protein rich | 14 | 28 | Lentils, green, brown | 5 | 30 |
| Frosted Flakes | 15 | 55 | Oatmeal cookie | 9 | 57 | Vermicelli | 16 | 35 | Lima, boiled | 10 | 32 |
| Grapenuts | 15 | 67 | Pizza, cheese and tomato sauce | 16 | 60 | | | | Navy | 12 | 38 |
| Life | 16 | 66 | Pizza Hut, supreme | 7 | 33 | | | | Pinto, boiled | 10 | 39 |
| Muesli, natural | 11 | 54 | Popcorn, light microwave | 6 | 55 | **Soups/vegetables** | | | Red lentils, boiled | 5 | 27 |
| Nutri-grain | 10 | 66 | Potato chips | 11 | 56 | Beets, canned | 5 | 64 | Soy, boiled | 1 | 16 |
| Oatmeal, old-fashioned | 11 | 48 | Pound cake | 15 | 54 | Black bean soup | 17 | 64 | | | |
| Puffed Wheat | 13 | 67 | Power bars | 24 | 58 | Carrots, fresh, boiled | 3 | 49 | **Breads** | | |
| Raisin Bran | 12 | 73 | Pretzels | 16 | 83 | Corn, sweet | 9 | 56 | Bagel, plain | 25 | 72 |
| Rice Chex | 23 | 89 | Saltine crackers | 12 | 74 | Green pea, soup | 27 | 66 | Baguette, French | 15 | 95 |
| Shredded Wheat | 13 | 67 | Shortbread cookies | 10 | 64 | Green pea, frozen | 4 | 47 | Croissant | 17 | 67 |
| Special K | 11 | 54 | Snickers bar | 15 | 41 | Lima beans, frozen | 10 | 32 | Dark rye | 10 | 76 |
| Total | 17 | 76 | Strawberry jam | 10 | 51 | Parsnips | 12 | 97 | Hamburger bun | 9 | 61 |
| | | | Vanilla wafers | 14 | 77 | Peas, fresh, boiled | 7 | 48 | Muffin, apple cinnamon | 13 | 44 |
| **Fruit** | | | | | | Split pea soup w/ham | 16 | 66 | Muffin, blueberry | 17 | 59 |
| | | | **Crackers** | | | Tomato soup | 6 | 38 | Pita | 10 | 57 |
| Apple | 6 | 38 | Graham | 14 | 74 | | | | Pizza, cheese | 16 | 60 |
| Apricots | 5 | 57 | Rice cakes | 17 | 80 | | | | Sourdough | 6 | 54 |
| Banana | 12 | 56 | Rye | 11 | 68 | **Drinks** | | | Rye | 6 | 64 |
| Cantaloupe | 4 | 65 | Soda | 13 | 72 | Apple juice | 12 | 40 | White | 10 | 70 |
| Cherries | 3 | 22 | | | | Colas | 16 | 65 | Wheat | 12 | 68 |
| Dates | 42 | 103 | **Cereal grains** | | | Gatorade | 12 | 78 | | | |
| Grapefruit | 3 | 25 | | | | Grapefruit juice | 11 | 48 | **Root crops** | | |
| Grapes | 8 | 46 | Barley | 11 | 25 | Orange juice | 13 | 46 | | | |
| Kiwi | 6 | 52 | Basmati white rice | 22 | 58 | Pineapple juice | 16 | 46 | French fries | 22 | 75 |
| Mango | 8 | 55 | Bulgar | 16 | 48 | | | | Potato, new, boiled | 12 | 59 |
| Orange | 5 | 43 | Couscous | 23 | 65 | **Milk products** | | | Potato, sweet | 16 | 52 |
| Papaya | 10 | 58 | Cornmeal | 9 | 68 | | | | Potato, white, boiled | 11 | 63 |
| Peach | 5 | 42 | Millet | 25 | 71 | Chocolate milk | 9 | 35 | | | |
| Pear | 4 | 40 | | | | Custard | 7 | 43 | Potato, white, mashed | 15 | 70 |
| Pineapple | 7 | 66 | **Sugars** | | | Ice cream, vanilla | 8 | 60 | Yam | 13 | 54 |
| Plums | 5 | 39 | | | | Skim milk | 4 | 32 | | | |
| Prunes | 10 | 15 | Fructose | 2 | 22 | Soy milk | 8 | 31 | | | |
| Raisins | 28 | 64 | Honey | 11 | 62 | Whole milk | 3 | 30 | | | |
| Watermelon | 4 | 72 | Maltose | 11 | 105 | Yogurt, fruit | 9 | 36 | | | |
| | | | Table sugar | 7 | 64 | Yogurt, plain | 3 | 14 | | | |

GL = Glycemic load.
GI = Glycemic index.

| Table 6.3 | Sample Substitutions for High-Glycemic-Index Foods | | |
|---|---|---|---|
| **High-Glycemic-Index Food** | **Low-Glycemic-Index Alternative** | **High-Glycemic-Index Food** | **Low-Glycemic-Index Alternative** |
| Bread, wheat | Oat bran, rye, or pumpernickel bread | Plain cookies and crackers | Cookies made with dried fruits and whole grains such as oats |
| Processed breakfast cereal | Unrefined cereal such as oats (either muesli or oatmeal) | Cakes and muffins | Cakes and muffins made with fruit, oats, or whole grains |
| Bananas | Apples | Potatoes | Pasta or legumes |

*Source:* Insel P., Turner R. E., and Ross D. *Nutrition,* 2nd ed. Sudbury, MA: Jones and Bartlett, 2004:149.

digested more slowly and cause a lower and more gradual change in blood sugar; therefore, they have a lower glycemic index  **Table 6.3** .

You should use caution when using the glycemic index for dietary purposes. At first glance, you can see that the values for the glycemic index are based on how quickly 50 grams of the carbohydrates from each food will turn into blood sugar. Fifty grams of carbohydrate is found in a slice of white bread, which is often used as the food to which all others are compared. Not all foods, in an average serving, contain 50 grams of carbohydrates. In fact, you'd have to eat about 1.5 pounds of carrots to consume 50 grams of carbohydrates!

To recognize this distinction, the glycemic load was created. The glycemic load takes into consideration the glycemic index of a food, plus the number of carbohydrates of that food you would eat in a typical serving. When reviewing the information in Table 6.2, use the following scale to guide you:

| Glycemic Load | Glycemic Index | Rating |
|---|---|---|
| More than 20 | More than 70 | High |
| 11–19 | 56–69 | Moderate |
| 10 or less | 55 or less | Low |

Both diabetes and heart disease have been associated with high-glycemic-index foods. Type 2 diabetes can be helped by lower-glycemic-index foods.

It is wise to eat minimally processed whole-grain products rather than highly processed grains, cereals, and sugars.

## Main Uses of Carbohydrates in Your Body

Your body uses carbohydrates as:

- Fuel in the form of glucose, the most important source of energy in our body. Glucose is stored in the liver and muscle as glycogen. The complex carbohydrates you eat are digested and broken down into simple sugars, mostly glucose, and then used by the muscles, brain, heart, and other organs for energy.
- Building blocks to make chemicals needed by the cells in the body.
- Chemical cement for repairing structures of the body.

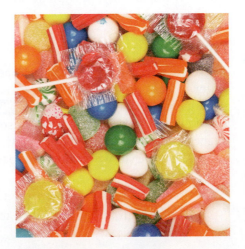

### The Inside Track
**Added Sugars**

Added sugars are put into foods and beverages during production (they are not the natural sugars in fruits and milk). Added sugars are found in candy, soft drinks, fruit drinks, pastries, and other manufactured sweets.

Added sugars should account for no more than 25% of your total calories. If your diet is high in added sugars, you will take in fewer essential nutrients.

**6**

| Table 6.4 | U.S. Department of Agriculture's Dietary Recommendations |

### Dietary Intake

| Nutrient | Calories per Gram | Grams Based on 2000-Calorie Diet | Percentage of Total Daily Calories |
|---|---|---|---|
| Protein | 4 calories per gram | 50–60 grams | 10–12% |
| Fats (total) Saturated fat | 9 calories per gram 9 calories per gram | Less than 65 grams Less than 20 grams | Less than 30% Less than 10% |
| Carbohydrates | 4 calories per gram | 225–325 grams | 45–65% |

### Daily Calorie Allowance

### Calories Required

| Activity Level | Men | Women |
|---|---|---|
| Resting | 12 per lb body weight | 13 per lb body weight |
| Sedentary | 16 per lb body weight | 14 per lb body weight |
| Light | 18 per lb body weight | 16 per lb body weight |
| Moderate | 21 per lb body weight | 18 per lb body weight |
| Active | 26 per lb body weight | 22 per lb body weight |

### Calorie Intake

| |
|---|
| 1600 calories per day for children, inactive women, and older adults |
| 2200 calories per day for moderately active women, inactive men, and teenage girls |
| 2800 calories per day for teenage boys, active women, and active men |
| 2200–2800 calories per day for pregnant and breastfeeding women |

## USDA Recommendations

The U.S. Department of Agriculture (USDA) makes the suggestions shown in (Table 6.4) for the average person's diet.

## Fiber

There are two categories of dietary fiber: soluble and insoluble. Insoluble fiber binds with water to help produce bowel movements. Good sources of insoluble fiber are wheat products, leafy vegetables, and fruits (Table 6.5). Soluble fiber is associated with reduced levels of cholesterol. Good sources of soluble fiber include oatmeal and beans. Evidence suggests that including fiber in your diet may help in the following ways:

- The fiber in wheat bran and oat bran is effective in relieving and preventing constipation.
- Insoluble fiber can lower the risk of diverticular disease.
- A diet high in fiber is linked to a lower risk of type 2 diabetes.

*What's the word...*

**dietary fiber** Nondigestible carbohydrates found in plants; two types are soluble and insoluble.

**insoluble fiber** Does not dissolve in water.

**soluble fiber** Partially dissolves in water.

| Table 6.5 | Foods Rich in Soluble and Insoluble Dietary Fiber | | |
|---|---|---|---|
| **Rich in Soluble Fiber** | **Rich in Insoluble Fiber** | **Rich in Soluble Fiber** | **Rich in Insoluble Fiber** |
| **Fruits** | | **Nuts and Seeds** | |
| Apples | Apples | Peanuts | Almonds |
| Cranberries | Bananas | Pecans | Sesame seeds |
| Grapefruit | Berries | Walnuts | Sunflower seeds |
| Mango | Cherries | **Legumes** | |
| Oranges | Pears | Most legumes | Most legumes |
| **Vegetables** | | **Grains** | |
| Asparagus | Broccoli | Oat bran | Brown rice |
| Broccoli | Green peppers | Oatmeal | Whole-wheat breads |
| Brussels sprouts | Red cabbage | Psyllium | Wheat-bran cereals |
| Carrots | Spinach | | |
| | Sprouts | | |

*Source:* Adapted from Shils M. E., Olson J. A., Shike M., and Ross A. C., eds. *Modern Nutrition in Health and Disease,* 9th ed. Philadelphia: Lippincott Williams & Wilkins, 1999.

- A high intake of fiber, especially that found in grains, has been linked to a lower risk of heart disease.
- Fiber in your diet promotes weight control by enhancing a full feeling.

Despite what many people think, large studies have not found a link between fiber and a reduced risk for colon cancer (Fuchs et al 1999).

The recommended daily intake for total fiber per day is 20 to 35 grams.

## Vitamins

You must get vitamins from food or a daily multiple vitamin because your body cannot make them. In the body, vitamins:

- Release energy from carbohydrates, lipids, and proteins
- Help grow and repair tissue
- Maintain and support reproductive functions
- Produce the immune response

### Types of Vitamins

*Fat-soluble* vitamins dissolve in fat, can be stored in the body, and are not excreted in the urine. They include four vitamins: A, D, E, and K.

*Water-soluble* vitamins dissolve in water and cannot be stored by the body in significant amounts. They include vitamin C and eight B vitamins: thiamin ($B_1$), riboflavin ($B_2$), niacin ($B_3$), pyridoxine ($B_6$), cobalamin ($B_{12}$), folate, pantothenic acid, and biotin. Excess amounts are excreted in the urine.

### Vitamin Excesses and Deficiencies

A healthy, balanced diet provides most of the vitamins your body needs. Taking large doses of vitamin supplements can (if fat soluble) result in an accumulation in the body excessive enough to cause you harm. Conversely, not getting enough of the right kinds of vitamins in your diet can cause health problems as well  Table 6.6 .

**Ask Yourself**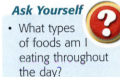

- What types of foods am I eating throughout the day?
- Where do my calories come from?

**What's the word. . .**

**vitamin** Nutrient necessary for normal functioning of the body; two types are water soluble and fat soluble.

## Table 6.6 — Major Vitamins

| Vitamin | Major Functions | Rich Food Sources | Deficiency Signs/Symptoms | Toxicity Signs/Symptoms |
|---|---|---|---|---|
| A and provitamin A (beta-carotene) | Vision in dim light, growth, reproduction, maintains immune system and skin, antioxidant | Liver, milk, dark green and leafy vegetables, carrots, sweet potatoes, mangos, oatmeal, broccoli, apricots, peaches, romaine lettuce | Poor vision in dim light, dry skin, blindness, poor growth, respiratory infections | Intestinal upset, liver damage, hair loss, headache, birth defects, death (beta-carotene is less toxic than vitamin A) |
| D | Bone and tooth development and growth | Few good food sources other than fortified milk and eggs | Weak, deformed bones (rickets) | Growth failure, loss of appetite, weight loss, death |
| E | Antioxidant: protects cell membranes | Vegetable oils, whole grains, wheat germ, sunflower seeds, almonds | Anemia (rarely occurs) | Intestinal upset, bleeding problems |
| C | Scar formation and maintenance, immune system functioning, antioxidant | Citrus fruits, berries, potatoes, broccoli, peppers, cabbage, tomatoes, fortified fruit drinks | Frequent infections, bleeding gums, bruises, poor wound healing, depression (scurvy) | Diarrhea, nosebleeds, headache, weakness, kidney stones, excess iron absorption and storage |
| Thiamin | Energy metabolism | Pork, liver, nuts, dried beans and peas, whole-grain and enriched breads and cereals | Heart failure, mental confusion, depression, paralysis (beriberi) | No toxicity has been reported |
| Riboflavin | Energy metabolism | Milk and yogurt, eggs and poultry, meat, liver, whole-grain and enriched breads and cereals | Enlarged, purple tongue; fatigue; oily skin; cracks in the corners of the mouth | No toxicity has been reported |
| Niacin | Energy metabolism | Protein-rich foods, peanut butter, whole-grain and enriched breads and cereals | Skin rash, diarrhea, weakness, dementia, death (pellagra) | Painful skin flushing, intestinal upset, liver damage |
| Vitamin $B_6$ | Protein and fat metabolism | Liver, oatmeal, bananas, meat, fish, poultry, whole grains, fortified cereals | Anemia, skin rash, irritability, elevated homocysteine levels | Weakness, depression, permanent nerve damage |
| Folate (folic acid) | DNA production | Leafy vegetables, oranges, nuts, liver, enriched breads and cereals | Anemia, depression, spina bifida in developing embryo, elevated homocysteine levels | Hides signs of vitamin $B_{12}$ deficiency; may cause allergic response |
| $B_{12}$ | DNA production | Animal products | Pernicious anemia, fatigue, paralysis, elevated homocysteine levels | No toxicity has been reported |

Source: Alters S. and Schiff W. *Essential Concepts of Healthy Living,* 3rd ed. Sudbury, MA: Jones and Bartlett, 2003:212.

## Daily Multivitamin Supplement

Walter Willett (2001), who is with the Harvard School of Public Health, says that most people in the United States get enough vitamins to prevent the classic deficiency diseases. He also states that although we may prevent the classic deficiency diseases, most of us do not get enough of five key vitamins that may be associated in preventing several chronic diseases:

- Folic acid
- Vitamin $B_6$
- Vitamin $B_{12}$
- Vitamin D (see **Figure 6.1**)
- Vitamin E

A standard, store-brand, 100% RDA-level multivitamin can supply you with enough of these vitamins. Such a supplement cannot replace healthy eating, but it is an inexpensive way of providing a nutritional safety net. See **Table 6.7** for newly recognized findings on vitamins.

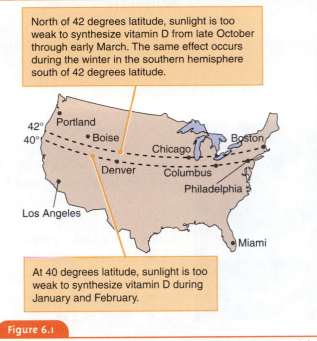

North of 42 degrees latitude, sunlight is too weak to synthesize vitamin D from late October through early March. The same effect occurs during the winter in the southern hemisphere south of 42 degrees latitude.

At 40 degrees latitude, sunlight is too weak to synthesize vitamin D during January and February.

**Figure 6.1**

Mapping vitamin D synthesis. Vitamin D synthesis halts for part of the winter if sunlight is too weak. In Los Angeles and Miami, the sunlight is strong enough to synthesize vitamin D year-round, even in January.

| Table 6.7 | Newly Recognized Findings on Vitamins | |
|---|---|---|
| **Vitamin** | **New or Suspected Roles in Health and Disease** | **Daily Optimal Intake** |
| A | Stimulates production and activity of white blood cells, takes part in remodeling bone, helps maintain health of endothelial cells (those lining the body's interior surfaces), regulates cell growth and division | 5000 IU for men; 4000 IU for women |
| $B_6$ | May help fight heart disease and some types of cancer | 1.3 to 1.7 mg |
| $B_{12}$ | May help fight heart disease and some types of cancer; may help those with dementia or Alzheimer's disease | 6 $\mu$g |
| Folic acid | Reduces chances of mothers having children with birth defects (spina bifida or anencephaly); may help fight heart disease and some types of cancer | 400 $\mu$g |
| C | Controls infections; neutralizes harmful free radicals; helps make collagen, which is needed for healthy bones, teeth, gums, and blood vessels | 90 mg for men; 75 mg for women (add extra 35 mg for smokers); as evidence unfolds, 200 to 300 mg |
| D | Helps body absorb and retain calcium and phosphorus, both critical for building bone; keeps cancer cells from growing and dividing; prevents risk of fractures; low intake increases risks of prostate, breast, colon, and other cancers | 5 $\mu$g up to age 50 years; 10 $\mu$g between ages 51 and 70 years; 15 $\mu$g after age 70 years |
| E | Thought to prevent heart attacks (further studies are needed) | 15 mg from food or 22 IU from natural source or 33 IU of synthetic form; may need 400 IU or more for optimal health |
| K | Helps make 6 of the 13 proteins needed for blood clotting; involved in building bone; reduces risk of hip fracture | 80 $\mu$g for men; 65 $\mu$g for women |

*Source:* Adapted from Willett W. C. *Eat, Drink, and Be Healthy.* New York: Fireside, 2001.

**6**

## Minerals

Minerals are essential for a variety of important bodily functions. They regulate fluid balance, conduct nerve impulses, and contract muscles (see ⬤ Table 6.8 ).

Minerals are classified according to the body's needs. At least 6 macrominerals are essential to health (e.g., sodium, chloride, potassium, calcium, phosphorus, and magnesium).

Microminerals are trace minerals (e.g., iron, zinc, copper, manganese, molybdenum, selenium, iodine, and fluoride).

Two of the most important minerals for keeping yourself healthy are calcium and iron. Calcium is especially important for women, to help them ward off osteoporosis in later life. Iron is important for women to prevent anemia.

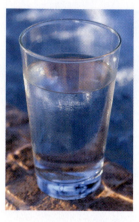

## Water

Water in the body serves many important purposes:

- Excrete wastes
- Maintain blood circulation throughout the body
- Maintain body temperature
- Digest and absorb nutrients

### Table 6.8    Some Essential Minerals

| Mineral | Roles | Rich Food Sources | Deficiency Signs/Symptoms | Toxicity Signs/Symptoms |
|---------|-------|-------------------|---------------------------|-------------------------|
| Calcium | Builds and maintains bones and teeth, regulates muscle and nerve function, regulates blood pressure and blood clotting | Milk products; fortified orange juice, tofu, and soy milk; fish with edible small bones such as sardines and salmon; broccoli; hard water | Poor bone growth, weak bones, muscle spasms, convulsions | Kidney stones, calcium deposits in organs, mineral imbalances |
| Potassium | Maintains fluid balance, necessary for nerve function | Whole grains, fruits and vegetables, yogurt, milk | Muscular weakness, confusion, death | Heart failure |
| Sodium | Maintains fluid balance, necessary for nerve function | Salt, soy sauce, luncheon meats, processed cheeses, pickled foods, snack foods, canned and dried soups | Muscle cramping, headache, confusion, coma | Hypertension |
| Magnesium | Regulation of enzyme activity, necessary for nerve function | Green leafy vegetables, nuts, whole grains, peanut butter | Loss of appetite, muscular weakness, convulsions, confusion, death | Rare |
| Zinc | Component of many enzymes and the hormone insulin, maintains immune function, necessary for sexual maturation and reproduction | Meats, fish, poultry, whole grains, vegetables | Poor growth, failure to mature sexually, improper healing of wounds | Mineral imbalances, gastrointestinal upsets, anemia, heart disease |
| Selenium | Component of a group of antioxidant enzymes, immune system function | Seafood, liver, and vegetables and grains grown in selenium-rich soil | May increase risk of heart disease and certain cancers | Hair and nail loss |
| Iron | Oxygen transport involved in the release of energy | Clams, oysters, liver, red meats, and enriched breads and cereals | Fatigue, weakness, iron-deficiency anemia | Iron poisoning, nausea, vomiting, diarrhea, death |

*Source:* Alters S. and Schiff W. *Essential Concepts of Healthy Living,* 3rd ed. Sudbury, MA: Jones and Bartlett, 2003:214.

## Tipping Point

- Drink 8.5 cups of water each day to stay properly hydrated. Even with all of the coffee and soda we drink, it is still important to drink water.

About 60% of your total body weight is water. If you lose even 4% of your body weight through sweat, you will lose the ability to make decisions, concentrate, or do physical work. If you lose as much as 20%, you will die.

Water is lost:

- From breathing
- From sweating
- In urine and stool

Water is taken in from:

- Eating food (e.g., fruits, vegetables, soups, meats, grains)
- Water in beverages (e.g., water itself, fruit juices, milk, sport drinks)
- The metabolism process or chemical breakdown of foods

If you lose more water than you take in, you become dehydrated. Dehydration can happen if you are:

- Not drinking enough fluids daily
- Working or exercising in a hot or cold environment
- Living at high altitude
- Drinking too much alcohol

Clear urine is a sign that you are well hydrated. The more dehydrated you are, the darker (and smellier) your urine will be, although medications, vitamins, and diet can affect color.

You can restore lost fluids by drinking water. Eating foods high in water content also helps restore fluids (adapted from American College of Sports Medicine position stand).

Before exercise:

- Drink about 16 ounces (2 cups) of fluid about 2 hours before exercise to promote adequate hydration and allow time for excretion of excess water.

During exercise:

- Drink fluids at regular intervals to replace water lost through sweating.
- Drink fluids cooler than the ambient temperature (between 60 and 72 °F)—they are absorbed better.

During exercise lasting more than 1 hour:

- A sports drink (containing carbohydrates and/or electrolytes) might be considered when exercising more than 1 hour.
- For exercise lasting less than 1 hour, it does not matter if you are drinking water or a sports drink.

After exercise:

- Consider weighing yourself before and after exercising to determine how much fluid you have lost—for every pound of weight lost, you should drink at least 16 ounces of fluid (2 cups).
- If you feel thirsty, chances are dehydration has begun.

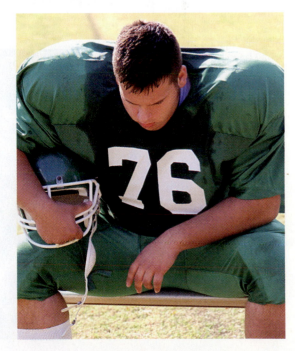

**6**

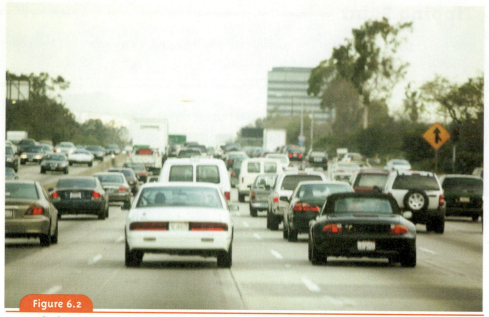

**Figure 6.2**

Free radical production is increased by exposure to cigarette smoke, exhaust fumes, and radiation.

## Free Radicals and Antioxidants

Normal metabolism creates free radicals. Free radicals can damage cell membranes and mutate genes.

Free radical production is increased by cigarette smoke, exhaust fumes, radiation, too much sunlight, some drugs, and too much stress **Figure 6.2**.

Antioxidants do battle with free radicals, and undo the damage they cause.

Get your antioxidants by eating a variety of fruits and vegetables. If you take supplements instead:

- The health benefits of phytochemicals come from working in combination **Table 6.9**.

- Isolated phytochemicals may cause more harm than good if taken in high doses.

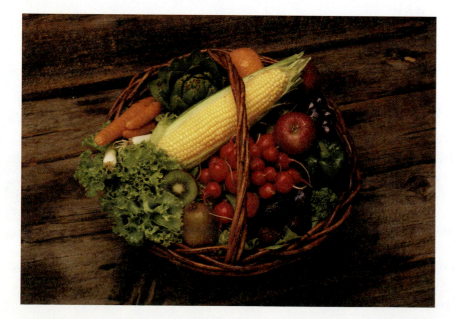

| Table 6.9 | Phytochemicals in Fruits and Vegetables and Their Possible Benefits | |
|---|---|---|
| **Food** | **Phytochemicals** | **Possible Benefits** |
| **Berries** Blueberries, strawberries, raspberries, blackberries, currants | Anthocyanides, ellagic acid | Antioxidants, cancer prevention |
| **Chili Peppers** | Capsaicin | Possible antioxidant, topical pain relief |
| **Citrus Fruits** Oranges, grapefruit, lemons, limes | Flavanones (tangeretic, nobiletin, hesperitin), carotenoids | Antioxidants |
| **Cruciferous Vegetables** Broccoli, kale, cauliflower, brussels sprouts, cabbage, mustard greens | Indoles, isothiocyanates, sulphoraphane, carotenoids | Antioxidants, anticancer properties |
| **Garlic Family** Garlic, onions, shallots, leeks, chives, scallions | Allylic sulfides, flavonoids (quercetin) | Anticancer properties |
| **Soy** | Daidzein, equol, genestein, entero-lactone, and other plant estrogens | Reduce risk of breast cancer, prostate cancer, and heart disease |

*Source:* Edlin G. and Golanty E. *Health and Wellness,* 8th ed. Sudbury, MA: Jones and Bartlett, 2004:99.

# Put Your Diet into Action

Is your diet meeting your nutrient needs? Answering this question is not an exact science, but useful guidelines are available.

## Comparison to Dietary Reference Intakes

The Institute of Medicine (IOM) of the National Academies changed the way nutritionists and nutrition scientists evaluate the diets of healthy people by creating the Dietary Reference Intakes (DRIs) Table 6.10 .

The DRI goal was not only to prevent nutritional deficiencies, but also to reduce the risk of chronic diseases such as osteoporosis, cancer, and cardiovascular disease.

## Comparison to Dietary Guidelines for Americans

The Dietary Guidelines for Americans offer a general picture of your dietary habits. They do not identify specific foods to eat. They promote food and lifestyle choices that reduce risk for chronic disease through the three basic messages seen in Figure 6.3 . In January 2005 new dietary guidelines were released, emphasizing a healthy approach to choosing a nutritious diet, maintaining a healthy weight, achieving adequate exercise, and "keeping food safe" to avoid food-borne illness. Appendix A contains the 2005 Dietary Guidelines for Americans.

## Table 6.10     Dietary Reference Intakes (DRI)

The Food and Nutrition Board of the National Academy of Sciences determines recommended nutrient intakes that apply to healthy individuals. Beginning in 1997, the Food and Nutrition Board (with the involvement of Health Canada) began releasing updated recommendations under a new framework called the Dietary Reference Intakes (DRI). In these revisions, target intake levels for healthy individuals in the United States and Canada are listed as either Adequate Intake (AI) levels or Recommended Dietary Allowances (RDA). Also, the DRI values include a set of Tolerable Upper Intake Levels (UL), which are levels of nutrient intake that should not be exceeded due to the potential for adverse effects from excessive consumption.

### Dietary Reference Intakes (DRI) for Vitamins and Minerals

| Life Stage Group | Vitamin A (μg/d)[1] | Vitamin D (μg/d)[2] | Vitamin E (mg/d)[3] | Vitamin K (μg/d) | Thiamin (mg/d) | Riboflavin (mg/d) | Niacin (mg/d)[4] | Pantothenic Acid (mg/d) | Biotin (μg/d) | Vitamin B6 (mg/d) | Folate (μg/d)[5] | Vitamin B12 (μg/d) | Vitamin C (mg/d) |
|---|---|---|---|---|---|---|---|---|---|---|---|---|---|
| **Infants** | | | | | | | | | | | | | |
| 0–6 mo | 400* | 5* | 4* | 2.0* | 0.2* | 0.3* | 2* | 1.7* | 5* | 0.1* | 65* | 0.4* | 40* |
| 7–12 mo | 500* | 5* | 5* | 2.5* | 0.3* | 0.4* | 4* | 1.8* | 6* | 0.3* | 80* | 0.5* | 50* |
| **Children** | | | | | | | | | | | | | |
| 1–3 y | 300 | 5* | 6 | 30* | 0.5 | 0.5 | 6 | 2* | 8* | 0.5 | 150 | 0.9 | 15 |
| 4–8 y | 400 | 5* | 7 | 55* | 0.6 | 0.6 | 8 | 3* | 12* | 0.6 | 200 | 1.2 | 25 |
| **Males** | | | | | | | | | | | | | |
| 9–13 y | 600 | 5* | 11 | 60* | 0.9 | 0.9 | 12 | 4* | 20* | 1.0 | 300 | 1.8 | 45 |
| 14–18 y | 900 | 5* | 15 | 75* | 1.2 | 1.3 | 16 | 5* | 25* | 1.3 | 400 | 2.4 | 75 |
| 19–30 y | 900 | 5* | 15 | 120* | 1.2 | 1.3 | 16 | 5* | 30* | 1.3 | 400 | 2.4 | 90 |
| 31–50 y | 900 | 5* | 15 | 120* | 1.2 | 1.3 | 16 | 5* | 30* | 1.3 | 400 | 2.4 | 90 |
| 51–70 y | 900 | 10* | 15 | 120* | 1.2 | 1.3 | 16 | 5* | 30* | 1.7 | 400 | 2.4[7] | 90 |
| >70 y | 900 | 15* | 15 | 120* | 1.2 | 1.3 | 16 | 5* | 30* | 1.7 | 400 | 2.4[7] | 90 |
| **Females** | | | | | | | | | | | | | |
| 9–13 y | 600 | 5* | 11 | 60* | 0.9 | 0.9 | 12 | 4* | 20* | 1.0 | 300 | 1.8 | 45 |
| 14–18 y | 700 | 5* | 15 | 75* | 1.0 | 1.0 | 14 | 5* | 25* | 1.2 | 400[6] | 2.4 | 65 |
| 19–30 y | 700 | 5* | 15 | 90* | 1.1 | 1.1 | 14 | 5* | 30* | 1.3 | 400[6] | 2.4 | 75 |
| 31–50 y | 700 | 5* | 15 | 90* | 1.1 | 1.1 | 14 | 5* | 30* | 1.3 | 400[6] | 2.4 | 75 |
| 51–70 y | 700 | 10* | 15 | 90* | 1.1 | 1.1 | 14 | 5* | 30* | 1.5 | 400 | 2.4[7] | 75 |
| >70 y | 700 | 15* | 15 | 90* | 1.1 | 1.1 | 14 | 5* | 30* | 1.5 | 400 | 2.4[7] | 75 |
| **Pregnancy** | | | | | | | | | | | | | |
| ≤18 y | 750 | 5* | 15 | 75* | 1.4 | 1.4 | 18 | 6* | 30* | 1.9 | 600 | 2.6 | 80 |
| 19–30 y | 770 | 5* | 15 | 90* | 1.4 | 1.4 | 18 | 6* | 30* | 1.9 | 600 | 2.6 | 85 |
| 31–50 y | 770 | 5* | 15 | 90* | 1.4 | 1.4 | 18 | 6* | 30* | 1.9 | 600 | 2.6 | 85 |
| **Lactation** | | | | | | | | | | | | | |
| ≤18 y | 1200 | 5* | 19 | 75* | 1.4 | 1.6 | 17 | 7* | 35* | 2.0 | 500 | 2.8 | 115* |
| 19–30 y | 1300 | 5* | 19 | 90* | 1.4 | 1.6 | 17 | 7* | 35* | 2.0 | 500 | 2.8 | 120 |
| 31–50 y | 1300 | 5* | 19 | 90* | 1.4 | 1.6 | 17 | 7* | 35* | 2.0 | 500 | 2.8 | 120 |

This table presents Recommended Dietary Allowances (RDA) and Adequate Intakes (AI). An asterisk (*) indicates AI. RDAs and AIs may both be used as goals for individual intake.

[1]As retinol activity equivalents (RAE).

[2]As cholecalciferol.

[3]As α-tocopherol.

[4]As niacin equivalents (NE).

[5]As dietary folate equivalents (DFE).

[6]In view of evidence linking folate intake with neural tube defects in the fetus, it is recommended that all women capable of becoming pregnant consume 400 μg of folic acid from supplements or fortified foods in addition to intake of food folate from a varied diet.

[7]Because 10% to 30% of older people may malabsorb food-bound vitamin $B_{12}$, it is advisable for those older than 50 years to meet their RDA mainly by consuming foods fortified with vitamin $B_{12}$ or a supplement containing vitamin $B_{12}$.

| Choline (mg/d) | Calcium (mg/d) | Phosphorus (mg/d) | Magnesium (mg/d) | Iron (mg/d) | Zinc (mg/d) | Selenium (μg/d) | Iodine (μg/d) | Copper (μg/d) | Manganese (mg/d) | Fluoride (mg/d) | Chromium (μg/d) | Molybdenum (μg/d) |
|---|---|---|---|---|---|---|---|---|---|---|---|---|
| 125* | 210* | 100* | 30* | 0.27* | 2* | 15* | 110* | 200* | 0.003* | 0.01* | 0.2* | 2* |
| 150* | 270* | 275* | 75* | 11 | 3 | 20* | 130* | 220* | 0.6* | 0.5* | 5.5* | 3* |
| 200* | 500* | 460 | 80 | 7 | 3 | 20 | 90 | 340 | 1.2* | 0.7* | 11* | 17 |
| 250* | 800* | 500 | 130 | 10 | 5 | 30 | 90 | 440 | 1.5* | 1* | 15* | 22 |
| 375* | 1300* | 1250 | 240 | 8 | 8 | 40 | 120 | 700 | 1.9* | 2* | 25* | 34 |
| 550* | 1300* | 1250 | 410 | 11 | 11 | 55 | 150 | 890 | 2.2* | 3* | 35* | 43 |
| 550* | 1000* | 700 | 400 | 8 | 11 | 55 | 150 | 900 | 2.3* | 4* | 35* | 45 |
| 550* | 1000* | 700 | 420 | 8 | 11 | 55 | 150 | 900 | 2.3* | 4* | 35* | 45 |
| 550* | 1200* | 700 | 420 | 8 | 11 | 55 | 150 | 900 | 2.3* | 4* | 30* | 45 |
| 550* | 1200* | 700 | 420 | 8 | 11 | 55 | 150 | 900 | 2.3* | 4* | 30* | 45 |
| 375* | 1300* | 1250 | 240 | 8 | 8 | 40 | 120 | 700 | 1.6* | 2* | 21* | 34 |
| 400* | 1300* | 1250 | 360 | 15 | 9 | 55 | 150 | 890 | 1.6* | 3* | 24* | 43 |
| 425* | 1000* | 700 | 310 | 18 | 8 | 55 | 150 | 900 | 1.8* | 3* | 25* | 45 |
| 425* | 1000* | 700 | 320 | 18 | 8 | 55 | 150 | 900 | 1.8* | 3* | 25* | 45 |
| 425* | 1200* | 700 | 320 | 8 | 8 | 55 | 150 | 900 | 1.8* | 3* | 20* | 45 |
| 425* | 1200* | 700 | 320 | 8 | 8 | 55 | 150 | 900 | 1.8* | 3* | 20* | 45 |
| 450* | 1300* | 1250 | 400 | 27 | 13 | 60 | 220 | 1000 | 2.0* | 3* | 29* | 50 |
| 450* | 1000* | 700 | 350 | 27 | 11 | 60 | 220 | 1000 | 2.0* | 3* | 30* | 50 |
| 450* | 1000* | 700 | 360 | 27 | 11 | 60 | 220 | 1000 | 2.0* | 3* | 30* | 50 |
| 550* | 1300* | 1250 | 360 | 10 | 14 | 70 | 290 | 1300 | 2.6* | 3* | 44* | 50 |
| 550* | 1000* | 700 | 310 | 9 | 12 | 70 | 290 | 1300 | 2.6* | 3* | 45* | 50 |
| 550* | 1000* | 700 | 320 | 9 | 12 | 70 | 290 | 1300 | 2.6* | 3* | 45* | 50 |

*Sources:* Data compiled from *Dietary Reference Intakes for Calcium, Phosphorus, Magnesium, Vitamin D, and Fluoride.* Washington, DC: National Academy Press, 1997. *Dietary Reference Intakes for Thiamin, Riboflavin, Niacin, Vitamin B₆, Folate, Vitamin B₁₂, Pantothenic Acid, Biotin, and Choline.* Washington, DC: National Academy Press, 1998. *Dietary Reference Intakes for Vitamin C, Vitamin E, Selenium, and Carotenoids.* Washington, DC: National Academy Press; 2000. *Dietary Reference Intakes for Vitamin A, Vitamin K, Arsenic, Boron, Chromium, Copper, Iron, Manganese, Molybdenum, Nickel, Silicon, Vanadium, and Zinc.* Washington, DC: National Academy Press, 2001. These reports may be accessed via http://nap.edu.

6

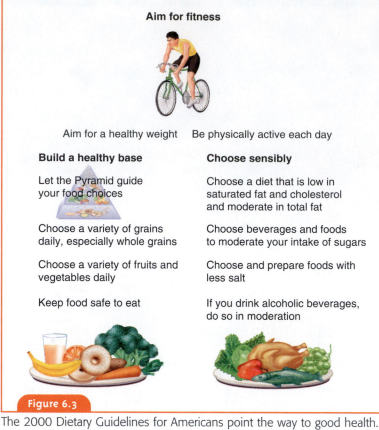

**Aim for fitness**

Aim for a healthy weight    Be physically active each day

**Build a healthy base**          **Choose sensibly**

Let the Pyramid guide            Choose a diet that is low in
your food choices                saturated fat and cholesterol
                                 and moderate in total fat

Choose a variety of grains       Choose beverages and foods
daily, especially whole grains   to moderate your intake of sugars

Choose a variety of fruits and   Choose and prepare foods with
vegetables daily                 less salt

Keep food safe to eat            If you drink alcoholic beverages,
                                 do so in moderation

**Figure 6.3**

The 2000 Dietary Guidelines for Americans point the way to good health. (*Source:* U.S. Department of Agriculture, Agriculture Research Service, Dietary Guidelines Advisory Committee. *Nutrition and Your Health: Dietary Guidelines for Americans, 2000,* 5th ed. Home and Garden Bulletin No. 232. Washington, DC: 2000.)

## MyPyramid

Early in 2005, the USDA released a new guide to healthy eating called MyPyramid **Figure 6.4**. MyPyramid, which is a revision of the original Food Guide Pyramid of the early 1990s, is designed to serve as a guide to healthful daily eating for Americans. The symbolism behind MyPyramid represents the individual nature of diet and physical activity. It acknowledges that each person is unique in his or her needs and, as such, each person's dietary needs may be slightly different.

The six colors in MyPyramid represent the different food groups: blue for milk, purple for meat and beans, orange for grains, green for vegetables, red for fruit, and yellow for oils. The widths of the bands of color represent a proportional daily need. For example, the orange grain band is the widest, indicating that these foods should make up the greatest part of your diet. Oils, a very slender yellow band, should be a small part of your diet. Finally, the icon going up the stairs on the left side of the pyramid reminds you of the importance of physical activity.

Please take a moment in your day to visit www.nutrition.gov. It offers a guidance program that will advise you based on your age, height, and activity level what you should be eating. Also, this site provides tips, menu ideas, and information on calories in the foods you eat.

A marked improvement in MyPyramid from the previous guides is its development of the daily amount of each food group required based on caloric need. This information

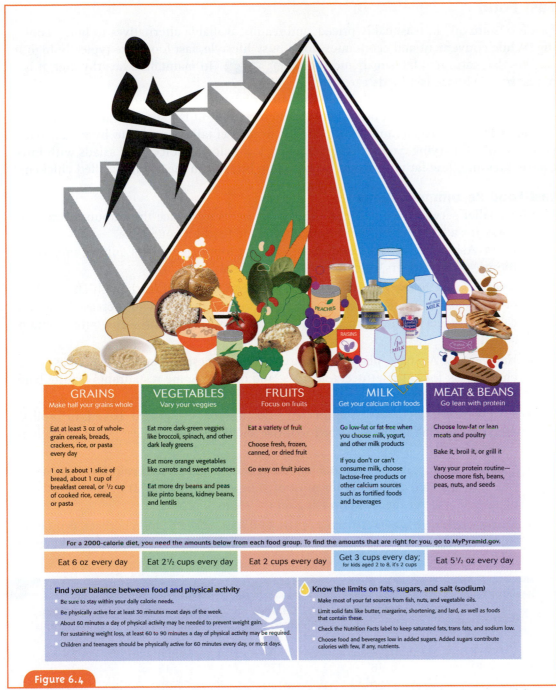

GRAINS
Make half your grains whole

VEGETABLES
Vary your veggies

FRUITS
Focus on fruits

MILK
Get your calcium rich foods

MEAT & BEANS
Go lean with protein

Eat at least 3 oz of whole-grain cereals, breads, crackers, rice, or pasta every day

1 oz is about 1 slice of bread, about 1 cup of breakfast cereal, or ½ cup of cooked rice, cereal, or pasta

Eat more dark-green veggies like broccoli, spinach, and other dark leafy greens

Eat more orange vegetables like carrots and sweet potatoes

Eat more dry beans and peas like pinto beans, kidney beans, and lentils

Eat a variety of fruit

Choose fresh, frozen, canned, or dried fruit

Go easy on fruit juices

Go low-fat or fat free when you choose milk, yogurt, and other milk products

If you don't or can't consume milk, choose lactose-free products or other calcium sources such as fortified foods and beverages

Choose low-fat or lean meats and poultry

Bake it, broil it, or grill it

Vary your protein routine— choose more fish, beans, peas, nuts, and seeds

For a 2000-calorie diet, you need the amounts below from each food group. To find the amounts that are right for you, go to MyPyramid.gov.

Eat 6 oz every day

Eat 2½ cups every day

Eat 2 cups every day

Get 3 cups every day; for kids aged 2 to 8, it's 2 cups

Eat 5½ oz every day

**Find your balance between food and physical activity**
- Be sure to stay within your daily calorie needs.
- Be physically active for at least 30 minutes most days of the week.
- About 60 minutes a day of physical activity may be needed to prevent weight gain.
- For sustaining weight loss, at least 60 to 90 minutes a day of physical activity may be required.
- Children and teenagers should be physically active for 60 minutes every day, or most days.

**Know the limits on fats, sugars, and salt (sodium)**
- Make most of your fat sources from fish, nuts, and vegetable oils.
- Limit solid fats like butter, margarine, shortening, and lard, as well as foods that contain these.
- Check the Nutrition Facts label to keep saturated fats, trans fats, and sodium low.
- Choose food and beverages low in added sugars. Added sugars contribute calories with few, if any, nutrients.

**Figure 6.4**

The USDA's MyPyramid is a research-based guidance system that helps consumers put the Dietary Guidelines into action. It shows how many servings to eat from each food group every day. (*Source:* U.S. Department of Agriculture/U.S. Department of Health and Human Services).

will assist individuals in making choices to keep their diet balanced throughout the day. Critics say that while MyPyramid is a better model than the original Food Guide Pyramid, it does not give enough information to make truly informed decisions regarding diet, doesn't reflect the Dietary Guidelines for Americans, and relies too heavily on the ability to access and utilize the Internet. Also, as the Harvard School of Public Health points out on its website, MyPyramid has been heavily influenced by the lobbying efforts of groups trying to protect their section of the pyramid.

**6**

## Fast Food

Fast foods are quick, reasonably priced, and readily available alternatives to home cooking. While convenient and economical for a busy lifestyle, fast foods are typically high in calories, fat, saturated fat, sugar, and salt ( **Table 6.11** ). To maintain a healthy diet, it is necessary to choose fast foods carefully.

In general, people with high blood pressure, diabetes, and heart disease must be very careful in choosing fast food because of the high content of fat, sodium, and sugar.

Many fast-food restaurants have switched from beef tallow or lard to hydrogenated vegetable oils for frying. Some restaurants offer low-calorie choices like salads with low-calorie dressing, low-fat milkshakes, whole-grain buns, lean meats, and grilled chicken.

### Fast-Food Recommendations

Choose smaller servings. Consider splitting some items to reduce the amount of calories and fat. Ask for a "doggy bag," or simply leave some food on your plate.

- *Pizza:* Ask for less cheese, and choose low-fat toppings such as onions, mushrooms, green peppers, tomatoes, or other vegetables.
- *Sandwiches:* Choose regular- or junior-size lean roast beef, turkey, chicken breast, or lean ham. Extras such as bacon, cheese, or mayonnaise will increase fat and calories. Select whole-grain breads over croissants or biscuits—the latter contain added fat.
- *Hamburgers:* A single, plain meat patty without cheese and sauces is the best choice. Ask for extra lettuce, tomatoes, and onions. Some restaurants feature hamburgers without buns.
- *Meat, Chicken, and Fish:* Look for items that are roasted, grilled, baked, or broiled. Avoid meats that are breaded or fried. Use small portions of heavy sauces, such as gravy, if at all.
- *Salads:* Dressing, bacon bits, and shredded cheese add fat and calories. Choose lettuce and assorted vegetables for most of your salad. Use low-fat or fat-free salad dressings. Ask for the salad dressing on the side.
- *Desserts:* Choose low-fat frozen yogurt, fruit ices, sorbets, and sherbets. But occasional indulgent desserts can add fun to a carefully selected, well-balanced diet.

| Table 6.11 | Partial Composition of Selected Fast-Food Items | | | | |
|---|---|---|---|---|---|
| Food | Total Calories | Total Fat (grams) | Calories from Fat | Cholesterol (milligrams) | Sodium (milligrams) |
| Big Mac | 560 | 31 | 280 | 85 | 1070 |
| Burrito Supreme | 440 | 18 | 170 | 45 | 1220 |
| French fries (medium/salted) | 370 | 20 | 180 | 00 | 240 |
| Turkey sub sandwich | 273 | 4 | 34 | 19 | 1391 |
| Fried chicken breast | 400 | 24 | 220 | 135 | 1116 |
| Pizza (slice) | 300 | 14 | 120 | 25 | 610 |
| Caesar salad (no dressing) | 240 | 13 | 120 | 25 | 780 |
| Caesar salad (with dressing) | 520 | 43 | 390 | 40 | 1420 |
| Chocolate shake (medium) | 320 | 7 | 60 | 20 | 230 |

*Source:* Edlin G. and Golanty E. *Health and Wellness,* 8th ed. Sudbury, MA: Jones and Bartlett, 2004:105.

# Vegetarian Diets

Nutrients that may be lacking in a **vegetarian diet** are protein, vitamin B$_{12}$, vitamin D, riboflavin, calcium, zinc, and iron.

Vegetarians who limit or omit animal products from their diets may need to take supplements (e.g., calcium, vitamin B$_{12}$). The various classifications of vegetarian include **lacto-**, **lacto-ovo-**, and **semi- or partial vegetarian**.

**Vegan diets** require careful planning to obtain adequate amounts of required nutrients. Refer to Tables 6.6 and 6.8 for alternative sources of these nutrients suitable for the vegetarian lifestyle. Obtaining adequate amounts of vitamins D and B$_{12}$ will require supplementation.

# Mediterranean Diet

The Mediterranean diet is based on the dietary traditions of the countries surrounding the Mediterranean Sea (Crete, Greece, southern Italy, and North Africa). The people who live there exhibit strikingly lower rates of chronic disease.

The traditional diets of the Mediterranean region are mainly based on the foods from a rich diversity of plant sources, and include fruits, vegetables, whole grains, beans, nuts, and seeds. Fruits and vegetables are locally grown and often consumed raw or processed very little. This factor may be significant in determining their potential value for fiber and antioxidants.

- In North Africa, couscous, vegetables, and legumes are the core of the diet.
- In southern Europe, the diet includes rice, polenta, pasta, and potatoes, along with vegetables and legumes.
- In the eastern Mediterranean, bulgur and rice, together with vegetables and legumes such as chickpeas, are the main part of many meals.
- Throughout the Mediterranean, bread is a staple eaten without butter or margarine.

## Characteristics of the Mediterranean Diet

**Fish, Poultry, and Red Meat**  Red meat (associated with colon cancer, prostate cancer, and heart disease) is eaten sparingly. In addition to poultry, only about 15 ounces of red meat per week is consumed. Fish consumption varies from one country to another, but averages 5 to 15 ounces per week.

**Dairy Products**  Cheese and yogurt from goats, sheep, buffalo, cows, and camels are traditionally consumed in low to moderate amounts. In the entire region, very little fresh milk is drunk. Butter and cream are used only on special occasions. The bacterial cultures of yogurt may contribute to good health.

**Wine with Meals**  Throughout the Mediterranean, wine is consumed in moderation and is usually taken with meals. For men, moderation is two glasses per day, for women one glass per day.

**Olive Oil and Total Fat**  Olive oil, which is high in monounsaturated fat, is a good source of antioxidants. It is the main source of fat in the Mediterranean diet. Current research suggests that olive oil may actually increase HDL (good) cholesterol, but has little effect on LDL (bad) cholesterol.

**Physical Activity**  The people of the Mediterranean engage in physical activity in their everyday lives and consider it vital to maintaining good health and proper weight.

---

**What's the word...**

**vegetarian diet** Diet in which vegetables are the foundation and meat products are restricted or eliminated.

**lacto-vegetarian** Person who includes some or all dairy products in his or her diet.

**lacto-ovo-vegetarian** Person who includes milk, dairy products, and eggs in his or her diet.

**semi- or partial vegetarian** Person who eats no red meat, but may include chicken or fish, dairy products, and eggs in his or her diet.

**vegan** Person who eats only foods of plant origin.

## Other Ethnic Diets

Every ethnic diet has its healthy and unhealthy foods, sauces, and preparation. The guidelines for healthy eating given in this chapter can be applied to any diet.

The suggestions that follow are based on recommendations from the National Institutes of Health and the American Dietetic Association **Table 6.12**.

| **Table 6.12** | **Ethnic Diet Recommendations** |
| --- | --- |
| **Good** | **Not as Good** |
| **Chinese**<br>Steamed, poached, boiled, roasted, barbecued, or lightly stir-fried fresh fish and seafood, skinless chicken, or tofu; with mixed vegetables, Chinese greens, steamed rice, steamed spring rolls, or soft noodles; with hoisin sauce, oyster sauce, wine sauce, plum sauce, velvet sauce, or hot mustard | Crab Rangoon, crispy duck or chicken, or anything breaded or deep-fried, including fried rice, fried wontons, egg rolls, and fried or crispy noodles |
| **Thai**<br>Dishes barbecued, sautéed, broiled, boiled, steamed, braised, or marinated; skewered and grilled meats; with fish sauce, basil sauce, or hot sauces; bean thread noodles; Thai salad | Coconut milk soup; peanut sauce or dishes topped with nuts; crispy noodles; red, green, and yellow curries containing coconut milk |
| **Japanese**<br>Dishes boiled or made in boiling broth, steamed, simmered, broiled, or grilled; with mixed rice, steamed rice, or buckwheat, wheat, or rice noodles | Dishes battered and fried or deep-fried; fried pork cutlet, fried tofu |
| **Mexican**<br>Fish marinated in lime juice; soft corn or wheat tortillas, burritos, fajitas, enchiladas, soft tacos, tamales filled with beans, vegetables, or lean meats; with refried beans, nonfat or low-fat rice and beans; with salsa, enchilada sauce, or picante sauce; gazpacho, menudo, or black bean soup; fruit or flan | Crispy fried tortillas; fried dishes such as chile rellenos, chimichangas, flautas, or tostadas; nachos and cheese, chili con queso, and other dishes made with cheese or cheese sauce; guacamole, sour cream; refried beans made with lard; fried ice cream |
| **Italian**<br>Pasta primavera or pasta, polenta, risotto, or gnocchi; with marinara, red or white wine sauce, red or white clam sauce, light mushroom sauce; dishes grilled or made with tomato-based sauce, broth and wine sauce, or lemon sauce; seafood stew; vegetable, minestrone, or bean soups | Cheese or smoked meats; dishes prepared alfredo, carbonara, fried, creamed, or with cream; veal scallopini; chicken, veal, or eggplant parmigiana; Italian sausage, salami, or prosciutto; buttered garlic bread; cannoli |
| **French**<br>Fresh fish, shrimp, scallops, mussels, or skinless chicken, steamed, skewered, and broiled or grilled; without sauces; clear soups | Dishes prepared in cream sauce, baked with cream and cheese, or in a pastry crust; drawn butter, hollandaise sauce, or mayonnaise-based sauce |
| **Indian**<br>Dishes prepared with curry and roasted in a clay oven or pan-roasted; kabobs; yogurt and cucumber salad, and other yogurt-based dishes and sauces; lentils and basmati rice; baked bread | Any fried or coconut-milk–based dishes; meat in cream sauce; clarified butter; fried breads |

# Challenges for Special Populations

## College Students

College students often eat on the run, eat fast food, and are served from dining hall or cafeteria lines. The circumstances of college life make it all too easy to eat food that is not very nutritious or to skip meals, especially breakfast. Think about how, what, and when you eat.

- Don't skip breakfast.
- Take your time when you eat.
- Be conscious of food choices in the dining hall line or at a fast-food restaurant.
- For snacks, eat granola bars, raw veggies, fruit, low-fat cheese, low-fat yogurt, plain popcorn (no butter!), and soup.
- Drink plenty of water.

Some great ideas for preparing quick, healthy meals can be found at websites such as meals.com.

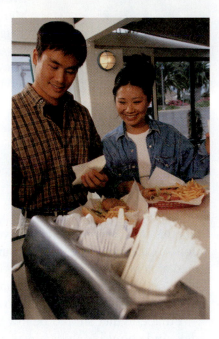

## Athletes

Carbo loading builds and maintains stores of glycogen for muscles, which extends endurance and delays fatigue. If you are an endurance athlete:

- A few days before an event, gradually increase the amount of complex carbohydrates you are eating to about 70% of your total calories.
- At the same time, gradually decrease the amount of workout time.
- Two to four hours before the event, eat a light meal of bagels, pasta, or breads and cereals.
- Afterward, eat a meal with carbs, protein, and fat to help repair and rebuild muscle.

It is rare that everyday exercise would require this dietary pattern. In fact, not all athletes find that carbo loading helps their performance. Test the effects of the carbo-load diet when you are not preparing for competition.

There is no need to take in extra protein; the average American already takes in 50% more calories than needed. As an athlete, you need only 12% protein in your overall daily intake of calories.

Legal supplements (vitamins, minerals, protein, certain amino acids) most likely don't help.

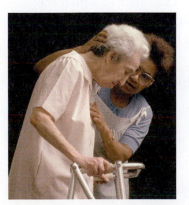

## Women

Because they tend to be smaller than men, women require less protein and fewer calories. Women should concentrate on getting enough of the right nutrients, especially:

- *Calcium* to head off osteoporosis, a special aging hazard for women, and
- *Iron* to avoid anemia, another special hazard for females who menstruate.

Women can get the nutrients they need from nonfat and low-fat dairy, orange juice, fortified cereal, lean red meat, and green leafy vegetables.

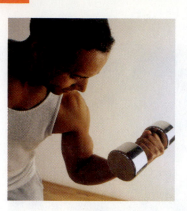

### Men

Men are at risk for heart disease, cancer, and later-life weight gain, because they tend to eat more red meat and fewer grains, vegetables, and fruits than recommended. They can get the necessary vitamins, minerals, fiber, and phytochemicals from grains, vegetables, and fruit.

### Diabetics

Diabetics must watch their diets very carefully, because they must maintain just the right blood sugar level at all times during the day. If the level falls, they must take immediate remedial action, such as drinking orange juice, to bring it up.

Diabetics must take a blood sugar measurement several times during each day. New instruments that make it easier to do so are now available.

A diabetic diet should be low in simple sugars and high in foods with a high glycemic index, and should include a reasonable amount of nonsaturated fats.

### Older People

People older than age 50 are usually less active, so they need to consume fewer calories to balance their calorie output.

The absorption of nutrients in the older digestive tract is less than it was when the person was younger, so it is a good idea to eat foods fortified with vitamin $B_{12}$, or to take vitamin $B_{12}$ supplements.

Older individuals should also make sure they include foods high in fiber in their diet, because constipation is more of a problem in this age group.

## Smart Food Choices

### Looking at Labels

On a food label's Nutrition Facts panel, manufacturers are required to provide information on certain nutrients in a certain order **Figure 6.5**:

- If a claim is made about any of the optional components, or if a food is fortified or enriched with any of them, nutrition information for these components is mandatory.
- The required nutrients address today's health concerns. The order in which the information must appear is the priority of current dietary recommendations.

### Dietary Supplement Labels

Supplement labels are limited by law in what they can and cannot say **Figure 6.6**. They:

- Identify the supplement
- Give the quantity (e.g., 40 capsules)
- Give directions for using and storing
- Show warnings, if needed
- List standardization levels, in some cases
- List an address from which to obtain more information

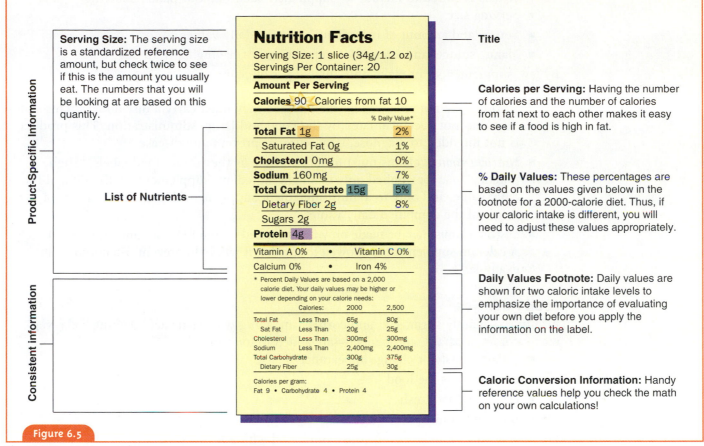

**Product-Specific Information**

**Serving Size:** The serving size is a standardized reference amount, but check twice to see if this is the amount you usually eat. The numbers that you will be looking at are based on this quantity.

**List of Nutrients**

**Consistent information**

**Nutrition Facts**

Serving Size: 1 slice (34g/1.2 oz)
Servings Per Container: 20

**Amount Per Serving**

**Calories** 90   Calories from fat 10

% Daily Value*

| | |
|---|---|
| **Total Fat** 1g | **2%** |
| Saturated Fat 0g | 1% |
| **Cholesterol** 0mg | 0% |
| **Sodium** 160mg | 7% |
| **Total Carbohydrate** 15g | **5%** |
| Dietary Fiber 2g | 8% |
| Sugars 2g | |
| **Protein** 4g | |

| | | | |
|---|---|---|---|
| Vitamin A 0% | • | Vitamin C 0% | |
| Calcium 0% | • | Iron 4% | |

* Percent Daily Values are based on a 2,000 calorie diet. Your daily values may be higher or lower depending on your calorie needs:

| | | Calories: | 2000 | 2,500 |
|---|---|---|---|---|
| Total Fat | Less Than | | 65g | 80g |
| Sat Fat | Less Than | | 20g | 25g |
| Cholesterol | Less Than | | 300mg | 300mg |
| Sodium | Less Than | | 2,400mg | 2,400mg |
| Total Carbohydrate | | | 300g | 375g |
| Dietary Fiber | | | 25g | 30g |

Calories per gram:
Fat 9 • Carbohydrate 4 • Protein 4

**Title**

**Calories per Serving:** Having the number of calories and the number of calories from fat next to each other makes it easy to see if a food is high in fat.

**% Daily Values:** These percentages are based on the values given below in the footnote for a 2000-calorie diet. Thus, if your caloric intake is different, you will need to adjust these values appropriately.

**Daily Values Footnote:** Daily values are shown for two caloric intake levels to emphasize the importance of evaluating your own diet before you apply the information on the label.

**Caloric Conversion Information:** Handy reference values help you check the math on your own calculations!

**Figure 6.5**

The Nutrition Facts panel.

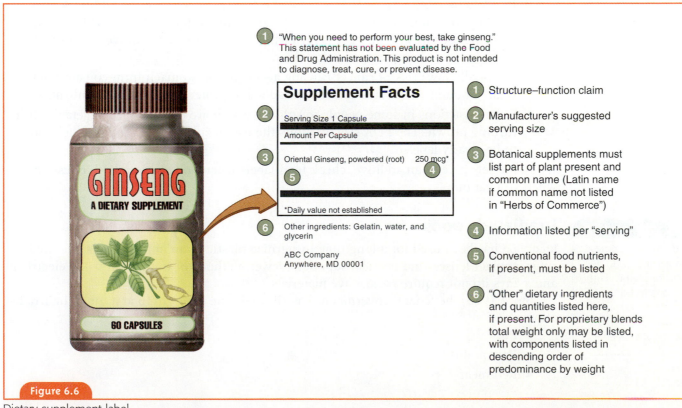

1. "When you need to perform your best, take ginseng." This statement has not been evaluated by the Food and Drug Administration. This product is not intended to diagnose, treat, cure, or prevent disease.

**Supplement Facts**

Serving Size 1 Capsule

Amount Per Capsule

Oriental Ginseng, powdered (root)   250 mcg*

*Daily value not established

Other ingredients: Gelatin, water, and glycerin

ABC Company
Anywhere, MD 00001

1. Structure–function claim
2. Manufacturer's suggested serving size
3. Botanical supplements must list part of plant present and common name (Latin name if common name not listed in "Herbs of Commerce")
4. Information listed per "serving"
5. Conventional food nutrients, if present, must be listed
6. "Other" dietary ingredients and quantities listed here, if present. For proprietary blends total weight only may be listed, with components listed in descending order of predominance by weight

**GINSENG**
**A DIETARY SUPPLEMENT**
**60 CAPSULES**

**Figure 6.6**

Dietary supplement label.

**6**

They are also required to include a "supplement facts" box or panel, showing:

- Serving size
- Source and amount of ingredients assigned daily values
- Name, source, and amount of ingredients not having daily values

By law, supplements can make only three types of claims:

- *Structure–function* claims (e.g., "Specially formulated to make you feel on top of the world!") are not reviewed by the FDA, so they must carry a disclaimer: "This statement has not been evaluated by the Food and Drug Administration. This product is not intended to diagnose, treat, cure, or prevent any disease."

- *Nutrient content* claims must mean the same as they do on food labels. "High potency" may be applied only to single-ingredient supplements with 100% of the daily value, and only to a multi-ingredient supplement if it has a minimum of two thirds of the combined daily values.

- *Disease* claims may be made only if authorized by the FDA or some other such body. A calcium supplement is allowed to say that it will help prevent osteoporosis, for example.

### Food Additives

Additives—mainly sugar, salt, and corn syrup, along with citric acid, baking soda, vegetable colors, mustard, and pepper—are added to food to:

- Enhance taste or change appearance
- Help process the food
- Keep the food fresh
- Boost nutritional value

Possible health problems from consuming food with additives include:

- Spells of sweating and a rise in blood pressure for some people after eating food in which monosodium glutamate (MSG) is used as a flavor enhancer.

- Possibly increased (but still low) risk of certain cancers from the additives butylated hydroxyanisole (BHA) and butylated hydroxytoluene (BHT), which are used to keep foods fresh. The FDA is reviewing the use of these additives, and some manufacturers have stopped using them.

- A (usually low) risk of cancer-causing agents in the stomach from consuming the small amounts of nitrates and nitrites added to protect meats from botulism.

- Severe reactions in some people to sulfites, which are used to keep vegetables from turning brown. The FDA strictly limits the use of sulfites and requires such foods to be clearly labeled.

If you are sensitive to an additive, check food labels when you shop and ask questions when you eat out.

### *What's the word...*

**irradiation** Treatment with gamma rays, x-rays, or high-voltage electrons to kill pathogens and, in the case of food, to increase shelf life.

### Irradiated Foods

Irradiation has been used for a long time to sterilize plastic wrap, milk cartons, teething rings, contact lenses, and medical supplies. Newer methods of irradiation using electricity and x-rays do not require radioactive materials.

Since 1963, the federal government has allowed, one food group at a time, the irradiation of:

- Pork
- Raw poultry
- Red meat

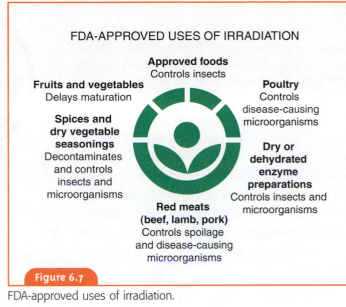

**Figure 6.7**

FDA-approved uses of irradiation.

- Fruits
- Vegetables
- Wheat and flour
- White potatoes
- Herbs and spices

All primary irradiated foods have the radura symbol ⬤ Figure 6.7 and a brief information label. Irradiation kills most pathogens, but does not completely sterilize a product. Proper handling is still necessary.

Not many irradiated foods are available, because consumers are skeptical or fearful of them. But when consumers have information about irradiation and its benefits, most want to purchase these products.

## Genetically Modified Foods

How do you modify an organism genetically? You insert genes from one organism into another to introduce new traits or enhance existing ones. Why would you do this? Well, for one thing, it makes crops:

- Be more resistant to disease, heat, and frost
- Last longer
- Be better tasting and more nutritious
- Require less fertilizer and pesticides

This process could save billions in costs, because such crops are more productive. This would help feed the hungry in the developing world.

What is the downside? We don't know if genetic modification of food crops will:

- Create previously unknown "transgenic" organisms that might have adverse effects on us and our environment
- Cross-pollinate and destroy other plants
- Create superweeds that resist herbicides

Whether you know it or not, you have been eating genetically modified foods since 1996, if what you eat comes from a supermarket. So far, such modification seems to be benign and helpful. Only time will tell.

*What's the word...*

**genetic modification**
Manipulating the DNA of an organism to change some of its characteristics.

**6**

## Organic Foods

Concerned about Frankenfood? Don't want to eat meat from cattle fed on growth hormone, or vegetables and fruit sprayed with so many pesticides that even bugs won't eat them? Look for the USDA organic label ( Figure 6.8 ). Foodstuffs can't carry it unless:

- Crops meet strict limits on pesticide spraying
- No sewage sludge is mixed into the soil
- Cattle are allowed outdoors and fed only organic feed
- No antibiotics or growth hormones are used
- No genetic engineering or ionizing radiation takes place

There are degrees of organic, however, so check the small print:

- "100% organic" means all organic ingredients; can carry USDA label
- "Organic" means 95% organic ingredients; can still carry label
- "Made with organic ingredients" means 70% organic; no label allowed

**USDA ORGANIC**

**Figure 6.8**

USDA organic label.

## Assessing and Changing Your Diet

How can you tell whether you are getting the right amounts of the essential nutrients to meet your needs? Complete Lab 6-1 to find out.

### Stay on the Healthy Path

Now you know what and how to eat so as to keep yourself healthy. Help yourself stay on the right path: Dust off and apply the self-management skills you learned from Chapter 1.

Use the MyPyramid and the Dietary Guidelines to help you figure out what is good to eat and what to avoid. Then, follow these tips:

- Cook at home.
- Plan ahead when you shop for food.
- Consume only small amounts of meat.
- Have a few meatless meals each week.

### Benefits of Food

If you are thinking you should take supplements to get the vitamins you need, think again. You lose out on other essential nutrients if you eat a diet high in calories, fat, and sodium and think you can make up for it with supplements.

Fruits and vegetables also have much more antioxidants and phytochemicals than supplements:

- Three fourths of a cup of cooked kale (with a lot less of vitamins E and C) will neutralize as many free radicals as approximately 80 times as much vitamin E or more than 50 times as much vitamin C in supplement form.
- Other sources of antioxidants high in oxygen radical absorbance capacity (ORAC) units include blueberries, blackberries, strawberries, prunes, plums, raisins, beets, and red bell peppers—even brussels sprouts, if you like them.

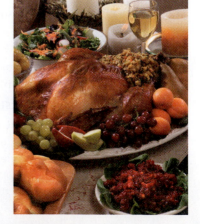

If you do take supplements, look for the U.S. Pharmacopoeia (USP) symbol on the bottle. The supplement should dissolve completely in less than 45 minutes. Supplements that take longer to dissolve won't go into the bloodstream and can't do you any good.

## Physical Performance

If physical activity is your thing—especially if you're a competitive athlete—you are always looking for an edge. Our advice? Skip the supplements and do this instead:

- Drink enough water.
- Know and consume a well-balanced diet, with enough fruits and vegetables and variety, and you'll get all the vitamins and minerals you need without taking supplements.
- Skip the protein-rich diet. It is unlikely to build bigger muscles. Even worse, it may dehydrate you and take away calcium.
- Include no more than 30% of your total calories in fat.
- Starchy foods high in complex carbohydrates are what your body prefers for fuel.
- Avoid sugary foods. You won't get the same energy boost.

## Nutritional Quackery

If you read a typical fitness magazine, you will see no shortage of nutrition advertisements. Popular claims by nutrition quacks (pretenders to medical skill) are that their products and services will:

- Take off body fat and lower weight
- Build muscle
- Boost energy
- Enhance endurance
- Fight fatigue
- Relieve muscle soreness

### Fad Diets

Billions of dollars are made annually in the sale and promotion of fad diets. What is a fad diet? Dietary plans that are more trend than science. Dietary plans that attempt to convince a consumer that one particular food is to blame for his or her weight problem. Dietary plans that promote "fast and simple" weight loss.

The truth is, people don't become overweight in a short time, and they can't return to good form in a short time. Diets don't work for the long term, but lifestyle changes do! You must be willing to persist. If it sounds too good to be true, it probably is. See the Time Out feature after this chapter for a summary of the most popular fad diets, their claims, and pros and cons for each approach.

### Dietary Supplements

Just about anything can be sold as long as it is called a "dietary supplement." The FDA considers dietary supplements to be food, so they are not evaluated for safety and effectiveness. People tend to believe that the products on the market have been researched, tested, and inspected.

Avoid buying products with claims like "fat burner," "fat metabolizer," "energy enhancer," "performance booster," "strength booster," "ergogenic aid," "anabolic optimizer," or "genetic optimizer."

### How Is Nutritional Quackery Harmful?

- Buying into quackery may increase health risks by preventing you from seeking adequate medical care.
- Products and services by quacks are usually expensive.
- Products and services may detract from scientific nutrition recommendations.
- False claims may promote distrust of the medical community.

## Reflect >>>> Reinforce >>>> Reinvigorate

### Knowledge Check

*Answers in Appendix D*

1. Anyone vigorously exercising for more than 1 hour should:

   A. Consider drinking an electrolyte/carbohydrate drink
   B. Drink only water
   C. Feel it is fine to drink soda pop to replace fluids
   D. Tough it out

2. For best absorption of fluids by the body, which temperature is best?

   A. Cooler than ambient temperature
   B. Warmer than ambient temperature
   C. Same as ambient temperature
   D. Temperature does not matter

3. Susan lives a very busy life and is on the go most waking hours of the day. Her three children seem to be involved in every sport and activity available through their school and community. Susan exercises daily. She belongs to a book club, volunteers at the local hospital, and is active in her church's programs. She brings home fast-food meals several times each week. She is considering giving vitamin supplements to her family, since she has little time to prepare well-balanced meals at home. Which is the recommended method for Susan to determine whether she needs to give her family a vitamin supplement?

   A. Compare the foods eaten by her family to dietary standards—namely, the Dietary Reference Intakes (DRIs)
   B. Have anthropometric measures made
   C. Obtain a biochemical assessment of their body fluids (e.g., blood, urine)
   D. Have a clinical nutrition examination of their hair, nails, and skin

4. Which vegetarian diet contains no animal products?

   A. Lacto-vegetarian
   B. Lacto-ovo-vegetarian
   C. Vegan
   D. Semi-vegetarian

5. Vegetarians limiting or omitting animal products from their diets may need to take:

   A. Vitamin $B_{12}$
   B. Calcium supplements
   C. Iron supplements
   D. All the above

6. What is the difference between complete and incomplete proteins?

   A. Only complete proteins assist in body structure.
   B. Only complete proteins possess all the essential amino acids.
   C. Only incomplete proteins build red blood cells.
   D. Only incomplete proteins are found in animal products.

7. The numerical value given to a food based on how quickly the body turns it to sugar based on the number of carbohydrates in one serving is called its:

   A. Vitamin output
   B. Glycemic index
   C. Nutritional content
   D. Glycemic load

8. Which of the following, if taken in excess, will the body retain?
   A. Vitamin $B_2$
   B. Vitamin $B_{12}$
   C. Vitamin C
   D. Vitamin E

9. Which of the following nutrients is known for fighting osteoporosis?
   A. Calcium
   B. Iron
   C. Sodium
   D. Magnesium

10. Which of the following is the USDA's calorie recommendation for active men and women?
    A. 1600 calories
    B. 2200 calories
    C. 2800 calories
    D. 3200 calories

## Modern Modifications

- Try granola bars, raw vegetables, fruit, and plain popcorn (no butter) for snacks.
- Drink plenty of water.
- Try to stick with meat dishes that are grilled, baked, roasted, or broiled.
- Have your salad dressing in a separate dish and dip your fork in it before the salad.
- Have sorbet or frozen yogurt instead of ice cream.
- Have a sandwich on whole-grain bread.

## Critical Thinking

Abby is a 20-year-old sophomore at State College. She has been making statements for some time regarding being "unhappy" about her weight, but has yet to take any action on it. She has been thinking about her diet, but she is unsure what to change. Yesterday her intake was as follows:

Breakfast: 2 eggs scrambled, 3 slices of bacon, 2 pieces of toast with butter

Lunch: peanut butter sandwich, Big Grab bag of Doritos, milk

Dinner: spaghetti with meat sauce, 4 bread sticks with butter and garlic, Coke, pie slice

Other: chocolate granola bar, 2 more Cokes, hot wings with friends, "a couple" of beers

Based on this menu, what areas of Abby's diet would you characterize as nutritionally adequate? Excessive? Lacking? How would you adapt Abby's diet to better conform to the Food Guide Pyramid (MyPyramidPlan.com)? The Healthy Eating Pyramid?

## Going Above and Beyond

### Websites

American Dietetic Association
*http://www.eatright.org*

Mayo Clinic Diet and Nutrition Resource Center
*http://www.mayohealth.org/mayo/common/htm/dietpage.htm*

Consumer Information Center: Food
*http://www.pueblo.gsa.gov/food.htm*

FDA Center for Food Safety and Applied Nutrition
*http://vm.cfsan.fda.gov*

Gateways to Government Nutrition Information
*http://www.nutrition.gov* or *http://www.foodsafety.gov*

MedlinePlus: Nutrition
*http://www.nlm.nih.gov/medlineplus/nutrition.html*

National Cancer Institute 5-a-Day Program
*http://www.5aday.gov*

USDA Food and Nutrition Information Center
*http://www.nal.usda.gov/fnic*

Nutrition Analysis Tool, University of Illinois, Urbana/Champaign
*http://www.nat.uiuc.edu*

Center for Science in the Public Interest
*http://cspinet.org*

Office of Dietary Supplements
*http://dietary_supplements.info.nih.gov*

Fast Food Finder
*http://www.olen.com/food*

Glycemic Index—University of Sydney
*http://www.glycemicindex.com*

## References and Suggested Readings

American Dietetics Association (ADA). Vegetarian diets: Position of the American Dietetics Association. *Journal of the American Dietetics Association* 1997; 7:1317–1321.

Clark K. Water, sports drinks, juice, or soda? *ACSM Health and Fitness Journal* 1998; 2:41.

Connor, S. L., Gustafson J. R., and Artaud-Wild, S. M. The Cholesterol-saturated Fat Index for Coronary Prevention: Background, use, and a comprehensive table of foods. *Journal of the American Dietetic Association* 1989; 89:807–816.

Foster-Powell K. et al. International table of glycemic index and glycemic load values: 2002. *American Journal of Clinical Nutrition* 2002; 76:5–56.

Fuchs C. S., Giovannucci E. L., Colditz G. A., Hunter D. J., Stampfer M. J., Rosner B., Speizer F. E., and Willett W. Dietary fiber and the risk of colorectal cancer and adenoma in women. *N Engl J Med* 1999; 340:169–176.

Insel P., Turner R. E., and Ross D. *Discovering Nutrition.* Sudbury, MA: Jones and Bartlett, 2003.

———. *Nutrition.* Sudbury, MA: Jones and Bartlett, 2002.

*J Am Diet Assoc.* 1989; 89:807–816.

Manner M. M. Vitamins and minerals, part I: How much do you need? *ACSM Health and Fitness Journal* 2001; 5:33–36.

———. Vitamins and minerals, part II: Who needs supplements? *ACSM Health and Fitness Journal* 2001; 5:33–36.

———. Vitamins and minerals, part III: Can you get too much? *ACSM Health and Fitness Journal* 2001; 5:26–28.

Mendosa D. Revised international table of glycemic index (GI) and glycemic load (GL) values—2002. [Accessed at http://diabetes.about.com/library/mendosagi/ngilists.htm, March 12, 2005.]

Willett W. C. *Eat, Drink, and Be Healthy.* New York: Fireside, 2001.

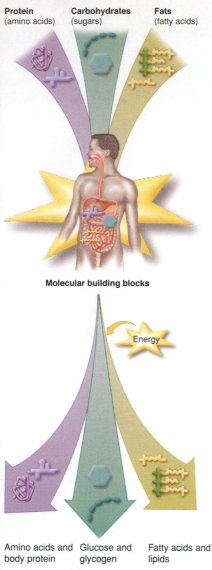

EXTRACTION OF ENERGY

Protein (amino acids)   Carbohydrates (sugars)   Fats (fatty acids)

**Molecular building blocks**

Energy

Amino acids and body protein   Glucose and glycogen   Fatty acids and lipids

BIOSYNTHESIS

Cells use metabolic reactions to extract energy from food and to form building blocks for biosynthesis.

### What's the word. . .

**metabolism** The rate at which your body uses energy.

**adenosine triphosphate (ATP)** The only form of energy used in the human body.

**aerobic** Using oxygen.

**anaerobic** Without using oxygen.

# Energy Production

You need energy to move. When you are doing nothing, your metabolic rate is low. If you start moving, your metabolism increases.

How do you get the energy to move around—or run a marathon? You get it from the carbohydrates, fats, and proteins in food.

During digestion, most carbohydrates are converted to glucose. Some glucose remains in the blood, where it can be used as a quick source of energy. The rest of the glucose is converted to glycogen and stored in the liver, muscles, and kidneys. When glycogen stores are full, leftover glucose is converted to body fat Figure TOI-1.

Protein is used mainly to build tissue. But some protein may also be stored as body fat. When other energy fuels run out, the body uses the protein in body fat for energy.

Your body cells convert glucose, glycogen, and fat to adenosine triphosphate (ATP). When a cell needs energy, it breaks down ATP.

When you exercise, your body mobilizes its stores of fat to increase ATP production.

ATP can be used in two ways: with oxygen (aerobic) or without oxygen (anaerobic).

ATP contracts your muscles during exercise. The amount of ATP needed depends on how long and how hard your body works.

## Aerobic and Anaerobic Activity

If a movement is quick, occurring at the beginning of exercise and at high points of exercise intensity, the body uses the small amount of ATP in the cells (e.g., sprinting; a clean-and-jerk weight lift).

If the movement must be sustained over time, during prolonged but low to relatively moderate exercise (e.g., jogging or running for a distance), the body must create the supply of ATP.

## The Energy Systems

Three different energy systems create energy: immediate energy system, anaerobic energy system, and aerobic energy system. Each system is defined by the way it produces and uses ATP Table TOI-1

### Immediate Energy System

ATP is the immediate source of energy within all cells of our body for activities such as sprinting. There are small stores of ATP within skeletal muscle, and these energy stores provide immediate energy to sustain physical activities for a short time. Once the ATP is used, it breaks down into adenosine diphosphate (ADP). For regeneration of ADP into ATP for more energy, creatine phosphate (CP) is needed. CP regenerates ATP. Without CP, ATP could provide energy for only a few seconds. With CP, the ATP-CP system can provide energy for about 10 seconds before other energy systems must take over.

### Anaerobic Energy System

When vigorous-intensity exercise continues beyond 30 seconds, the only way to continue providing ATP to the exercising muscle is by using glucose in the muscle. Glucose is obtained from glycogen. However, in the process of generating ATP from glucose, lactic

| Table TO1-1 | Characteristics of the Body's Energy Systems | | |
|---|---|---|---|
| | **ENERGY SYSTEM*** | | |
| | Immediate | Nonoxidative | Oxidative |
| **Duration of activity for which system predominates** | 0–10 seconds | 10 seconds–2 minutes | >2 minutes |
| **Intensity of activity for which system predominates** | High | High | Low to moderately high |
| **Rate of ATP production** | Immediate, very rapid | Rapid | Slower but prolonged |
| **Fuel** | Adenosine triphosphate (ATP), creatine phosphate (CP) | Muscle stores of glycogen and glucose | Body stores of glycogen, glucose, fat, and protein |
| **Oxygen used?** | No | No | Yes |
| **Sample activities** | Weight lifting, picking up a bag of groceries | 400-meter run, running up several flights of stairs | 1500-meter run, 30-minute walk, standing in line for a long time |

*For most activities, all three systems contribute to energy production; the duration and intensity of the activity determine which system predominates.

*Source:* Adapted from Brooks G. A., et al. *Exercise Physiology: Human Bioenergetics and Its Application,* 3rd ed. Mountain View, CA: Mayfield, 2000 Copyright © 2002. Mayfield Publishing Co.

acid is formed. Normally, only a small amount of lactic acid is present in the blood and muscle. When lactic acid begins to accumulate in the muscle and then blood, it is a sign of muscular fatigue.

## Aerobic Energy System

The aerobic system provides energy to support long-term steady-state exercise, such as long-distance running or swimming. Muscles can use both glucose and fatty acids for energy. These fuel sources can be taken from the circulating blood and from stores within the muscle. Glucose is stored as glycogen and fatty acids are stored as triglycerides in the muscle. When long-duration activities are performed at a slow pace, more "fat," in the form of fatty acids, is used for energy than muscle glycogen.

## Role of Energy Systems in Exercise

All three energy systems are involved during most types of exercise. When exercise duration increases, a shift occurs from anaerobic energy to aerobic energy. See Table 1 in Appendix A to see how each system contributes to energy needs.

Fit individuals use more stored fat than persons who are less active, so they can exercise longer.

As the intensity and duration of your workout increases, more energy is needed to sustain that level of activity, so more oxygen is required.

The more aerobically fit you are, the higher your $VO_{2max}$, and the more energy you produce. This increases your ability to exercise at a higher level of intensity and for longer periods.

Being aware of how your body produces and uses energy helps you make the connection between nutrition and exercise.

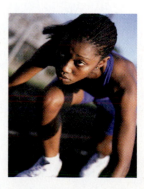

# Time Out 2

## Fad Diets

Have you ever heard the saying, "If it sounds too good to be true, then it probably is"? When it comes to dieting, you can count on it. Fad diets have been around for as long as people have been eating, but now they represent a formidable industry. Billions of dollars are made every year on products designed to help people lose weight.

Most of the diet plans on the market fail to actually teach people how to eat correctly. They promise fast weight loss, and sometimes even deliver on that claim. Of course as soon as the individual stops the diet, he or she invariably returns to the old dietary patterns and the weight piles on again.

In general, fad diets are flawed in the following ways:

- Most propose a diet that places people at risk for coronary heart disease.

| Table TO2.1 | Fad Diets | | |
|---|---|---|---|
| Diet | Date | Author | Premise |
| **Weight Watchers** | 1963 | Jean Nidetch, housewife | General goal of 10 percent weight loss with a "points" system to simplify calorie counting. |
| **Atkins** | *Dr. Atkins' Diet Revolution,* first published in 1972 | Dr. Robert C. Atkins, cardiologist | Achieve a "metabolic advantage" with a four-phase diet low in carbohydrates and high in protein. |
| **Pritikin** | First Longevity Center opened in 1976 | Nathan Pritikin, engineer | "Caloric Density Solution"—a disciplined low-fat approach designed to fight heart disease and high blood pressure. |
| **Ornish** | Studies of the theory started in the late 1970s; *Eat More, Weigh Less* published in 1993 | Dr. Dean Ornish, professor of medicine at the University of California | "Eat more, weigh less" with a diet high in fiber, low in fat. |
| **South Beach** | Developed in 1996; *The South Beach Diet* published in 2003 | Dr. Arthur Agatston, cardiologist | "Lose belly fat first" with this three-phase plan. |
| **Eat, Drink, and Be Healthy** | *Eat, Drink, and Be Healthy* published in 2001 | Dr. Walter C. Willett, chairman of Department of Nutrition at Harvard School of Public Health | Revise the food pyramid for healthy living. |

*Source:* Courtesy of FRONTLINE/WGBH Educational Foundation. Copyright © 2005. WGBH/Boston

- Most describe some specific food or combination of foods as "fat-burning" foods. No scientific evidence exists to support this claim.

- Most fad diets require extremely restrictive dietary patterns—patterns that most people cannot maintain for long periods of time. Significant restrictions on the consumption of macronutrients (fats, carbohydrates, proteins) tend to trigger strong cravings for the missing component.

- Highly imbalanced diets can eventually lead to ketosis, a state where the body believes it is starving and begins to metabolize muscle mass instead of fat.

- Almost none of the fad diets encourage physical activity or even discuss the importance of physical activity in weight management.

**Table T02.1** lists some of the more popular diets and offers a brief analysis of their content.

| Logic | Criticism | Sample Dinner |
|---|---|---|
| Every food is assigned a point value based on calories, total fat, and dietary fiber to meet a daily targeted points range. Weekly meetings create supportive and educational community. There is an emphasis on exercise and making the diet part of a long-term lifestyle change. | Some members shy away from the weekly weigh-ins and meetings. | Chinese vegetables with chicken, tossed salad, brown rice (10 points) |
| By reducing the intake of carbohydrates, you will burn excess body fat for fuel, and feel satiated on a diet that emphasizes fats and protein. Essential nutrients come from low-carbohydrate vegetables. | Critics, who range from vegetarians like Dr. Dean Ornish to proponents of cardiac health such as Nathan Pritikin, argue that the long-term effects of a diet high in protein and saturated fats are unknown. | From the (preliminary) "induction" phase: broiled steak, oven-fried turnips, arugula and Boston lettuce salad |
| Strict adherence to low-fat, low-cholesterol diet, along with exercise, leads to better health and weight loss. | Early criticism was directed at what at the time seemed like an unscientific approach to fight heart disease. Today, proponents of good fats, like Dr. Walter Willett criticize the diet's severe restriction on vegetable oils. Others question whether the diet is too severe and hard to follow. | Salmon paella, baked plantain, onion basket stuffed with carrots and spinach, steamed asparagus |
| Fiber and soy reduce insulin and cholesterol levels, and eating less fat means less total calories consumed. Emphasis on anti-oxidants and avoidance of animal fats promotes overall health. | Like Pritikin, some critics feel that the diet is so low in fat, it's not practical for long-term maintenance. Others believe "good" fats, such as vegetable oils and omega-3 fatty acids, are unnecessarily avoided. | Rigatoni with tomato mushroom sauce, arugula fennel salad with cucumber and chick peas |
| Initial restriction of carbohydrates trains the body not to crave them. Mono- and polyunsaturated fats, whole-grain carbs, and fiber will improve blood chemistry, lower weight and reduce bad cholesterol. Focus on realistic exercise plan. | Skeptics claim that all diets are tough to stick to, and despite its popularity, South Beach is no different. The Florida Citrus industry is fighting against the diet's restriction of orange juice. | From Phase One: Fish kabobs, oven-roasted vegetables, sliced cucumber with olive oil |
| Inverts USDA food pyramid by creating a foundation of "good fats" and whole-grain carbohydrates in combination with exercise. Emphasizes fruits, vegetables, and nuts, while putting refined starches at the top of the pyramid. Lose weight by reducing caloric intake in this regimen. | Critics argue Willett's "good" fats, such as olive oil, are laden with calories. Meanwhile, Atkins advocates, such as Gary Taubes, do not agree with the good fat/bad fat distinction, saying that the risks from saturated fat are overblown. | Pork tenderloin with pistachio-gremolata crust, wild rice pilaf, steamed asparagus. |

*For most activities, all three systems contribute to energy production; the duration and intensity of the activity determine which system predominates.

## CHAPTER 7

# Maintaining a Healthy Body Composition and Body Weight

## Objectives

After reading this chapter, you should be able to:

- Differentiate between essential body fat and storage fat.
- Define overweight and obesity, and explain their causes.
- Recognize different body shapes and their associated risks.
- Recognize the different ways to assess body composition.
- Identify strategies for effective weight management.
- Explain how to safely gain weight.
- Describe various eating disorders and their treatment.

# What Is Body Composition?

Nothing is more personal than your own body. And nothing has a greater influence over how long that body functions properly than its composition. Body composition is the ratio of muscle mass to fat mass. *Muscle mass* is composed of muscle, bone, organs, and other tissues of the body. *Fat mass* is the total amount of essential and storage fat in the body.

## Essential Body Fat

Your essential body fat resides in your nerve cells, muscles, and bone marrow, as well as in your lungs, heart, liver, and intestines. It has many important functions:

- Keeps your physiological activity normal (e.g., nerve conduction)
- Helps keep your body warm
- Protects your organs from injury
- Stores energy needed when your body is active or when you are injured or ill

The desirable amount of essential fat for a healthy person is:

- Adult women: 10% to 12% of total body weight
- Adult men: 3% to 5% of total body weight

Women have more essential body fat in their hips, thighs, breasts, and uterus.

## Storage Fat

Some fat beyond what is essential is also desirable. Besides organ protection and body insulation, storage fat supplies energy: 3500 calories per pound of adipose tissue

**Figure 7.1**. A variety of methods exist for determining whether body composition places a person at risk for disease. Some methods are simple calculations and are based on the relationship between the person's height and weight. Other methods look specifically at the fat contained in the body.

<aside>
**What's the word. . .**

**body composition** Proportion of fat, muscle, bone, and other tissues in the body.

**essential body fat** Minimum amount of body fat needed for good health.

**storage fat** Excess fat deposited in adipose tissue (fat cells) that protects organs and insulates the body.
</aside>

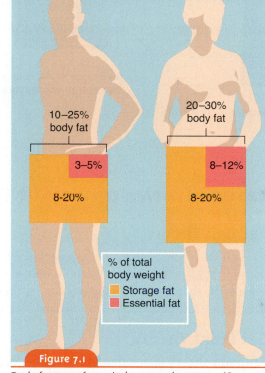

**Figure 7.1**

Body fatness of a typical man and woman. (*Source:* Data compiled from Nutrition for physical fitness and athletic performance for adults—Position of ADA and the Canadian Dietetic Association. *Journal of the American Dietetic Association* 1993; 93:691–697. Reprinted with permission from the American Dietetic Association.)

# What Causes Weight Gain?

Your weight changes depend on a simple rule:

When the number of calories consumed is not equal to the number of calories used, the following occurs:

Calories Consumed > Calories Used = **Weight Gain**

Calories Consumed < Calories Used = **Weight Loss**

Calories Consumed = Calories Used = **No Weight Gain**

See **Figure 7.2**.

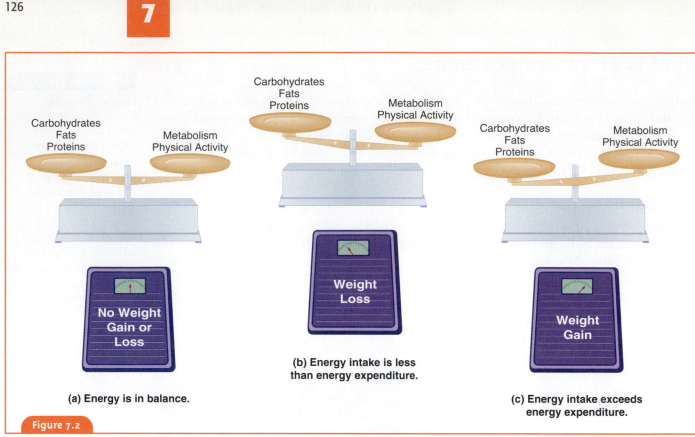

**Figure 7.2**

The balance between energy intake and expenditure controls weight management.

# Early Theories of Weight Gain

### Fat Cell Theory

Fat cell theory says that obesity is related to too many fat cells and enlarged fat cells (see 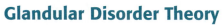 Figure 7.3). People with an above-average number of fat cells may have been born with them or may have developed them at certain times because of overeating. Restricting calories decreases only the size of fat cells, not the number.

### Set Point Theory

Set point theory states that obese individuals are "programmed" to carry a certain amount of weight. This programming originates from a weight regulatory mechanism in the brain's hypothalamus. Even if you lose weight, your body strives to get back to its set point. To lose weight, you must change the set point.

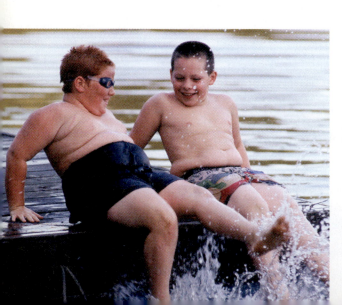

### Glandular Disorder Theory

Hypothyroidism is the cause of only 1% to 2% of all overweight (Insel, Turner, and Ross 2002).

# Current Theories of Weight Gain

Many factors influence weight gain. Some may emerge very early in life.

### Genetics

Some individuals are genetically (and sometimes culturally) pre-disposed to gain weight more easily than others or to store fat around the abdomen and chest. Children of overweight or obese

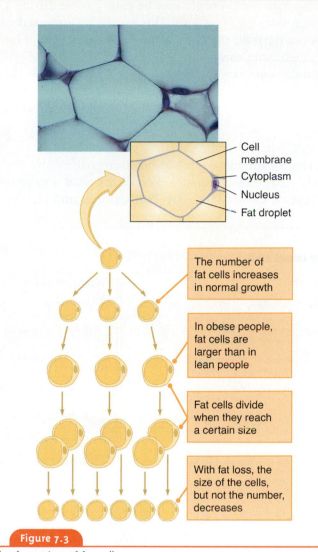

Cell membrane
Cytoplasm
Nucleus
Fat droplet

The number of fat cells increases in normal growth

In obese people, fat cells are larger than in lean people

Fat cells divide when they reach a certain size

With fat loss, the size of the cells, but not the number, decreases

**Figure 7.3**

The formation of fat cells.

parents, particularly the biological mother, are more likely to develop weight problems, for example (NCCDPHP 2001).

## Diseases and Drugs

Some illnesses may lead to obesity or weight gain, including Cushing's disease, and polycystic ovary syndrome. Drugs such as steroids and some antidepressants may also cause weight gain. A doctor is the best source to tell you whether illnesses or medications are contributing to weight gain or making weight loss difficult (NCCDPHP 2001).

## Calorie Consumption

In the United States, a changing environment has expanded our food options and broadened our eating habits. Grocery stores stock their shelves with a greater selection of products. Prepackaged foods, fast-food restaurants, and soft drinks are readily accessible. While such foods are fast and convenient, they tend to be high in fat, sugar, and calories. Choosing many foods from these categories can contribute to an excessive calorie intake. Some foods are marketed as healthy, low fat, or fat free but may contain a lot of calories. It is important to read food labels for nutritional information and to eat in moderation (NCCDPHP 2001).

Portion size has also increased. People may be eating more during a meal or snack because of larger portion sizes **Figure 7.4**. This results in increased calorie consumption. If the body does not burn off the extra calories consumed from larger portions, fast food, or soft drinks, weight gain can occur.

How do portions today compare to portions sizes 20 years ago? They are larger! The National Institutes of Health (NIH) has developed a website (see the list of websites at the end of this chapter) to inform people about the increasing portion sizes.

## Calories Used

Our bodies need calories for functions such as breathing, digestion, and daily activities. Weight gain occurs when calories consumed exceed this need. For example, to lose 1 pound, you must decrease caloric intake by 3500 calories and maintain the same

### Portion Distortion

As portions have grown larger over the past 40 years, so have North Americans. Studies show that the more food put in front of people, the more they eat.

Since the 1960s, the serving sizes of foods sold in stores and restaurants—from candy bars to burgers and soda—have become much bigger. For example, bagels used to be 2 to 3 ounces (about 200 calories); today they are 5 to 6 ounces (more than 400 calories, depending on the type and equivalent to five pieces of bread)

"Super-size" portions are partially to blame for Americans' overweight explosion. It could also be that many people are innocently overeating. Nutritionists observe that most Americans overestimate how much food makes up a serving size.

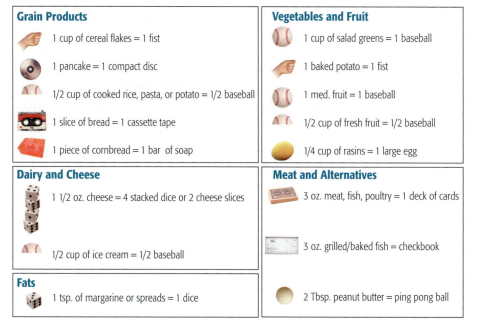

### 1 Serving Looks Like . . .

**Grain Products**

1 cup of cereal flakes = 1 fist

1 pancake = 1 compact disc

1/2 cup of cooked rice, pasta, or potato = 1/2 baseball

1 slice of bread = 1 cassette tape

1 piece of cornbread = 1 bar of soap

**Dairy and Cheese**

1 1/2 oz. cheese = 4 stacked dice or 2 cheese slices

1/2 cup of ice cream = 1/2 baseball

**Fats**

1 tsp. of margarine or spreads = 1 dice

**Vegetables and Fruit**

1 cup of salad greens = 1 baseball

1 baked potato = 1 fist

1 med. fruit = 1 baseball

1/2 cup of fresh fruit = 1/2 baseball

1/4 cup of rasins = 1 large egg

**Meat and Alternatives**

3 oz. meat, fish, poultry = 1 deck of cards

3 oz. grilled/baked fish = checkbook

2 Tbsp. peanut butter = ping pong ball

*Source:* Department of Health and Human Services/National Institutes of Health, 2005.

A "portion" is the amount of a specific food you **choose** to eat for a meal or snack. Portions can be bigger or smaller than the recommended food servings.

A "serving" is a unit of measure used to describe the amount of food **recommended** from each food group. It is the amount of food listed on the Nutrition Facts panel on packaged food or the amount of food recommended in the Food Guide Pyramid and the *Dietary Guidelines for Americans.*

Healthy eating plans use certain numbers of servings of fruits, vegetables, carbohydrates, etc. But exactly how much is a serving of broccoli or a serving of cheese?

Estimating serving sizes is easier than you think—just use a familiar object for a reference. At **http://hin.nhlbi.nih.gov/portion/ servingcard7.pdf** you can download a Serving Size card shown here to help you recall what a standard food serving looks like. Print and cut out the card and laminate it for longtime use.

Rather than cutting carbs, fats, or proteins, using the familiar objects helps you become aware of how much you are eating. For example, a 3-ounce serving of meat is the size of a deck of cards.

There is no need to go hungry, you can increase the portions of some foods such as fruits and vegetables. You can eat lots of broccoli, green beans, deep-green lettuce, apples, and strawberries without eating too many additional calories. Besides, most people do not eat enough fruits and vegetables to meet the dietary guidelines.

**Figure 7.4**

amount of activity, or increase physical activity so that it burns 3500 calories. Physical activity plays a key role in energy balance because it uses up calories consumed.

Despite all the benefits of being physically active, most Americans are sedentary. Technology has created many time- and labor-saving products. Some examples include cars, elevators, computers, dishwashers, and televisions. Cars are used to run short-distance errands instead of walking or riding a bicycle. As a result, these recent lifestyle changes have reduced the overall amount of energy expended in our daily lives (NCCDPHP 2001). According to the Behavioral Risk Factor Surveillance System, in 2000 more than 26% of adults reported no leisure-time physical activity.

The belief that physical activity is limited to exercise or sports may keep people from being active. Another myth is that physical activity must be vigorous to achieve health benefits. Physical activity is any bodily movement that results in an expenditure of energy. Moderate-intensity activities such as household chores, gardening, and walking can also provide health benefits.

## Socioeconomic, Age, and Gender Factors

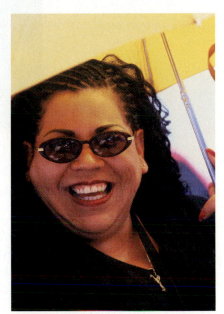

- Age: Fatness increases during adulthood and declines in the elderly.
- Gender: Obesity is more prevalent in women than men.
- Culture: People in developed countries have more body fat than those in developing societies.
- Race/ethnicity: Obesity is more prevalent in African American, Hispanic, Native American, and Pacific Islander people.
- Income: Obesity is more prevalent in lower-income women.
- Education: Less-educated women have a higher incidence of obesity.
- Employment: Unemployed women have a higher incidence of obesity.
- Marriage: Married men have a higher incidence of obesity.
- Residence: Rural women have a higher incidence of obesity.
- Region: People living in the Southern states have a higher incidence of obesity (Insel, Turner, and Ross 2002).

## Psychological Factors

- Weight cycling: This is a pattern of losing and regaining weight, over and over again (yo-yo dieting). Experts believe that despite potential risks, any successful effort to lose pounds, even if temporary, can have potential benefits.
- Restrained eaters: This involves trying to reduce food intake by fasting or avoiding food as long as possible, usually by skipping meals or delaying eating. When emotionally stressed, the restrained eater overeats without realizing it.
- Binge eaters: This involves compulsive overeating, sometimes for days. Such behavior is common among people in weight-loss programs (Insel, Turner, and Ross 2002).

# Determining Recommended Body Composition

Using weight as the primary determinant is not necessarily a good indicator of how healthy you are. What is important is the ratio of body fat to lean body mass in your body composition.

For instance, a female bodybuilder may weigh more than a standard chart says she should. But she may have only about 8% to 13% of her body weight in total fat. This is probably the least amount of body fat a woman can have and still be healthy.

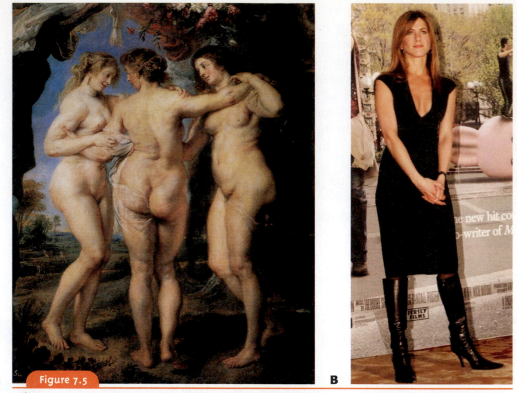

**Figure 7.5**

A    B

Voluptuous women were once considered the female ideal **(A)**; in today's society Jennifer Aniston embodies a popular standard **(B)**.

What society deems as a desirable or ideal body differs in different time periods, usually depending on trends in fashion. It used to be—and still is in some cultures—that women with a good bit of nonessential fat were considered physically attractive and sexually desirable. Today the skinny fashion-model body type is "in"  Figure 7.5  .

Methods exist for determining body composition by using both weight and body fat.

# Assessing Body Composition Using Weight

You can assess your body composition by comparing yourself to a weight-to-height table or by measuring your body mass index.

- Use a scale to measure your weight.
- Use a tape measure to measure your height.

## Height–Weight Tables

Many versions of height–weight tables are available, all with different weight ranges. Some tables take into account a person's frame size and age; others do not.

Body composition measured on a table does not show the proportion of body fat to lean muscle mass. Athletes may be overweight as measured by the table, but not unhealthy.

Height–weight tables may serve as an excellent way for doctors to make sure babies are growing normally, but are not generally useful for adults as a measure of personal health.

## Body Mass Index

The body mass index (BMI), based on an individual's height and weight (see  Table 7.1  ), is a simple estimate of body composition. A BMI number is *not* a certain percentage of body fat.

**Table 7.1  Body Mass Index Table**

Body Weight (pounds)

| Height (inches) | Normal |  |  |  |  |  | Overweight |  |  |  |  | Obese |  |  |  |  |  |  |  |  |  | Extreme Obesity |  |  |  |  |  |  |  |  |  |  |  |  |  |  |
|---|---|---|---|---|---|---|---|---|---|---|---|---|---|---|---|---|---|---|---|---|---|---|---|---|---|---|---|---|---|---|---|---|---|---|---|---|
| **BMI** | 19 | 20 | 21 | 22 | 23 | 24 | 25 | 26 | 27 | 28 | 29 | 30 | 31 | 32 | 33 | 34 | 35 | 36 | 37 | 38 | 39 | 40 | 41 | 42 | 43 | 44 | 45 | 46 | 47 | 48 | 49 | 50 | 51 | 52 | 53 | 54 |
| 58 | 91 | 96 | 100 | 105 | 110 | 115 | 119 | 124 | 129 | 134 | 138 | 143 | 148 | 153 | 158 | 162 | 167 | 172 | 177 | 181 | 186 | 191 | 196 | 201 | 205 | 210 | 215 | 220 | 224 | 229 | 234 | 239 | 244 | 248 | 253 | 258 |
| 59 | 94 | 99 | 104 | 109 | 114 | 119 | 124 | 128 | 133 | 138 | 143 | 148 | 153 | 158 | 163 | 168 | 173 | 178 | 183 | 188 | 193 | 198 | 203 | 208 | 212 | 217 | 222 | 227 | 232 | 237 | 242 | 247 | 252 | 257 | 262 | 267 |
| 60 | 97 | 102 | 107 | 112 | 118 | 123 | 128 | 133 | 138 | 143 | 148 | 153 | 158 | 163 | 168 | 174 | 179 | 184 | 189 | 194 | 199 | 204 | 209 | 215 | 220 | 225 | 230 | 235 | 240 | 245 | 250 | 255 | 261 | 266 | 271 | 276 |
| 61 | 100 | 106 | 111 | 116 | 122 | 127 | 132 | 137 | 143 | 148 | 153 | 158 | 164 | 169 | 174 | 180 | 185 | 190 | 195 | 201 | 206 | 211 | 217 | 222 | 227 | 232 | 238 | 243 | 248 | 254 | 259 | 264 | 269 | 275 | 280 | 285 |
| 62 | 104 | 109 | 115 | 120 | 126 | 131 | 136 | 142 | 147 | 153 | 158 | 164 | 169 | 175 | 180 | 186 | 191 | 196 | 202 | 207 | 213 | 218 | 224 | 229 | 235 | 240 | 246 | 251 | 256 | 262 | 267 | 273 | 278 | 284 | 289 | 295 |
| 63 | 107 | 113 | 118 | 124 | 130 | 135 | 141 | 146 | 152 | 158 | 163 | 169 | 175 | 180 | 186 | 191 | 197 | 203 | 208 | 214 | 220 | 225 | 231 | 237 | 242 | 248 | 254 | 259 | 265 | 270 | 278 | 282 | 287 | 293 | 299 | 304 |
| 64 | 110 | 116 | 122 | 128 | 134 | 140 | 145 | 151 | 157 | 163 | 169 | 174 | 180 | 186 | 192 | 197 | 204 | 209 | 215 | 221 | 227 | 232 | 238 | 244 | 250 | 256 | 262 | 267 | 273 | 279 | 285 | 291 | 296 | 302 | 308 | 314 |
| 65 | 114 | 120 | 126 | 132 | 138 | 144 | 150 | 156 | 162 | 168 | 174 | 180 | 186 | 192 | 198 | 204 | 210 | 216 | 222 | 228 | 234 | 240 | 246 | 252 | 258 | 264 | 270 | 276 | 282 | 288 | 294 | 300 | 306 | 312 | 318 | 324 |
| 66 | 118 | 124 | 130 | 136 | 142 | 148 | 155 | 161 | 167 | 173 | 179 | 186 | 192 | 198 | 204 | 210 | 216 | 223 | 229 | 235 | 241 | 247 | 253 | 260 | 266 | 272 | 278 | 284 | 291 | 297 | 303 | 309 | 315 | 322 | 328 | 334 |
| 67 | 121 | 127 | 134 | 140 | 146 | 153 | 159 | 166 | 172 | 178 | 185 | 191 | 198 | 204 | 211 | 217 | 223 | 230 | 236 | 242 | 249 | 255 | 261 | 268 | 274 | 280 | 287 | 293 | 299 | 306 | 312 | 319 | 325 | 331 | 338 | 344 |
| 68 | 125 | 131 | 138 | 144 | 151 | 158 | 164 | 171 | 177 | 184 | 190 | 197 | 203 | 210 | 216 | 223 | 230 | 236 | 243 | 249 | 256 | 262 | 269 | 276 | 282 | 289 | 295 | 302 | 308 | 315 | 322 | 328 | 335 | 341 | 348 | 354 |
| 69 | 128 | 135 | 142 | 149 | 155 | 162 | 169 | 176 | 182 | 189 | 196 | 203 | 209 | 216 | 223 | 230 | 236 | 243 | 250 | 257 | 263 | 270 | 277 | 284 | 291 | 297 | 304 | 311 | 318 | 324 | 331 | 338 | 345 | 351 | 358 | 365 |
| 70 | 132 | 139 | 146 | 153 | 160 | 167 | 174 | 181 | 188 | 195 | 202 | 209 | 216 | 222 | 229 | 236 | 243 | 250 | 257 | 264 | 271 | 278 | 285 | 292 | 299 | 306 | 313 | 320 | 327 | 334 | 341 | 348 | 355 | 362 | 369 | 376 |
| 71 | 136 | 143 | 150 | 157 | 165 | 172 | 179 | 186 | 193 | 200 | 208 | 215 | 222 | 229 | 236 | 243 | 250 | 257 | 265 | 272 | 279 | 286 | 293 | 301 | 308 | 315 | 322 | 329 | 338 | 343 | 351 | 358 | 365 | 372 | 379 | 386 |
| 72 | 140 | 147 | 154 | 162 | 169 | 177 | 184 | 191 | 199 | 206 | 213 | 221 | 228 | 235 | 242 | 250 | 258 | 265 | 272 | 279 | 287 | 294 | 302 | 309 | 316 | 324 | 331 | 338 | 346 | 353 | 361 | 368 | 375 | 383 | 390 | 397 |
| 73 | 144 | 151 | 159 | 166 | 174 | 182 | 189 | 197 | 204 | 212 | 219 | 227 | 235 | 242 | 250 | 257 | 265 | 272 | 280 | 288 | 295 | 302 | 310 | 318 | 325 | 333 | 340 | 348 | 355 | 363 | 371 | 378 | 386 | 393 | 401 | 408 |
| 74 | 148 | 155 | 163 | 171 | 179 | 186 | 194 | 202 | 210 | 218 | 225 | 233 | 241 | 249 | 256 | 264 | 272 | 280 | 287 | 295 | 303 | 311 | 319 | 326 | 334 | 342 | 350 | 358 | 365 | 373 | 381 | 389 | 396 | 404 | 412 | 420 |
| 75 | 152 | 160 | 168 | 176 | 184 | 192 | 200 | 208 | 216 | 224 | 232 | 240 | 248 | 256 | 264 | 272 | 279 | 287 | 295 | 303 | 311 | 319 | 327 | 335 | 343 | 351 | 359 | 367 | 375 | 383 | 391 | 399 | 407 | 415 | 423 | 431 |
| 76 | 156 | 164 | 172 | 180 | 189 | 197 | 205 | 213 | 221 | 230 | 238 | 246 | 254 | 263 | 271 | 279 | 287 | 295 | 304 | 312 | 320 | 328 | 336 | 344 | 353 | 361 | 369 | 377 | 385 | 394 | 402 | 410 | 418 | 426 | 435 | 443 |

*Source:* Adapted from *Clinical Guidelines on the Identification, Evaluation, and Treatment of Overweight and Obesity in Adults: The Evidence Report.*

| Table 7.2 | Classification of BMI Values |
| --- | --- |
| **BMI** | **Classification** |
| Less than 18.5 | Underweight |
| 18.5 to 24.9 | Normal |
| 25 to 29.9 | Overweight |
| 30 or greater | Obese |

The BMI can help detect the potential for health or nutritional disorders. The BMI number alone is *not* diagnostic.

A healthy BMI for adults is between 18.5 and 24.9. BMI ranges are based on the effect body weight has on disease and death.

### What Does BMI Mean?

You can interpret BMI values for adults with one fixed number, regardless of age or gender, using the guidelines in   Table 7.2  .

People with a very low or high BMI have a higher relative mortality   Figure 7.6  .

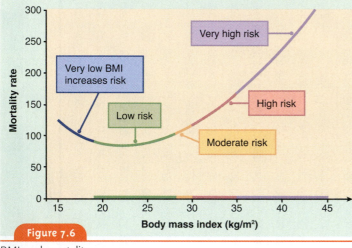

**Figure 7.6**

BMI and mortality.

# Assessing Body Fatness

Everyone needs a certain amount of fat for stored energy, heat insulation, shock absorption, and other functions. As a rule, women have more fat than men. Experts generally agree that men with more than 25% body fat and women with more than 30% body fat are obese.

The desirable ranges of body fat are:

- Adult women: 20% to 25% of total body weight
- Adult men: 12% to 20% of total body weight

Risk of chronic disease rises when the percentage of body fat:

- Exceeds 30% of total body weight in adult women
- Exceeds 25% of total body weight in adult men

Body fatness can be assessed by several methods. Very sophisticated methods such as dual energy X-ray absorptiometry (DEXA), isotope dilution, and computed tomography (CT) and magnetic resonance imaging (MRI) scans more accurately assess body composition; however, their expense may limit their usefulness on a large scale.

## Skinfold Measurements

Because half of your body's fat is located under your skin, you can estimate your percentage of body fat by measuring skinfold thickness. This requires some skill.

See Lab 7-1, Activity 4 for complete instructions on how to take a skinfold measurement.

## Bioelectrical Impedance Analysis

Body fat percentage can be measured using bioelectrical impedance analysis.

- Electrodes are attached to the wrist and ankle, and a small electrical impulse is sent through the body.

**What's the word. . .**

**body mass index (BMI)** A measure of body fatness, calculated by dividing your weight in pounds by your height in inches. Then divide that answer by your height in inches. Multiply the answer by 703.

**bioelectrical impedance** Measurement of the strength and speed of an electrical signal sent through the body.

- Current flows more easily through the parts of the body composed mostly of water (blood, urine, and muscle) than it does through bone, fat, or air.
- A computer measures the bioelectrical impedance of the signal and combines it with information such as height, weight, and gender to assess percentage of body fat.

## Procedure

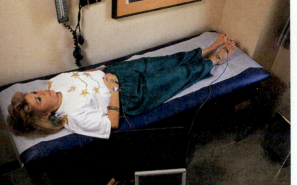

Bioelectrical impedance.

1. You stand with bare feet on a device resembling a conventional bathroom scale with two built-in footpad electrodes.

   OR

   You lie on a cot and spot electrodes are placed on your hands and bare feet and connected to a bio-electrical impedance machine.

2. A built-in computer measures your bioelectrical impedance, and then uses this number and your gender, height, fitness level, weight, and in some cases your age to assess your percentage of body fat.

## Caution

- You need to be adequately hydrated.
- If you are dehydrated, the amount of fat will likely be overestimated.
- People with pacemakers are not candidates for this method.

## Disadvantages

- Tends to overestimate your body fat if you are lean and athletic, unless the machine is equipped with an "athlete" mode.
- Does not take into account the location of body fat.

**What's the word...**

**hydrostatic (underwater) weighing** Measuring a person's weight while he or she is suspended in water.

# Hydrostatic (Underwater) Weighing

Hydrostatic (underwater) weighing is another method to measure body fat percentage.

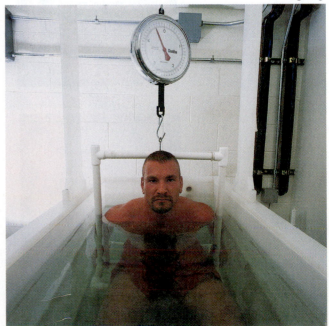

Underwater weighing.

## Procedure

1. You are weighed while suspended on a trapeze in the air.
2. You are then seated on a special scale and totally submerged in a pool or tank.
3. You exhale as much air as possible and remain motionless as your weight is recorded.
4. The procedure is repeated two to five times to get a dependable weight number.
- Because fat floats, a fat person will weigh less underwater than a lean person of the same body weight.
- Your percentage of body fat is calculated from equations based on density of body composition.

**Disadvantages**

- Underwater weighing requires expensive equipment.
- The procedure requires a well-trained technician.
- The calculation of body fat percentage is based on studies of young Caucasians. The formula may not fit all cases.
- Some people feel uncomfortable when they are fully submerged, leading to incorrect readings.
- There is always air left in the lungs. It is difficult to accurately correct for this.
- This method does not take into account the location of body fat.

Bod Pod.

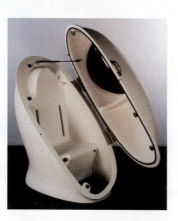

## Densitometry (Air Displacement)

Air displacement is more practical to use as a measure of body fat than water displacement. A new device, the Bod Pod, allows an individual to sit in a sealed chamber of known volume and displace a certain volume of air.

Apple shape.

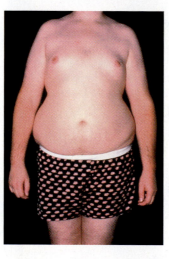

## Body Fat Distribution

It is not only how much fat an individual has, but where the fat is on the body that affects a person's health. Women usually collect fat in their hips and buttocks, giving their figures a "pear" shape. Men typically build up fat around their bellies, giving them more of an "apple" shape. This is not a hard-and-fast rule. Some men are pear shaped and some women become apple shaped, especially after menopause. Most people have a combination of both characteristics. It's healthier not to develop a beer belly.

Pear shape.

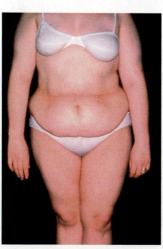

## Calculate Your Waist-to-Hip Ratio

Your waist-to-hip ratio (WHR) tells you where you store body fat **Figure 7.7** .

WHR = Waist Circumference (inches) ÷ Hip Circumference (inches)

Standard WHRs for:

- Men should be less than 0.95
- Women should be no more than 0.8

Ratios greater than these indicate a tendency toward central (torso) obesity. People who store excess fat centrally, as opposed to in their extremities, are at an increased risk for cardiorespiratory diseases and diabetes.

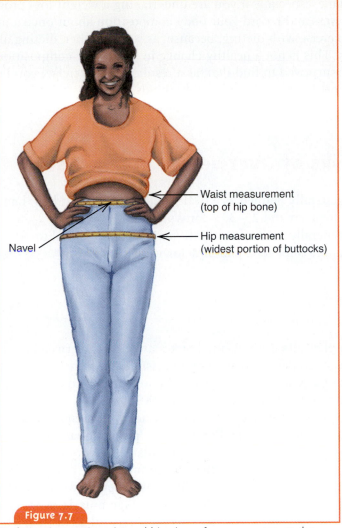

Waist measurement
(top of hip bone)

Hip measurement
(widest portion of buttocks)

Navel

**Figure 7.7**

To determine one's waist and hip circumferences, measure the waist directly above the hip bone; measure the hips at the widest point of the buttocks.

## Measure Your Waist Circumference

Some experts believe that measuring your waist is as good as the WHR, and is easier to do.

- See Lab 7-1, Activity 1 for detailed instructions on how to measure your waist circumference.
- Note that if an individual is less than 5 feet in height or has a BMI of 35 or greater, waist circumference standards used for the general population may not apply.

# Importance of Regular Assessment of Body Composition

As most people age, they lose lean body mass, and gain body fat.

From about the age of 25 years until 65 years, most people gain about 40 pounds. They also lose about 20 pounds of lean tissue mass.

That means they have actually gained 60 pounds of fat!

It is important, especially if you are undertaking a weight-loss program of diet and exercise, to reassess and record your body composition about once a month.

Combine exercise with dieting, because, as stated earlier, dieting alone can cost you lean body mass. This is not a healthy change in your body composition.

You will be surprised to find that, as a result of the exercise, you have gained more lean mass and lost body fat. If you lost 4 pounds, you may have gained 4 pounds of lean mass, meaning you lost 8 pounds of fat! Isn't that pretty encouraging?

# Health Risks of Overweight and Obesity

Overweight is generally defined as a BMI greater than 25 but less than 30, or body fat that is 20–25% for men and 25–30% for women.

Obesity is generally defined as a BMI greater than or equal to 30, or a body fat level that is more than 25% for men and 30% for women.

# Obesity

More than 60% of adults in the United States are either overweight or obese (NCHS 2004). The obesity epidemic covered on television and in newspapers did not occur overnight, of course. Obesity and overweight are chronic conditions. Indeed, a variety of factors play a role in obesity (NCCDPHP 2001).

Note that overweight may or may not be due to increases in body fat. It may also reflect an increase in lean muscle. For example, professional athletes may be very lean and muscular with very little body fat, yet they may weigh more than individuals of the same height. While they may qualify as "overweight" due to their large muscle mass, they are not necessarily "overfat," regardless of their BMI (NCCDPHP 2004).

Concerns regarding body fat include both the distribution of fat throughout the body and the size of the adipose tissue deposits. Body fat distribution can be estimated by skinfold measures, waist-to-hip circumference ratios, or techniques such as ultrasound, CT, or MRI scans (NCCDPHP 2004).

# Health Risks of Too Much Body Fat

The main concern about overweight and obesity is one of health and not appearance Figure 7.8 . Too much storage fat is unhealthy.

Obese people are at a higher risk for diabetes, heart disease, stroke, high blood pressure, and premature death. They are also prone to gallbladder disease, arthritis, varicose veins, and shortness of breath Table 7.3 .

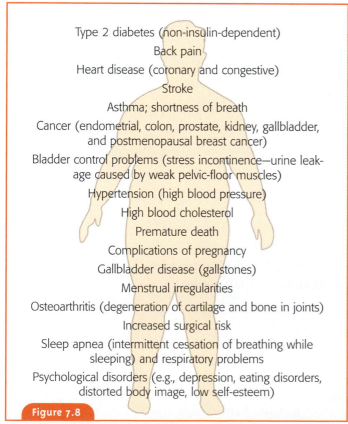

Type 2 diabetes (non-insulin-dependent)
Back pain
Heart disease (coronary and congestive)
Stroke
Asthma; shortness of breath
Cancer (endometrial, colon, prostate, kidney, gallbladder, and postmenopausal breast cancer)
Bladder control problems (stress incontinence—urine leakage caused by weak pelvic-floor muscles)
Hypertension (high blood pressure)
High blood cholesterol
Premature death
Complications of pregnancy
Gallbladder disease (gallstones)
Menstrual irregularities
Osteoarthritis (degeneration of cartilage and bone in joints)
Increased surgical risk
Sleep apnea (intermittent cessation of breathing while sleeping) and respiratory problems
Psychological disorders (e.g., depression, eating disorders, distorted body image, low self-esteem)

Figure 7.8

Health risks for overweight and obese people.

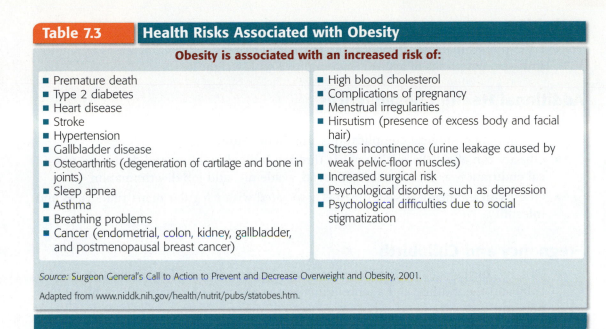

| Table 7.3 | Health Risks Associated with Obesity |
| --- | --- |

**Obesity is associated with an increased risk of:**

- Premature death
- Type 2 diabetes
- Heart disease
- Stroke
- Hypertension
- Gallbladder disease
- Osteoarthritis (degeneration of cartilage and bone in joints)
- Sleep apnea
- Asthma
- Breathing problems
- Cancer (endometrial, colon, kidney, gallbladder, and postmenopausal breast cancer)

- High blood cholesterol
- Complications of pregnancy
- Menstrual irregularities
- Hirsutism (presence of excess body and facial hair)
- Stress incontinence (urine leakage caused by weak pelvic-floor muscles)
- Increased surgical risk
- Psychological disorders, such as depression
- Psychological difficulties due to social stigmatization

*Source:* Surgeon General's Call to Action to Prevent and Decrease Overweight and Obesity, 2001.

Adapted from www.niddk.nih.gov/health/nutrit/pubs/statobes.htm.

## Premature Death

- The risk of premature death rises with increasing weight.
- Obese individuals are at a 50% to 100% increased risk of death from all causes.

## Heart Disease

- High blood pressure is twice as common in obese adults.
- Obesity is associated with elevated triglycerides (blood fat) and decreased HDL (good) cholesterol.
- Heart disease (heart attack, congestive heart failure, sudden cardiac death, chest pain, and abnormal heart rhythm) is increased in those who are overweight or obese.

## Diabetes

- More than 80% of people with type 2 diabetes are overweight or obese.
- A weight gain of 11 to 18 pounds increases a person's risk of developing type 2 diabetes to twice that of individuals who have not gained weight.

## Cancer

- Overweight and obesity are associated with an increased risk for some types of cancer, including endometrial (cancer of the lining of the uterus), colon, gallbladder, prostate, kidney, and postmenopausal breast cancer.
- Women gaining more than 20 pounds from age 18 to midlife double their risk of postmenopausal breast cancer.

## Breathing Problems

- Sleep apnea (interrupted breathing while sleeping) is more common in obese persons.
- Obesity is associated with a higher prevalence of asthma.

## Arthritis

For every 2-pound increase in weight, the risk of developing arthritis increases by 9% to 13%. However, symptoms of arthritis can improve with weight loss.

## Additional Health Consequences

- Overweight and obesity are associated with increased risks of gallbladder disease, incontinence, surgical complications, and depression.
- Obesity can affect the quality of life through limited mobility and decreased physical endurance, as well as through social, academic, and job discrimination.
- Obesity in premenopausal women is associated with irregular menstrual cycles and infertility.

## Pregnancy and Childbirth

- Obesity during pregnancy is associated with increased risk of death in both the baby and the mother, and a tenfold increase in the risk of maternal high blood pressure.
- Obese women are more likely to have gestational diabetes and problems with labor and delivery.
- Infants born to women who are obese during pregnancy are more likely to have a high birth weight and low blood sugar (associated with brain damage and seizures).
- Obesity during pregnancy is associated with increased risk of birth defects, particularly neural tube defects such as spina bifida.

## Children and Adolescents

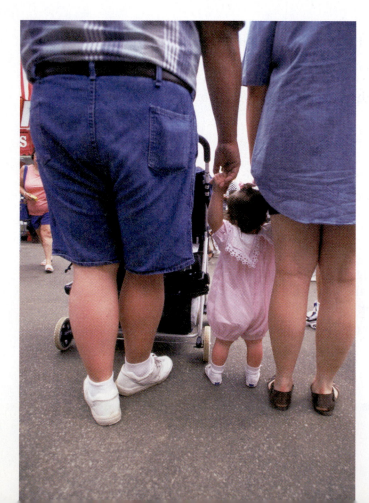

- The Centers for Disease Control and Prevention (CDC) estimates that 16% of all children 6 to 19 years old are overweight **Figure 7.9**. That is a 45% increase in the last 10 years.
- Risk factors for heart disease, such as high cholesterol and high blood pressure, occur with increased frequency in overweight children and adolescents compared to those with a healthy weight.
- The incidence of type 2 diabetes (non-insulin-dependent), previously considered an adult disease, has increased dramatically in children and adolescents. Overweight and obesity are closely linked to type 2 diabetes.
- Overweight adolescents have a 70% chance of becoming overweight or obese adults. This risk increases to 80% if one or more parent is overweight or obese.
- Obese people are more likely to have accidents, because they can't move easily.
- Obese people are socially and occupationally stigmatized, and generally have lower self-esteem.

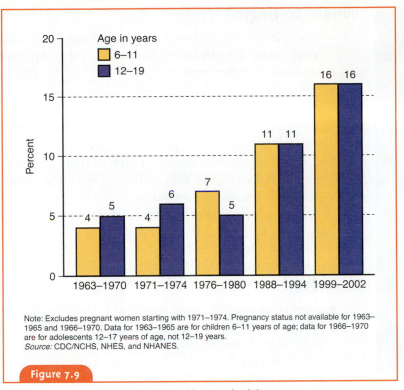

Note: Excludes pregnant women starting with 1971–1974. Pregnancy status not available for 1963–1965 and 1966–1970. Data for 1963–1965 are for children 6–11 years of age; data for 1966–1970 are for adolescents 12–17 years of age, not 12–19 years.
*Source:* CDC/NCHS, NHES, and NHANES.

**Figure 7.9**

Prevalence of overweight among children and adolescents ages 6 to 19 years.

## Weight Management

Worldwide, the number of overweight or obese people has increased markedly in recent years. More than 60% of Americans are now overweight or obese. Health problems from excess body fatness are a major concern. Obesity is a risk factor for many chronic diseases, including heart disease, cancer, hypertension, and diabetes. Surveys show that nearly half of all American women and one third of men are trying to slim down. Weight management is an annual multibillion-dollar business (ADA 1997; ACSM 2001).

Losing weight permanently is difficult. Studies show that 95% of all dieters regain their lost weight and go on to add more pounds. However, lessons can be learned from those who have been successful. Their successes prove that anyone can lose weight.

A *Consumer Reports* (2002) survey of more than 32,000 dieters on long-term weight-loss maintenance found that ordinary people can be successful without using expensive commercial diet programs, special foods, dietary supplements, or drugs. Long-term weight loss is a result of lifetime healthful living.

Most successful long-term dieters chose walking, and a sizable number added weight lifting. They also consumed lean protein with judicious amounts of healthful fats.

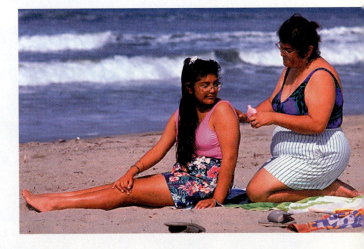

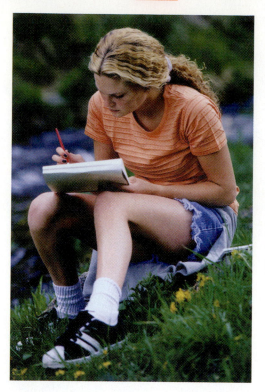

## Where to Begin?

- Complete the body composition assessments in Lab 7-1. Take your photo in tight-fitting clothes. Attach a date to it. Keep this on hand as motivation.
- Set a realistic weight-loss goal. Most experts say it is reasonable to lose half a pound to 2 pounds per week. Some people lose more; some lose less. You have to burn 3500 calories more than you consume to lose 1 pound.

Studies show that dieters lose about 10% of their starting weight in the first 3 to 6 months (ACSM 2001; NHLBI 1998). For those who weigh 200 pounds, that is about 20 pounds.

- Keep a food diary. Write down what you ate, how much you ate, when you ate, and whether you think you were overeating. Dieters who keep a daily food record usually lose more weight.

## Exercise

- Increasing exercise while eating the same number of calories is not very effective for losing weight in the short term. To lose even a small amount of weight just by exercising, you have to exercise a lot. For example, to burn 1 pound of fat, you have to briskly walk or run 35 miles.
- The National Academies' Institute of Medicine's activity guideline (2002) says that, although health benefits are achieved from 30 minutes of activities, it takes 1 hour or more to prevent weight gain. Sedentary individuals can meet this goal by using moderate-intensity activity (e.g., walking at 4 miles per hour) for a total of 60 minutes on most days of the week, or engaging in a high-intensity activity (e.g., jogging, running) for 20 to 30 minutes 4 to 7 days per week.
- While vigorous exercise uses calories at a higher rate, any physical activity burns calories. For example, a 140-pound person can burn 175 calories in 30 minutes of moderate bicycling, and 322 calories in 30 minutes of moderate jogging. The same person can also burn 105 calories by vacuuming or raking leaves for the same amount of time.
- Evidence clearly shows the need for activity in a weight-reduction program. Dieting can lead to weight loss, but the loss accompanies a greater loss of protein (lean tissue) and water. When lean tissue is lost, the body becomes less able to burn calories and more fat weight is eventually gained.

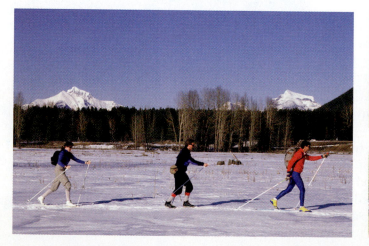

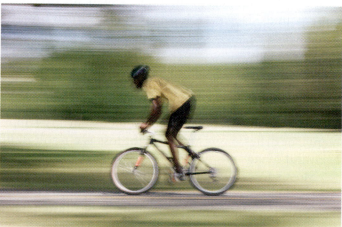

- Studies show that weight loss with exercise maximizes the removal of fat, minimizes the loss of protein, and helps maintain the metabolic rate. Dieting alone is seldom effective over the long term. Most weight-loss diets fail and the person has more weight and fat than before the dieting began.

Certain cautions should be taken by overweight and obese persons during exercising:

- For maximum benefit and minimum risk, choose low- to moderate-intensity activities.
- Ease into an exercise program. Increase the duration and frequency of exercise before increasing the intensity.
- Include strength training to build or maintain lean muscle.

**The Inside Track**

**Use a Step Counter**

For several years, researchers and public-health officials have encouraged people to walk at least 10,000 steps per day, which is roughly 5 miles. Children should be moving even more. But most Americans take an average of 5300 steps in a day.

Those who are overweight tend to walk 1500 to 2000 steps per day fewer than those who are not overweight. Moving 2000 steps per day, which is about 1 mile and should take about 15 to 20 minutes, burns 100 calories (depending on your height) (NHLBI 1998; Hill et al. 2004).

## Eat Fewer Calories

Your diet should be low in calories, but not too low (e.g., less than 800 kcal/day). Diets lower than 800 kcal/day have been found to be no more effective than low-calorie diets in producing weight loss.

To lose weight, try to eat 300 to 500 fewer calories than you need and to exercise 30 to 60 minutes on most days of the week. **Table 7.4** is a general guide to the number of calories you might want to consume if you are trying to lose 0.5 to 2 pounds per week.

| Table 7.4 | Guide for Losing Weight |
| --- | --- |
| **Starting Weight (in pounds)** | **Number of Daily Calories** |
| <180 | 1500 |
| 180–215 | 1600 |
| 216–250 | 1800 |
| 250> | 2000 |

## Cut Back on Sugars (Carbohydrates)

The body's use of carbohydrates seems to be the key to weight mangement. Eating foods that make your blood-sugar and insulin levels shoot up and then crash may contribute to weight gain. Such foods include white bread, white rice, other highly processed grain products, and potatoes. As an alternative, choose foods that have a gentler effect on blood sugar (refer to the discussion of glycemic load in Chapter 6 for more information). These include whole grains such as whole-grain breads and pasta, oats, as well as beans, nuts, fruits, and vegetables.

## Eat Lean Protein

Eating lean protein includes reduced-fat dairy products, egg whites, fish, chicken, and lean cuts of beef and pork. Adding protein to the diet slows the absorption of food—blood sugar will rise more slowly. You will not be as hungry.

Eating more protein and fewer carbohydrates has become a popular dieting approach. The long-term effects of eating this way on weight and overall health need further study. Such a diet might cause kidney damage in some people and rob bones of calcium. Avoid protein containing saturated and trans fats.

## Eat Fruits and Vegetables

Fruits and vegetables are clearly an important part of a good diet. Almost everyone can benefit from eating more of them. They also provide fiber. Some experts recommend at least nine servings per day rather than the often-recommended five servings. Choose a variety that includes dark-green, leafy vegetables; yellow, orange, and red fruits and vegetables; cooked tomatoes; and citrus fruits. Try to avoid fruit drinks because they are high in calories.

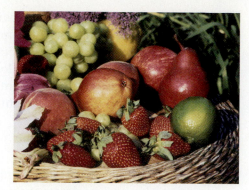

## Eat High-Fiber Grains and Legumes

This type of eating includes oatmeal, brown rice, whole-wheat bread, and lentils. You can trick your stomach into feeling full before you have eaten too many calories. Examples of foods with the lowest energy density include water-rich fruits and vegetables, whole grains, and lean meats.

## Include Small Amounts of Healthful Fats

Examples of healthful fats are olive oil, avocadoes, nuts, olives, and fatty fish (e.g., salmon). Fat in a meal or in snacks such as nuts helps you feel full. Actually, eating certain healthful kinds of fats—mono- and polyunsaturated vegetable oils, nuts, and fish oil—seems to protect people against heart disease. Once again, avoid saturated and trans fats.

## Other Strategies

Avoid overeating by using these tactics:

- Limit or avoid desserts—anything with simple sugars and/or refined carbohydrates, because they are all calories and not much nutrition.
- Eat slowly; eat at regular times; enjoy your food.
- Eat smaller portions; use small plates and bowls.
- Keep a food log—know how many calories you are eating.
- Eat a healthy snack before mealtime to curb your appetite.
- Stop eating before you feel full; you do not have to eat everything.
- Keep tempting food out of sight.

## Weight-Loss Options to Avoid

### Using a Diet Book

Be wary of diet books, especially those recommending a single food, such as grapefruit or cabbage, or an imbalance of foods. The problem with following a special diet of the kind usually found in popular diet books is that it is difficult to stay with it. Once you backslide, you regain weight, and that can be really discouraging.

It is better to permanently change the way you eat, with balance and good sense. That is the kind of diet you are most likely to stay with, and be happy about your success.

### Diet Supplements

Diet supplements are the new snake oil. They promise the easy way out, but cannot guarantee success. In fact, they are sold as supplements precisely so that they can steer clear of government regulation, and some are unsafe.

Can you live the rest of your life on a diet drink? Not likely. To get a quick weight loss (mainly muscle mass), you are substituting a diet supplement for the range of nutrients you need and can get from a healthy, balanced diet.

There is no good shortcut to healthy and sustainable weight loss.

## Medical Help

If you are obese and need professional help, a hospital- or clinic-based program may be your best approach. There you will be put on a medically supervised and closely monitored diet designed to get you back to a healthy weight.

## Prescription Drugs

There are prescription drugs available that can help people lose weight. Only two of them are approved by the FDA: one to suppress appetite, and the other to block fat absorption in the small intestine. However, they are not intended to be taken for a lifetime. You'll still need to learn a positive way to eat!

Other drugs, such as those that increase the metabolic rate, are not recommended and may even be unsafe: Some weight-loss drugs have been found to cause potentially fatal heart problems. Even if safe, it is not a good idea to depend on drugs alone. Proper diet and exercise are still the real answer.

## Surgery

A growing number of people who find it impossible to change their eating and non-exercise habits have turned to surgery to change their bodies. The very obese who cannot control their appetites are often candidates. Due to the frequency and significance of complications, surgical approaches to weight control should be considered only as a last resort for the obese.

A popular but potentially risky procedure is gastric bypass **Figure 7.10A**. The stomach is divided into two parts, using staples, and one part is used as a small pouch for digesting food. The patient feels full after eating only a small amount, and cannot eat more without getting sick.

A related surgical technique is resectioning the intestines so that only a small amount of food is digested.

A third method is liposuction, in which subcutaneous fat is suctioned away **Figure 7.10B**. It is intended for body reshaping, not weight loss.

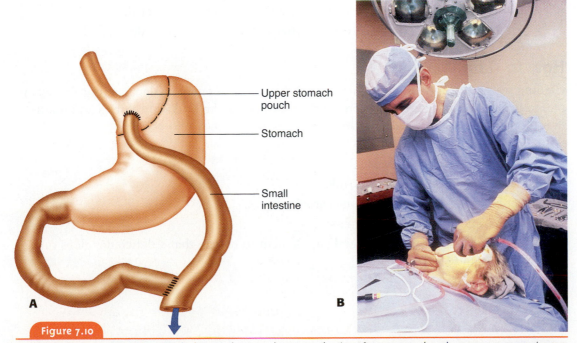

**Figure 7.10**

**A.** Gastric bypass surgery is a surgical procedure used to treat obesity. After surgery, the obese person experiences discomfort after overeating and is less likely to overeat. **B.** Liposuction has gained popularity in recent years.

# Health Risks of Too Little Body Mass

Dieting (or more simply, a change in your eating habits) should be combined with exercise to balance the intake and output of calories.

Another major reason to include exercise with dieting or controlled eating is to preserve and build lean body mass, essential for good health. Dieting alone to lose weight often results in unhealthy loss of lean body mass. Weight loss with exercise maximizes the removal of fat, minimizes the loss of protein, and helps maintain the metabolic rate.

It is easier to reduce caloric intake (refusing to eat a piece of cake with 250 calories) than it is to burn off the calories (jogging more than 2 miles at 110 calories per mile). Dieting alone uses deprivation to achieve weight loss, but with a greater loss of protein (lean tissue) and water. The body becomes less able to burn calories and more fat is eventually gained.

Dieting alone is seldom effective over the long term. Most weight-loss diets fail and the person ends up with more weight and fat than before dieting began.

## Underweight

**What's the word...**

**underweight** A BMI less than 19.

**eating disorder** A spectrum of abnormal eating patterns that eventually may endanger a person's health or increase the risk for other diseases. Generally, psychological factors play a key role.

Underweight is not as common as overweight. When being underweight is part of one's genetic make up, and diet and other health behaviors are fine, the health risk is not a problem.

If the cause is not hereditary, and underweight is the result of undernutrition, deficits in protein and other energy-producing nutrients can cause disorders such as fatigue, reproduction problems in women, and susceptibility to disease.

## Causes of Underweight

- Hereditary and metabolic factors
- Prolonged psychological and emotional stress
- Addiction to alcohol and illicit drugs
- Inadequate or bizarre diets
- Eating disorders, compulsive dieting, and compulsive overexercising
- An underlying disease (e.g., cancer) (Insel, Turner, and Ross 2002)

## How to Gain Weight

Gaining weight can be difficult, but the basic concepts of energy balance apply. For example, to gain 1 pound, you must increase daily caloric intake by 3500 calories and maintain the same amount of activity.

- Eat small frequent meals.
- Eat snacks between meals.
- Eat high-calorie foods and drinks.
- Eat extra servings of nutritious carbohydrates.
- Exercise to increase muscle mass.
- Use a balanced vitamin/mineral supplement to ensure that a deficiency does not contribute to poor appetite.

# Eating Disorders

Eating disorders are a severe psychological response to body image issues. They occur mainly among high-achievement–oriented girls and young women **Figure 7.11**.

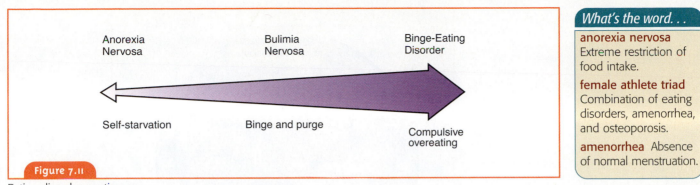

Anorexia          Bulimia          Binge-Eating
Nervosa          Nervosa          Disorder

Self-starvation          Binge and purge          Compulsive
                                                  overeating

**What's the word...**

**anorexia nervosa**
Extreme restriction of food intake.

**female athlete triad**
Combination of eating disorders, amenorrhea, and osteoporosis.

**amenorrhea** Absence of normal menstruation.

**Figure 7.11**

Eating disorder continuum.

Affected individuals see themselves as overweight even though they are dangerously thin. Unusual eating habits develop: avoiding food and meals, and picking out a few foods and eating these in small quantities.

## Anorexia Nervosa

Anorexia nervosa is an obsession for thinness manifested in self-imposed starvation. Those suffering from anorexia nervosa develop emaciated bodies. This condition can be fatal if left untreated. Also, about 25% of anorexics exercise compulsively to stay lean **Figure 7.12**.

Related to anorexia is female athlete triad, an increasingly common condition among female athletes **Figure 7.13**. The symptoms and results include amenorrhea and osteoporosis.

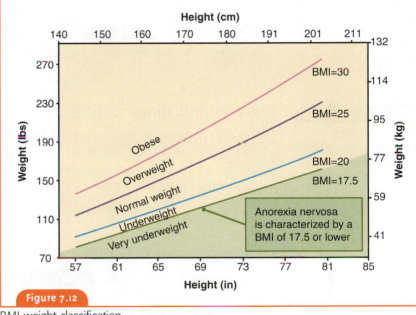

**Figure 7.12**

BMI weight classification.

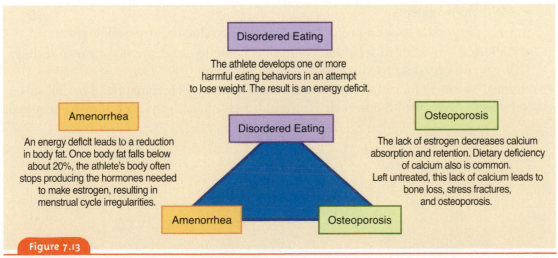

**Disordered Eating**

The athlete develops one or more harmful eating behaviors in an attempt to lose weight. The result is an energy deficit.

**Amenorrhea**

An energy deficit leads to a reduction in body fat. Once body fat falls below about 20%, the athlete's body often stops producing the hormones needed to make estrogen, resulting in menstrual cycle irregularities.

**Osteoporosis**

The lack of estrogen decreases calcium absorption and retention. Dietary deficiency of calcium also is common. Left untreated, this lack of calcium leads to bone loss, stress fractures, and osteoporosis.

**Disordered Eating**

**Amenorrhea**          **Osteoporosis**

**Figure 7.13**

Stress fractures are a red flag for female athlete triad.

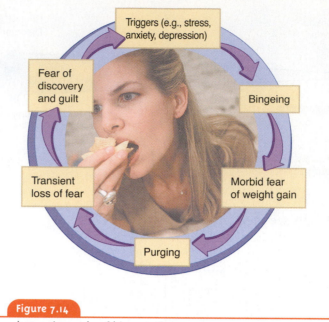

**Figure 7.14**

The destructive cycle of binge eating.

## Bulimia and Binge Eating

Bulimia and binge eating are often done by people who are depressed and impulsive, usually when they are angry, sad, bored, or worried **Figure 7.14**. In both of these conditions, people eat more food than is typically eaten.

Bulimics binge by periodically eating large amounts of food, then purge by forced vomiting or use of laxatives. Another method is bingeing one day and starving the next day.

## Treating Eating Disorders

Serious eating disorders (see **Table 7.5** ), such as anorexia and bulimia, are very difficult to treat successfully. People with eating disorders deny them and are secretive about them. If you are a friend or family member who wants to help, here is where to start:

- Tell the person you are concerned about their weight loss.
- Encourage the person to discuss with you any problems or anxieties.
- Make no judgments.
- Urge the person to see a professional—counselor, doctor, or psychologist.
- Talk to a counselor to see if intervention is possible—and about your own feelings, if you are very distressed yourself over the situation.

Professional treatment for eating disorders is a must. Usually a combination of overall supervision by a physician, medication such as an antidepressant, and psychotherapy are required.

Reward yourself when you have reached a body change goal. Tangible rewards may include going to a movie you want to see or buying a favorite music CD. Intangible rewards may include taking an afternoon off from work or school.

Numerous small rewards, given to yourself for meeting small goals, are more effective in motivating yourself than bigger rewards that require a longer, more difficult effort.

| Table 7.5 | Eating Disorders | | |
|-----------|-------------|---------------------|-----------|
| | **Characteristics** | **Related Health Issues** | **Treatment** |
| Anorexia | Intense fear of weight gain<br>Strict dietary restriction<br>Significant weight loss<br>Possible excessive exercise | Slow the heart rate<br>Lower blood pressure<br>Increasing risk of heart failure<br>Starvation<br>Damage to the brain<br>Hair and nails grow brittle<br>Skin may dry out, become yellow<br>Develop covering of soft hair<br>Anemia<br>Swollen joints<br>Reduced muscle mass<br>Light-headedness<br>Brittle bones | Restoring weight lost<br>Treating psychological disturbances such as distortion of body image, low self-esteem, and interpersonal conflicts<br>Achieving long-term remission and rehabilitation |
| Bulimia | Intense fear of weight gain<br>Consumption of large quantity of calories in single episode (binge)<br>Consumption followed by elimination of food from body (purge)<br>Guilt and shame associated with behavior | Acid in vomit can wear down the outer layer of the teeth<br>Inflame and damage the glands near the cheeks<br>Damage to the stomach<br>Irregular heartbeat<br>Heart failure<br>Chemical imbalances<br>Peptic ulcers<br>Pancreatitis<br>Long-term constipation | Reduce or eliminate binge eating and purging behavior<br>Nutritional rehabilitation<br>Psychosocial intervention<br>Establish a pattern of regular, non-binge meals<br>Improvement of attitudes related to the eating disorder<br>Encouragement of healthy exercise<br>Resolution of mood or anxiety disorders |
| Binge eating | Frequent compulsive overeating<br>No purge cycle<br>Eating occurs whether hungry or full<br>Guilt and shame associated with behavior | High blood pressure<br>High cholesterol level<br>Fatigue<br>Joint pain<br>Type 2 diabetes<br>Gallbladder disease<br>Heart disease | Similar to bulimia<br>Research is under way to study the effectiveness of different interventions |

*Source:* National Institute of Mental Health. Eating disorders: Facts about eating disorders and the search for solutions. 2001. www.nimh.nih.gov.

# Reflect ▸▸▸▸ Reinforce ▸▸▸▸ Reinvigorate

## Knowledge Check

*Answers in Appendix D*

1. Body composition consists of:

   A. Fat, muscle, bone, and other body tissues

   B. Storage fat

   C. Essential fat and muscle mass only

2. The risk of chronic disease rises when your body fat:

   A. Is found only in your legs

   B. Exceeds 12% (men) and 20% (women)

   C. Exceeds 25% (men) and 30% (women)

3. You are healthy only if:

   A. You are a bodybuilder whose weight matches your height on a standard chart

   B. Your body shape matches the ideal

   C. You have the right amount of body fat and lean body mass

**Scenario One:** During Megan's first year in college she gained 12 pounds. Because she didn't like the cafeteria food in her dorm, she ate one or more meals at various fast-food restaurants each day. Moreover, her college did not require a physical education class, so her physical activity involved walking to classes and little else.

4. Which is the most practical method for Megan to assess her *body weight*?

   A. Body mass index (BMI)

   B. Weight-to-height tables

   C. Underwater weighing

5. Which is the most practical method for Megan to assess her *body fat*?

   A. Underwater weighing

   B. Skinfold measurements

   C. Bioelectrical impedance analysis

**Scenario Two:** Patti has just discovered that her BMI is 27, which means she is considered overweight. She has decided that she will lose the necessary weight to lower her BMI to the healthy score of 23.

6. What is the most effective and healthy way for Patti to lower her BMI score?

   A. Exercising 3 times a week without changing her eating habits

   B. Going on a strict diet with no exercise

   C. Combining regular exercise and a healthy diet

7. How often should Patti be reassessing her body composition?

   A. Every 2 weeks

   B. Every 3 months

   C. Every month

8. When you are trying to lose weight, which of the following is the most effective way to shed unwanted pounds?

   A. Cut out all of the empty calories in your diet (candy, white bread, soda) and be involved in moderate activity (walking for 30 minutes 4 days per week)

   B. Exercise 4 days per week very intensely (30-minute jog) while keeping the same diet

   C. Do more household chores, such as vacuuming, raking, and washing dishes, while maintaining the same diet

9. While reading about the different reasons for weight gain, you learned about three different theories on excessive weight gain. Which theory says that everyone has a set number of fat cells and that when you lose weight you are not decreasing the number of fat cells, but the actual size of the fat cell?

   A. Glandular disorder theory
   B. Set point theory
   C. Fat cell theory

10. Diet books seem to come and go. You see people on talk shows talking about one fad diet or another, and that is exactly what they are: fads. Which of the following reasons is why most of these fad diets do not work?

    A. These diets do not generate the results that they claim they can.
    B. They often involve extreme changes to your lifestyle that are difficult (and possibly unsafe) to maintain.
    C. They don't take into account your caloric intake.

## Modern Modifications

How many times have you vowed to eat better and exercise more? Right. And how long did that effort last? Right again. Is there a way to keep yourself on track to shape up? Yes, there is: Use proven techniques to modify your behavior.

Monitor yourself by observing and recording each aspect of what you do:

- Amount of sedentary time spent per day
- Calories taken in each time you eat something
- Frequency, duration, and intensity of each exercise you do
- Changes in your body shape, composition, and weight as your program progresses

Monitoring is a continuous process of self-motivation. Focus on what matters. Keep records. Use the charts in the lab manual to track your progress.

### Keep a Food Diary

Track your eating habits for the next few days. Record:

- What you eat
- How much you eat
- When you eat: Try to associate it with an event (i.e., 3 PM break between classes)
- Why you eat: Was it lunch time? Were you just hungry? Were you stressed or bored?
- How did you feel after? Satisfied? Still hungry? Guilty?

## Critical Thinking

1. Paul is in his first year at State College. He has gained 17 pounds during the year. Paul carries 17 credit hours, and he works 20 to 25 hours each week. He does not believe he has enough time for exercise. Because of the hectic nature of his schedule and his dislike of residence hall food, Paul eats at least one meal at a fast-food restaurant each day. He has tried two popular magazine diets during the year, but has not kept the weight off. What is the most significant issue Paul faces? What is the most likely explanation for his weight gain? Describe a strategy for Paul to lose and keep off the extra weight. What are the long-term risks facing Paul if he continues this pattern?

**2.** Lateisha has decided to lose some extra body fat. What would be the most reasonable way for Lateisha to track her body fat? Where, in the university community, can she get this procedure done? How often should she have her body fat checked?

## Going Above and Beyond

### Websites

American Obesity Association
*http://www.obesity.org*

American Dietetic Association
*http://www.eatright.org*

Center for Science in the Public Interest
*http://www.cspinet.org*

Centers for Disease Control and Prevention, Obesity and Genetics
*www.cdc.gov/genomics/info/perspectives/obesity.htm*

Fast Food Facts: Interactive Food Finder
*http://www.olen.com/food*

Frontline on Fat
*http://www.pbs.org/wgbh/pages/frontline/shows/fat*

MedlinePlus on Obesity Weight Loss
*http://www.nlm.nih.gov/medlineplus/obesity.html*
*http://www.nlm.nih.gov/medlineplus/weightlossdieting.html*

National Association of Anorexia Nervosa and Associated Disorders (ANAD)
*http://www.anad.org*

National Eating Disorders Association
*http://www.nationaleatingdisorders.org*

National Institutes of Health
*hin.nhlbi.nih.gov/portion/*

Office of Dietary Supplements
*http://dietary_supplements.info.nih.gov*

Shape Up America!
*http://shapeup.org*

USDA Food and Nutrition Information Center
*http://www.nal.usda.gov/fnic*

Weight Control Information Network
*http://www.pueblo.gsa.gov/cic_text/health/weightloss4life/wtloss.htm*

Weightloss2000
*http://www.weightloss2000.com*

## References and Suggested Readings

ACSM. Position stand: Appropriate intervention strategies for weight loss and prevention of weight regain for adults. *Medicine and Science in Sports and Exercise* 2001; 33:2145–2156.

ADA. Weight management: Position of the American Dietetics Association. *Journal of the American Dietetics Association* 1997; 97:71–74.

Anderson R. E. Exercise, active lifestyle, and obesity: Making an exercise prescription work. *Physician and Sports Medicine* 1999; 27:41–50.

Foreyt J. P. An etiological approach to obesity. *Hospital Practice,* August 15, 1997: 123–148.

Hill J. O., et al. *The Step Diet Book.* New York: Workman Publishing Company, 2004.

Insel P., Turner R. E., and Ross D. *Discovering Nutrition.* Sudbury, MA: Jones and Bartlett, 2003:268–270.

————. *Nutrition.* Sudbury, MA: Jones and Bartlett, 2002:302–318.

Klem M. L., et al. A descriptive study of individuals successful at long-term maintenance of substantial weight loss. *American Journal of Clinical Nutrition* 1997; 66:239–249.

NCCDPHP. *Defining Overweight and Obesity.* Atlanta, GA: NCCDPHP, 2004. http://www.cdc.gov/nccdphp/dnpa/obesity/defining.htm [October 19, 2004].

————. *Factors Contributing to Obesity.* Atlanta, GA: NCCDPHP, 2001. http://www.cdc.gov/nccdphp/dnpa/obesity/contributing_factors.htm [October 19, 2004].

NCHS. *Prevalence of Overweight and Obesity Among Adults:* United States, 1999–2002. Hyattsville, MD: NCHS, 2004. http://www.cdc.gov/nchs/products/pubs/pubd/hestats/obese/obse99.htm [October 19, 2004].

NHLBI. Clinical guidelines on the identification, evaluation, and treatment of overweight and obesity in adults. NIH Publication No. 98-4083 (1998). http://www.nhlbi.nih.gov/guidelines/obesity/practgde.htm.

Rubinstein S. and Caballero B. Is Miss America an undernourished role model? *Journal of the American Medical Association* 2000; 283:1569.

The truth about dieting. *Consumer Reports* 2002; 67:26–31.

Stevens J., et al. The effect of age on the association between body-mass index and mortality. *New England Journal of Medicine* 1998; 338:1–7.

Wickelgren I. Obesity: How big a problem? *Science* 1998; 280:1364–1376.

Willett W. C. *Eat, Drink, and Be Healthy.* New York: Fireside, 2001:36–55.

————. Guidelines for healthy weight. *New England Journal of Medicine* 1999; 341:427–434.

————. Is dietary fat a major determinant of body fat? *American Journal of Clinical Nutrition* 1998; 76(suppl):556s–562s.

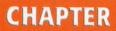

## CHAPTER 8

# Managing Stress

### Objectives

After reading this chapter, you should be able to:

- Explain stress, distress, and eustress.
- Identify common symptoms of stress.
- Describe common sources of stress.
- Describe strategies useful in coping with stress.

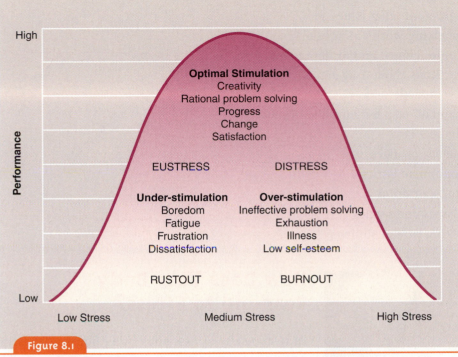

**Figure 8.1**

The stress continuum showing the effects of stress on performance.

# What Is Stress?

Demands on your body that cause stress can be threats or challenges. Good **stress** (**eustress**) helps you perform better. Bad stress (**distress**) upsets you or makes you sick **Figure 8.1** .

You feel distressed if you believe that:

- You have more problems than you can handle.
- You don't feel up to a task.

Exercising until you are exhausted is a physical **stressor**. Taking a tough exam is a mental stressor. Giving an in-class report is a social stressor. Being in a room filled with loud music is an environmental stressor. How you respond to the stressor is known as your **stress response**.

# Stress and College

There is no avoiding it: College students experience significant stress. How many of the following daily hassles are you confronted with? An article in the *College Student Journal* stated that students are more often challenged by daily hassles than by major life events, with the top five sources of stress being changes in sleeping habits, vacations/breaks, changes in eating habits, increased workload, and new responsibilities.

## Sources of Stress in Daily College Life

- Financial aid
- Decisions about sexuality
- Parental expectations

**8**

- Changes in sleep patterns
- Significant other issues
- Balancing work and school
- Homesickness and/or depression
- Decisions about drug and alcohol use
- Test anxiety
- Maintaining a family while in school
- Medical issues
- Dietary changes
- Roommate issues
- Transportation
- Classes and grades
- Taking care of siblings

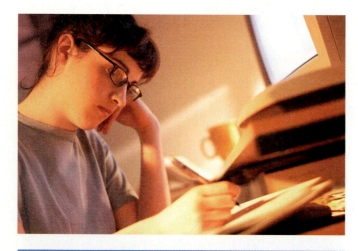

## How Does Your Body Respond to Stress?

In response to stress, your body pours adrenaline, a stimulant hormone, into your bloodstream. The effects are:

- You sweat to cool the extra body heat.
- You hear and see better, to assess the situation and act quickly.
- Your heart speeds up, to get more blood to the muscles, brain, and heart.
- Blood flow increases to your brain, heart, and muscles—most important in dealing with danger.
- Your muscles tense to prepare for action.
- Less blood flows to your skin, digestive tract, kidneys and liver—least needed in times of crisis.
- You breathe faster, to take in more oxygen.
- Your liver dumps extra sugar and fats into your bloodstream for quick energy.
- Platelets and blood-clotting factors rise to prevent hemorrhage in case of injury.
- Your body releases endorphins to mask pain.

**Endorphins** are believed to be a source of "runner's high," an example of eustress.

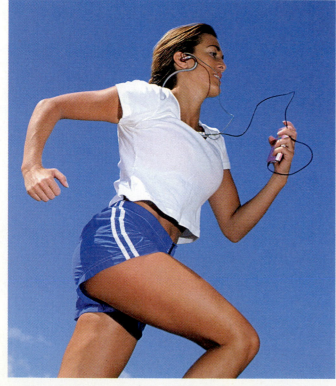

## How Does Your Nervous System React to Stress?

The **sympathetic nervous subsystem** of the **autonomic nervous system** triggers energy output to handle a crisis, including stress. It acts on almost all your organs, including your sweat glands, blood vessels, and muscles.

## How Does Your Endocrine System React to Stress?

The endocrine system releases hormones to control body functions. In response to a stressor, it releases extra hormones from the adrenal gland, giving rise to the stress response.

## What Is the Fight-or-Flight Response?

Adrenaline secreted into the bloodstream prepares the body for quick action during times of stress. The stress response is often called "fight-or-flight" because it gets you ready to take action either by staying and fighting or by running away from danger. Even in situations not requiring a physical response (e.g., being late for an in-class exam, having to stop at three red lights in a row, being unable to find a parking space), the fight-or-flight response may be activated.

## How Do You Return to Normal?

Once you have stopped stressing over something, the parasympathetic subsystem of your autonomic nervous system takes over and calms you down. It takes you back to homeostasis by bringing down your blood pressure, heart rate, and hormone levels; drying your sweaty palms; and slowing your breathing back to a normal pace.

# Personality Types and Stress

Certain kinds of behavior can aggravate the effects of stress. Extreme type-A people are at risk of coronary problems, unless they are able to channel their drive in constructive ways and keep themselves in good physical shape.

Type-B people take things easy, do not respond to pressure or hurry, and do not set deadlines for themselves. They have a secure sense of self-esteem. However, an extreme type-B person may be avoiding life's challenges and as a result may not accomplish much.

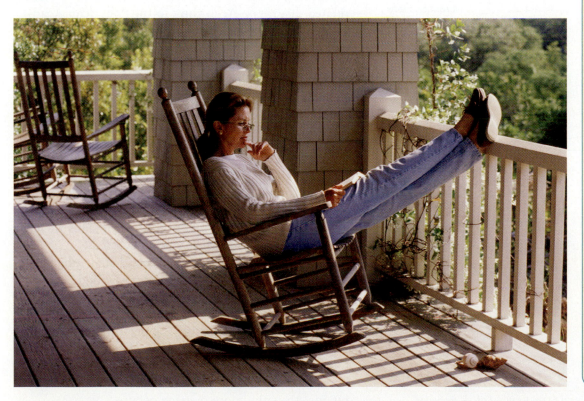

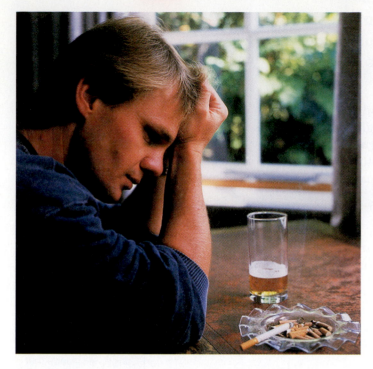

# Ineffective Responses to Stress

## Behavioral Responses

- Pacing and fidgeting, nail-biting, foot-tapping
- Overeating, smoking, drinking too much
- Crying, yelling, swearing, blaming other people and things
- Throwing things or hitting someone

## Mental Responses

- Decreased concentration and memory
- Mind racing or going blank, confusion, indecisiveness
- Loss of sense of humor

## Emotional Responses

- Anger and frustration, short temper, irritability, impatience
- Anxiety, nervousness, worry, fear
- Boredom, general fatigue, depression, low self-esteem

# Stress and Disease

Of all illnesses, 50% to 80% relate to stress. The top-selling drugs in the United States are for stress-related disorders. According to the American Academy of Family Physicians, two thirds of all medical office visits are for stress-related illnesses **Figure 8.2**.

## General Adaptation Syndrome

The general adaptation syndrome to stress (alarm, resistance, exhaustion) was first described by Dr. Hans Selye, a biologist **Figure 8.3**.

In the *alarm* stage, the first stage, the body prepares for quick action. The adrenal glands secrete adrenaline into the bloodstream, which prepares the body to deal physically with the stressor. This stage is where the fight-or-flight reaction occurs.

In the *resistance* stage, the second stage, the body attempts to regain internal balance. The body is no longer in the emergency state but continues to fight off unresolved stress in the individual. Adrenaline is no longer secreted, relieving the person's sense of urgency to respond to the stressor, but other stress related hormones remain present, breaking down the body's ability to fight off disease. The longer one retains stress the more damage occurs.

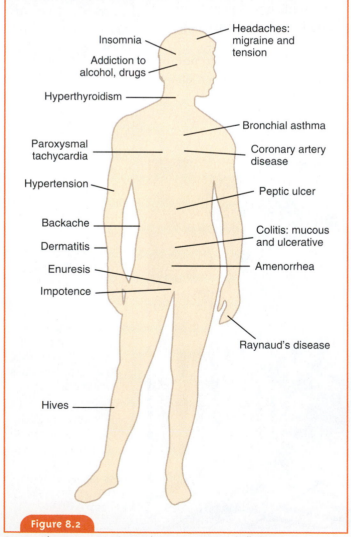

Insomnia

Addiction to alcohol, drugs

Hyperthyroidism

Paroxysmal tachycardia

Hypertension

Backache

Dermatitis

Enuresis

Impotence

Hives

Headaches: migraine and tension

Bronchial asthma

Coronary artery disease

Peptic ulcer

Colitis: mucous and ulcerative

Amenorrhea

Raynaud's disease

**Figure 8.2**

Stress relates to an estimated 50% to 80% of all diseases.

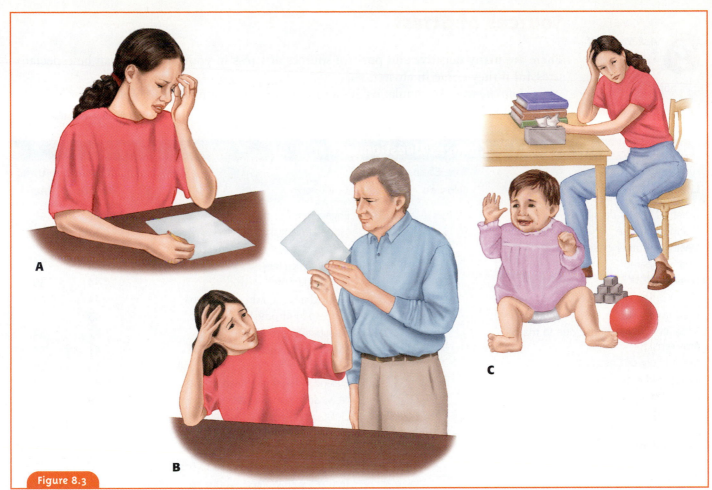

**Figure 8.3**

There are three stages of general adaptation syndrome. (a) In the alarm stage, the body's normal resistance to stress is lowered from the first interaction with the stressor. (b) In the resistance stage, the body adapts to the continued presence of the stressor and resistance increases. (c) In the exhaustion stage, the body loses its ability to resist the stressor any longer and becomes exhausted. The body's defenses are also weakened.

The *exhaustion* stage, the third stage, represents the wearing on the body that increases the risk of illness and premature death. Experts call the long-term wear of the stress response the allostatic load. When you are unable to cope with stress due to the allostatic load, you become more susceptible to illnesses.

## Psychoneuroimmunology

Depending on your body's and mind's ability to cope with stress, you can develop some serious health problems as a result of chronic stress, especially in your circulatory and immune systems:

- High blood pressure and arteriosclerosis leading to stroke or heart attack
- Increased susceptibility to colds, infections, rheumatoid arthritis, cancer, herpes, HIV

Other health problems from poor response to stress can include:

- Rapid or irregular heart rate, chest pains
- Muscle aches or stiffness (especially in neck, shoulders, and low back)
- Temporomandibular joint dysfunction (TMJ)
- Tension or migraine headaches
- Flushing or sweating, trembling, fatigue, cold extremities
- Nausea, abdominal cramps, irritable bowel syndrome, ulcers, and colitis
- Bronchial asthma, allergies, insomnia

### What's the word. . .

**general adaptation syndrome** A series of body changes that result from stress. The syndrome occurs in three stages: alarm, resistance, and exhaustion.

**allostatic load** The ongoing demand on the body from long-term exposure to stress hormones.

**psychoneuroimmunology** Study of nervous, endocrine, and immune systems interaction.

**8**

# Sources of Stress

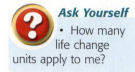

**Ask Yourself**
• How many life change units apply to me?

There are many negative and positive sources of stress in your life. They can be especially stressful if they come in clusters.

■ *Life changes:* Accumulating 300 or more life change units within 6 months or 500 life change units within 1 year shows a high degree of recent life stress  Table 8.1 .

| Table 8.1 | The Recent Life Changes Questionnaire |

| Life Event | Life Change Units | | Life Event | Life Change Units | |
|---|---|---|---|---|---|
| | Women | Men | | Women | Men |
| Death of son or daughter | 135 | 103 | Engagement to marry | 47 | 42 |
| Death of spouse | 122 | 113 | Moderate illness | 47 | 39 |
| Death of brother or sister | 111 | 87 | Loss or damage of personal property | 47 | 35 |
| Death of parent | 105 | 90 | Sexual difficulties | 44 | 44 |
| Divorce | 102 | 85 | Getting demoted at work | 44 | 39 |
| Death of family member | 96 | 78 | Major change in living conditions | 44 | 37 |
| Fired from work | 85 | 69 | Increase in income | 43 | 30 |
| Separation from spouse due to marital problems | 79 | 70 | Relationship problems | 42 | 34 |
| | | | Trouble with in-laws | 41 | 33 |
| Major injury or illness | 79 | 64 | Beginning or ending school or college | 40 | 35 |
| Being held in jail | 78 | 71 | Making a major purchase | 40 | 33 |
| Pregnancy | 74 | 55 | New, close personal relationship | 39 | 34 |
| Miscarriage or abortion | 74 | 51 | Outstanding personal achievement | 38 | 33 |
| Death of a close friend | 73 | 64 | Troubles with co-workers at work | 37 | 32 |
| Laid off from work | 73 | 59 | Change in school or college | 37 | 31 |
| Birth of a child | 71 | 56 | Change in your work hours or conditions | 36 | 32 |
| Adopting a child | 71 | 54 | Troubles with workers whom you supervise | 35 | 34 |
| Major business adjustment | 67 | 47 | Getting a transfer at work | 33 | 31 |
| Decrease in income | 66 | 49 | Getting a promotion at work | 33 | 29 |
| Parents' divorce | 63 | 52 | Change in religious beliefs | 31 | 27 |
| A relative moving in with you | 62 | 53 | Christmas | 30 | 25 |
| Foreclosure on a mortgage or a loan | 62 | 51 | Having more responsibilities at work | 29 | 29 |
| Investment and/or credit difficulties | 62 | 46 | Troubles with your boss at work | 29 | 29 |
| Marital reconciliation | 61 | 48 | Major change in usual type or amount of recreation | 29 | 28 |
| Major change in health or behavior of family member | 58 | 50 | General work troubles | 29 | 27 |
| Change in arguments with spouse | 55 | 41 | Change in social activities | 29 | 24 |
| Retirement | 54 | 48 | Major change in eating habits | 29 | 23 |
| Major decision regarding your immediate future | 54 | 46 | Major change in sleeping habits | 28 | 23 |
| | | | Change in family get-togethers | 28 | 20 |
| Separation from spouse due to work | 53 | 54 | Change in personal habits | 27 | 24 |
| An accident | 53 | 38 | Major dental work | 27 | 23 |
| Parental remarriage | 52 | 45 | Change of residence in same town or city | 27 | 21 |
| Change residence to a different town, city, or state | 52 | 39 | Change in political beliefs | 26 | 21 |
| | | | Vacation | 26 | 20 |
| Change to a new type of work | 51 | 50 | Having fewer responsibilities at work | 22 | 21 |
| "Falling out" of a close personal relationship | 50 | 41 | Making a moderate purchase | 22 | 18 |
| Marriage | 50 | 50 | Change in church activities | 21 | 20 |
| Spouse changes work | 50 | 38 | Minor violation of the law | 20 | 19 |
| Child leaving home | 48 | 38 | Correspondence course to help you in your work | 19 | 16 |
| Birth of grandchild | 48 | 34 | | | |

*Source:* Reprinted from *Journal of Psychosomatic Research,* vol. 43, Miller, M.A. and Rahe, R. H., Life changes scaling for the 1990s, 279-292, © 1997, with permission from Elsevier.

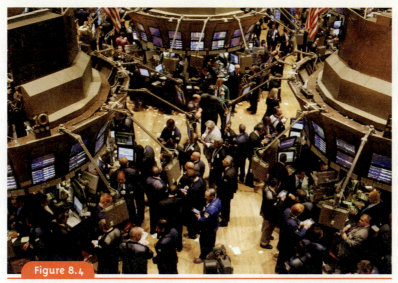

**Figure 8.4**

An extreme example of job-related stress is working on the New York Stock Exchange. So many people have heart attacks there every year that the exchange has installed a defibrillator near the phone banks.

- *Daily hassles:* Commuting, misplacing keys, mechanical breakdowns, money worries, arguments, lousy weather, waiting in long or slow lines, noise, bright lights, heat, violence, confined spaces.

- *College-life stress:* Adjusting to a new locale, making new friends, keeping up with tougher academic work, taking exams, meeting deadlines, too much caffeine, not enough sleep, overloaded schedule, worry about earning money to live on or taking on loans to pay expenses.

- *Job stress:* Rushed by tight schedules and deadlines; too much overtime taking away from personal life; concerns about job performance, job security, or money earned; interactions with co-workers, bosses, or customers; no input on how work is done; dealing with bureaucratic rules and regulations **Figure 8.4**.

- *Social stress:* Changes in relationships with family and old friends, aggressive behavior from others, negative community pressures from ethnic or lifestyle prejudice and discrimination, difficulties in using English as a second language.

- *Negative thought patterns:* Pessimistic thinking, self-criticism, over-analyzing situations and relationships.

- *Personality difficulties:* Unrealistic expectations, taking things too personally, exaggerating, all-or-nothing or rigid thinking.

# Key Strategies for Coping with Stress Effectively

Effective coping strategies are anything that helps change or reduce the stress or the perception of stress.

Of course, if you treat only the symptoms of your stress, you'll simply develop other symptoms. For example, if you get headaches when stressed, and your method of dealing with the stress is to take ibuprofin, you haven't addressed the cause of the stress. Odds are that you'll experience the headaches again. Over time, the continued exposure to unaddressed stress may lead to ulcers, depression, or even some forms of coronary artery disease or cancer.

## Time Management

- Rank tasks in order of importance. (See Lab 8-1, Activity 1 on time ranking.)
- Schedule tasks with a time period for each. Break your day into quarter-hour or half-hour segments. (See Lab 8-1, Activity 2 on scheduling.)
- List your deadlines on a calendar or daily planner so that you can allow time to meet them.
- Delegate. Ask for help. Involve others in doing your low-priority tasks.
- Say "no" if demands seem unreasonable or you do not have time for them.
- Have a place for everything and put everything in its place.
- Schedule personal time each day for exercise, a hobby, meditation, or some other activity that improves your quality of life.
- Watch less television (limit yourself to 1 hour each night).

## Healthy Diet

- Eat a well-balanced diet of milk, whole grains, fruits, vegetables, fish, and poultry; eat slowly; eat less junk food.
- Take in less caffeine (e.g., coffee, tea, colas, too much chocolate). Caffeine generates a stress reaction in the body.
- Avoid "stress-reducing" supplements, such as those containing vitamins and amino acid compounds. They do not help reduce the effects of stress.

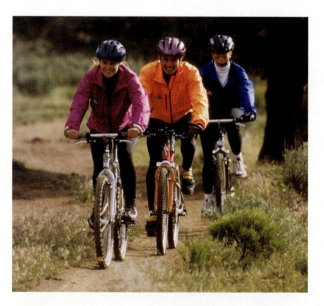

## Exercise

Exercise is a good way to dissipate stress. Get regular exercise (at least 30 minutes, three times per week). Take a brisk walk, a run, or a bike ride.

Cardiovascular exercise flushes stress hormones out of the body. Otherwise, they pool in the body and cause havoc (e.g., cortisol destroys white blood cells). Regular cardiovascular exercise may contribute to an overall sense of relaxation.

Exercise may also combat emotional problems, such as depression, by increasing the level of endorphins, chemicals in the brain that seem to enhance a sense of well-being and relieve anxiety.

## Sleep

Sleep reduces stress. Tired people do not cope well with stressful situations. If you get enough sleep, you feel better and are more resilient and adaptable.

Successful sleep is:
- Waking naturally
- Waking refreshed
- Having plenty of daytime energy

The "power nap" or catnap is short (5 to 20 minutes) and can be rejuvenating. Many people don't get enough sleep, some by choice. But bad things happen when you are sleep deprived:

- You doze off in class.
- You can't focus on an exam.
- You risk serious injury by dozing off while driving or working.

Lack of sleep also adversely affects your health:

- You are at a greater risk of infection.
- You become moody.
- You have problems with memory.

When are you getting enough sleep? When you wake up naturally without an alarm clock and feel alert during the day.

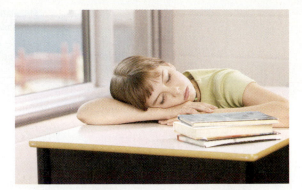

## Social Support

Keep your connections to family and friends strong. When you are feeling stressed, talk to a family member, friend, counselor, school advisor, teacher, or someone else whom you respect and trust. You'll be surprised how much better you feel after talking to someone.

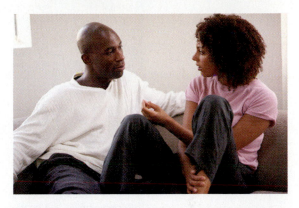

## Healthy Thought Patterns

Attitude is crucial to stress management. In sailing terms, *attitude* is how sails are set to take advantage of prevailing winds. Thus, what we believe determines how we react to stress.

Positive thinking can help you manage stress. If you say to yourself, "I will ace that exam," you are more likely to do well and feel less stressed.

## Communication: Managing Anger

Anger creates physical symptoms similar to stress: faster heartbeat and breathing, muscle tension, flushed face, and trembling. Out-of-control anger is bad for you. It hurts you and your relationships with others.

If you are angry:

- Reframe the situation. Maybe the cause isn't directed at you.
- Distract yourself. Count to 10. Imagine yourself in a peaceful place.
- Analyze the conflict. Listen to the other person's point of view. Negotiate a constructive solution.

If the other person is angry at you:

- Respond calmly.
- Ask why the person is angry.
- Focus on resolving the cause of the anger.
- If all else fails, disengage and try again later.

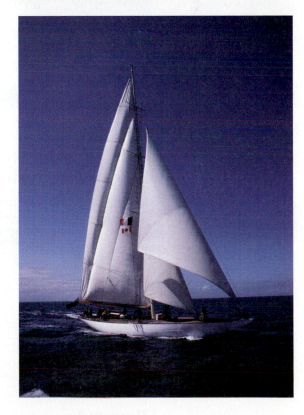

**8**

| Table 8.2 | Defense Mechanisms |

| Defense Mechanism | Positive or Negative? | Definition | Simple Example |
|---|---|---|---|
| Affiliation | Positive | Sharing your feelings of stress, without trying to make others take responsibility for it. | Talking with a close friend about the difficulties you are having with speaking in front of class. |
| Humor | Positive | Finding the humor or irony of a situation. Differs from sarcasm, which is an anger response. | At the end of a day filled with conflict, finding humor in the ridiculous odds that "all those things" could happen in the same day. |
| Denial | Negative | Pretending a stressor is minor or does not exist. | Failing to recognize the possibility one has an alcohol problem after receiving a third DUI citation. |
| Rationalization | Negative | Defending or justifying personal actions and feelings others find unacceptable. | "I only smoke when I drink, so I'm not really a smoker." |
| Splitting | Negative | Categorization of others in one's life; idolizing one group and disenfranchising the other. | After a major argument with all four roommates, ignoring and shutting out those who disagreed with you, while spending all your time with those who did agree. |
| Repression | Negative | Blocking disturbing thoughts or experiences from the conscious mind. | Often used by those having experienced physical, emotional, or sexual abuse as children so the upsetting thoughts are not always present. |

*Source:* Adapted from Levo L. M. Understanding defense mechanisms. *Lukenotes* 2003; 7.

## Defense Mechanisms

Defense mechanisms can be both positive and negative means of coping with stress. Sometimes we are aware that we are using a defense mechanism, and other times we may not be aware. **Table 8.2** describes some of the more common defenses.

# Additional Ways to Manage Stress

## Music

Listening to and creating music has a soothing effect. For most people, music is a popular way to relax. To be fully effective as a relaxation technique, music should be instrumental, without lyrics.

## Time-outs

Take time-outs to get away from the things that are bothering you. This will decrease your stress level.

Time-outs include power naps, meditation, daydreaming, a social conversation, a short walk, a refreshment break, or listening to music.

You have cycles throughout the day, peaks of energy and concentration interspersed with low energy and inefficiency. Watch for periods of low energy and take breaks when they occur.

A mid-morning break, lunch, a mid-afternoon break, and the evening meal divide a day into roughly 2-hour segments.

## Relaxation Exercises

An effective relaxation technique is anything that helps reduce sensory overload by redirecting positive sensations through the five senses. However, just like throwing a football, building with wood, or sewing, it is a skill and must be practiced for an individual to be good at it.

### The Relaxation Response

The relaxation response is your ability to put your body into a state of deep relaxation (Benson 2000). All parts of the stress reaction are reversed: Your pulse slows, your blood pressure falls, your breathing slows, and your muscles relax

**Figure 8.5**.

The stress reaction is automatic. The relaxation response needs to be done deliberately. There are many ways of doing this:

- Sit quietly.
- Breathe from your diaphragm.
- Pet a dog or cat.
- Lie down on something comfortable, like a hammock.

### Progressive Muscular Relaxation

Muscle tension is the most common symptom of stress. All ill people suffer from muscle tension. If you can reduce muscular tension, you become less susceptible to disease.

To combat stress, Edmund Jacobson developed a relaxation technique called progressive muscular relaxation (see Lab 8-2, Activity 1).

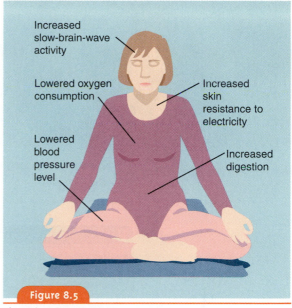

Increased slow-brain-wave activity

Lowered oxygen consumption

Increased skin resistance to electricity

Lowered blood pressure level

Increased digestion

**Figure 8.5**

The relaxation response.

**What's the word. . .**

**relaxation response** Reversal of stress symptoms.

**progressive muscular relaxation** Systematically tensing and relaxing the body's muscles from the feet to the head.

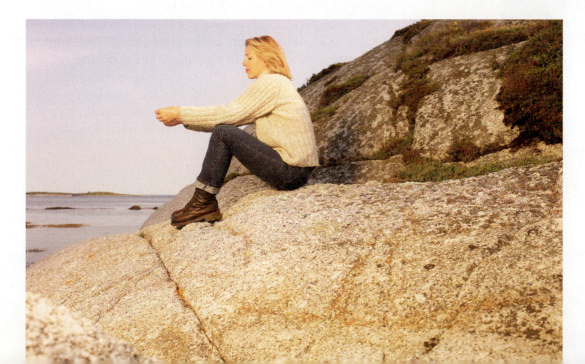

**8**

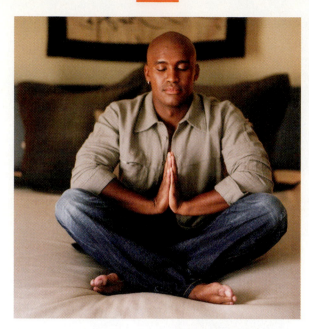

## Meditation

Relaxation achieved through meditation is actually more physiologically restful than sleep. As little as 20 minutes once or twice per day provides significant benefit.

Basic steps (see Lab 8-2, Activity 2 on the relaxation response) are as follows:

1. Find a quiet environment.
2. Take a comfortable position, usually sitting. Consciously relax the body's muscles.
3. Select a mental device (also known as a mantra). Try using the word *one*.
4. Close your eyes and inhale, then exhale. At the end of each exhalation say the mantra word (e.g., *one*) silently to yourself. Do this for 10 to 20 minutes.

### What's the word. . .

**asanas** Various postures used in doing yoga exercises.

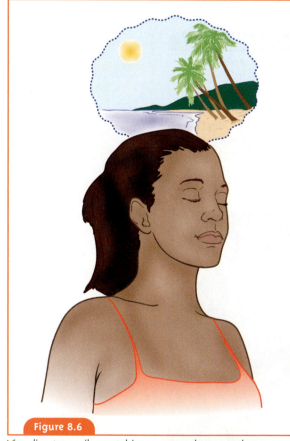

**Figure 8.6**

Visualize tranquil mental images to relax you when you are stressed.

## Mental Imagery

Imagination can produce feelings of relaxation. For example, visualize yourself feeling warm, calm, and relaxed. Picture a tranquil setting that appeals to you and create a mental picture of the details 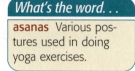.

- Mental imagery is generating images that have a calming, healing effect.
- Visualization is mental imagery consciously directed by yourself.
- In guided mental imagery, images are suggested by another person, either live or on tape.

Mental imagery can be used in a stressful situation (e.g., before making a public speech, at the start of an exam, while waiting in line, while sitting in a dentist's chair, during a meeting).

The technique can also be used to change your habits or improve your performance in various activities. Visualize, or imagine, yourself doing something differently or performing successfully.

## Yoga

Yoga, used since ancient times, can invigorate the body and calm the mind. Various postures, known as asanas, are performed in a specific sequence while breathing in a controlled manner. Yoga should be practiced for 15 to 45 minutes in a quiet place.

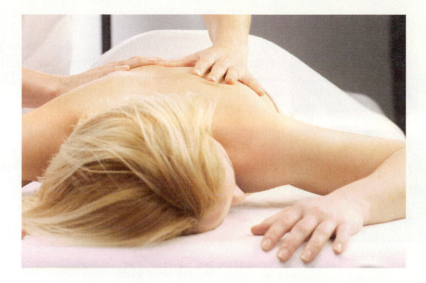

## Massage

Research indicates that human touch is vital for well-being. For example, infants require human touch to thrive. People of all ages need it as well.

All forms of massage tend to be both relaxing and invigorating. Massage requires the assistance of someone else to achieve full benefit.

Hydrotherapy (e.g., baths, hot tubs, jacuzzis, saunas) is another form of muscle massage.

## Pets

Animals can offer more than just friendship; they can decrease stress levels as well. You will often find that hospitals and dentists have aquariums—yes, even fish are capable of lowering our stress levels. The benefits of pet ownership have been studied a great deal. Numerous findings have confirmed that pets lower their owners' blood pressure.

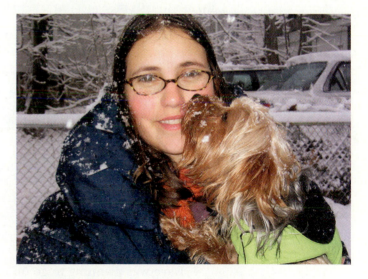

## Sense of Humor

Humor may be the ultimate stress reliever. Studies show that humor promotes mental, emotional, physical, and spiritual well-being.

The author Norman Cousins, suffering from a connective tissue disease, credits his recovery to deliberate efforts to apply humor to his situation.

When you try to find the humorous side of life, you can inoculate yourself against the hazards of stressful perceptions.

The average American laughs 15 times per day. Under stress, laughter drops to zero.

Think of some ways in which you can experience humor to lift your spirits (e.g., listening to a humorous radio program, sharing funny stories, reading cartoons).

## Hobbies

Hobbies promote clear thinking. They can help to take your mind off a problem and divert your attention to something else. When you return to the problem you will be better able to deal with it. Many people find that time spent pursuing hobbies helps generate solutions to life problems.

Hobbies provide pleasure and involve creativity. A hobby can boost self-esteem, which transfers to other areas of life.

## Reflect >>>> Reinforce >>>> Reinvigorate

### Knowledge Check

*Answers in Appendix D*

1. Good stress is called:

   A. Eustress
   B. Distress
   C. Stressful
   D. No stress

2. Which categories are manifest signs of stress?

   A. Physical (e.g., aches, stomach problems)
   B. Emotional (e.g., anxiety, boredom)
   C. Mental (e.g., indecisiveness, confusion)
   D. Behavioral (e.g., drinking, yelling, swearing)
   E. All of the above

3. What are the three stages of the general adaptation syndrome?

   A. Flight, fright, sleep
   B. Confusion, hallucination, procrastination
   C. Alarm, resistance, exhaustion
   D. Anger, criticism, guilt

4. Dave was planning to go on a rafting trip next month, but has just been told that his trip is cancelled. A travel agent recommended by a friend had arranged the trip. An appropriate way for Dave to reduce his stress would be to:

   A. Plan another vacation for the same time period
   B. Spend his vacation at home and read a book about river rafting
   C. Complain to his friend about his recommendation
   D. None of the above

5. Maria has four final exams and only 2 days left to study for them. An appropriate way for Maria to reduce her stress would be to:

   A. Take her mind off her own tests by helping a friend study
   B. Pick the hardest course and spend most of her time studying for that exam
   C. Set up a schedule so that she has some time to study for each test
   D. None of the above

## Prayer

Prayer is one of the oldest and most commonly used methods of coping with life problems. If you are religious, prayer can promote mental and physical health.

A prayer commonly associated with stress seeks divine guidance or divine intervention. Such prayers are used when you need help yourself or when you pray for help to be given to others.

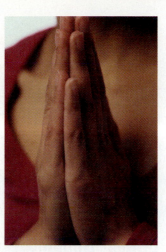

6. Greg lives across from an all-night service station and is disturbed by the traffic noise. An appropriate way for Greg to reduce his stress would be to:

   **A.** Turn up his music to block out the noise
   **B.** Take a sleeping pill to help get to sleep
   **C.** Stay up later so that he can fall asleep more easily
   **D.** None of the above

7. Joyce must speak to a large group of people. She is well prepared to give the speech. However, she keeps remembering another time when she gave a speech and forgot what she was supposed to say. An appropriate way for Joyce to reduce her stress would be to:

   **A.** Set aside some time to sit quietly before the speech
   **B.** Look directly at the audience while she gives her speech
   **C.** Keep her hands busy while she gives the speech
   **D.** None of the above

8. A personality characterized by perfectionism, competitiveness, and a constant sense of urgency is a:

   **A.** Type-A personality
   **B.** Type-B personality
   **C.** Type-C personality
   **D.** Mental illness, not a personality type

9. Secretions from the brain designed to relieve pain are called:

   **A.** Glands
   **B.** Adrenaline
   **C.** Endorphins
   **D.** Homeostasis

10. A type of stress that raises your awareness and excitement level, without causing negative responses is called:

    **A.** Distress
    **B.** Eustress
    **C.** Stressor
    **D.** Allostatic load.

## Modern Modifications

- Take 5 minutes each morning to visualize yourself being successful.
- Go for a brisk walk when you feel yourself becoming stressed during the day.
- Compile a CD with soothing music to listen to when you need to relax.
- Take a yoga class or rent a how-to video.
- Keep track of how many times you laugh in a day. If you are not laughing 15 times by the time you go to bed, try finding more humor in your life!

## Critical Thinking

James is 1 year away from completing his degree. His advisors in the business department tell him his GPA is good, but not great, and that he will have to do an excellent job of selling himself to employers during his senior year. James finds that his sleeping patterns have changed, and he's not as rested as he would like to be. His friends, who are also getting close to graduation, go out often, and James usually accompanies them. Lately, James has been feeling down and has had more colds than normal.

Assess James's stress situation. Develop a list of the stressors he is most likely facing. Are his sources of stress positive or negative? What forms of coping is James using? How can he get himself back on track? If you were James, how would you handle the situation?

## Going Above and Beyond

### Websites

American Institute of Stress
*http://www.stress.org*

American Psychological Association
*http://www.apa.org http://helping.apa.org*

The Humor Project
*http://www.humorproject.com*

National Institute for Occupational Safety and Health (NIOSH)
*http://www.cdc.gov/niosh/stresshp.html*

National Institute of Mental Health
*http://www.nimh.nih.gov*

National Sleep Foundation
*http://www.sleepfoundation.org*

## References and Suggested Readings

Benson H. *The Relaxation Response*. New York: Avon/Wholecare, 2000.

Boscarino J. S. Diseases among men 20 years after exposure to severe stress: Implications for clinical research and medical care. *Psychosomatic Medicine* 1997; 59:605–614.

Clements K. and Turpin G. Life event exposure, physiological reactivity, and psychological strain. *Journal of Behavioral Medicine* 2000; 23:73–94.

Friedman M. and Ulmer D. *Treating Type A Behavior and Your Heart*. New York: Knopf, 1984.

Laitinen J. E., et al. Stress-related eating and drinking behavior and body-mass index and predictors of this behavior. *Preventive Medicine* 2002; 34:29–39.

McKinney C. H., et al. Effects of guided imagery and music (GIM) therapy on mood and cortisol in healthy adults. *Health Psychology* 1997; 16:390–400.

Miller M. A. and Rahe R. H. Life changes scaling for the 1990s. *Journal of Psychosomatic Research* 1997; 43:279–292.

Pashkow F. J. Is stress linked to heart disease? The evidence grows stronger. *Cleveland Clinic Journal of Medicine* 1999; 66:75–77.

Ross S., Niebling B., and Heckert T. Sources of stress among college students. *College Student Journal* 1999.

Scheufele P. M. Effects of progressive relaxation and classical music on measurements of attention, relaxation, and stress responses. *Journal of Behavioral Medicine* 2000; 23:207–228.

Seaward B. L. *Managing Stress: Principles and Strategies for Health and Wellness*, 4th ed. Sudbury, MA: Jones and Bartlett, 2004.

Selye H. *The Stress of Life*, rev. ed. New York: McGraw-Hill, 1978.

Stephens T. Physical activity and mental health in the United States and Canada: Evidence from four population surveys. *Preventive Medicine* 1988; 17:35–47.

Steptoe A. M. and Joekes K. Task demands and the pressures of everyday life: Associations between cardiovascular reactivity and work blood pressure and heart rate. *Healthy Psychology* 2000; 19:46–54.

Williams R. and Williams V. *Anger Kills*. New York: HarperCollins, 1993.

## CHAPTER 9

# Cardiovascular Disease

## Objectives

After reading this chapter, you should be able to:

- Identify the major risk factors associated with cardiovascular disease.
- Differentiate between risk factors that can be changed and those that cannot be changed.
- Describe the major forms of cardiovascular disease.
- Describe healthy approaches for preventing the development of cardiovascular disease.

# Risk Factors for Cardiovascular Disease

There are many influences on the level of risk a person experiences for cardiovascular disease. Some of these influences you have personal control over through the daily choices you make and behaviors you exhibit. Other factors are beyond your personal control.

How would you know if you are at risk of developing cardiovascular disease? Know your history. Take the opportunity to discuss that family history with an elder in the family. Is there a history of:

- High blood pressure?
- Stroke?
- Heart attack?
- High cholesterol?
- Diabetes?
- Obesity?

It is also important to take a realistic look at your own personal behavior. Do you:

- Smoke?
- Avoid physical activity?
- Consume a diet high in fat?
- Consume a diet high in calories?
- Have high cholesterol?
- Have high blood pressure?
- Lack fruit in your diet?
- Lack vegetables in your diet?

For each question to which you answered "yes," the risk for developing cardiovascular disease is increased. The best way to learn your health status is to take a trip to your physician or a health center. To be informed you need to have the correct information. To determine your personal risk you should have an accurate measurement of your cholesterol level, blood pressure, and percentage of body fat. Your personal health-care professional can measure these things for you.

**What's the word. . .**
**sedentary** Little or no physical activity.

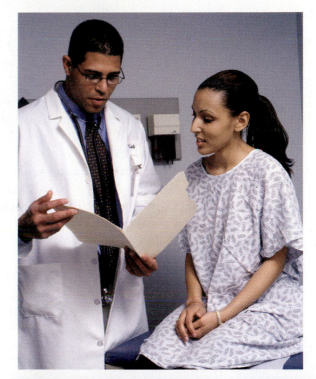

## What Are the Benefits of Knowing?

Having a thorough understanding of your level of risk for cardiovascular disease allows you to take action to become a healthier you! Identifying troublesome behaviors can set the stage for determining how ready you are to make positive changes in your daily life. Those daily changes can then help you to live a longer more satisfying life.

## What Can Be Individually Influenced?

### Sedentary Lifestyle

Sedentary is the term used to describe a lifestyle characterized by little to no physical activity. Finding time to be active is often cited as the reason for the lack of physical activity, particularly in the college environment. Trying to balance classes, homework, a part-time or full-time job, sleep, relationships, and family, while still finding time for yourself, is not always easy.

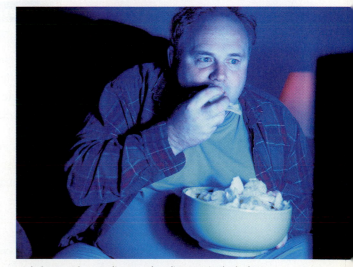

Risk factors for cardiovascular disease include being overweight, a sedentary lifestyle, and excessive alcohol consumption.

And when you do have "self-time," being physically active is not always at the top of the list of choices for things to do. Some suggestions to increase your activity are:

- Set aside 30 minutes each day (or two 15-minute blocks) to walk, work in the yard, stretch your muscles, play catch with a friend, or play with the dog—anything that gets your body moving.
- Limit your television time.
- Structure breaks in your studying, and use that time to be active, even if it means just walking up and down the hallway.
- At least three times each week, make sure your physical activity is intense enough to make you break a sweat for 30 minutes.

Some moderate-intensity activities to work into each day are listed in ( Table 9.1 ).

When choosing an exercise, pick one that's fun and convenient for you.

## Cholesterol

**Cholesterol** is a substance that travels throughout the body's bloodstream. It is necessary for the body to function correctly, particularly in terms of cell maintenance. The body itself makes some cholesterol, and some is added to the body through the consumption of food. Cholesterol comes in two main forms: **low-density lipoprotein (LDL)** and **high-density lipoprotein (HDL)**.

LDL is the more dense form of cholesterol. It promotes the buildup of cholesterol in arteries, causing blockage and damage, called atherosclerosis.

HDL is a protective form of cholesterol ("good" cholesterol) that carries excess LDL to the liver for elimination.

### What's the word...

**cholesterol** Waxy substance floating in the blood. In abundance, it causes heart disease.

**low-density lipoprotein (LDL)** Carrier of harmful cholesterol; "bad" cholesterol.

**high-density lipoprotein (HDL)** Carrier of cholesterol to the liver where it can be removed; "good" cholesterol.

| Table 9.1 | Moderate-Intensity Activities |
| --- | --- |
| **Common Chores** | **Sporting Activities** |
| Washing and waxing a car for 45–60 minutes | Playing volleyball for 45–60 minutes |
| Washing windows or floors for 45–60 minutes | Playing touch football for 45 minutes |
| Gardening for 30–45 minutes | Walking 2 miles in 30 minutes (1 mile in 15 minutes) |
| Wheeling yourself in a wheelchair for 30–40 minutes | Shooting baskets (basketball) for 30 minutes |
| Pushing a stroller 1.5 miles in 30 minutes | Dancing fast (social) for 30 minutes |
| Raking leaves for 30 minutes | Performing water aerobics for 30 minutes |
| Shoveling snow for 15 minutes | Swimming laps for 20 minutes |
| Stair walking for 15 minutes | Playing basketball for 15–20 minutes |
| | Jumping rope for 15 minutes |
| | Running 1.5 miles in 15 minutes (1 mile in 10 minutes) |

*Source:* National Heart, Lung, and Blood Institute, 2004.

What are the recommended levels for the various types of cholesterol?

- Overall cholesterol should stay below 200 milligrams per deciliter (mg/dL).
- LDL levels should stay below 100 mg/dL. An increased risk for heart disease begins when the LDL level exceeds 130 mg/dL.
- HDL should stay above 35 mg/dL to remain a protective force in the body.

## High Blood Pressure

Elevated blood pressure is called hypertension. Blood pressure measures the amount of force the heart is using to move blood throughout the circulatory system. You may recognize a reading such as 120/80 as a blood pressure reading. When blood pressures are elevated, the increase in force may cause damage to arteries over time. This damage can allow for plaque buildup and failure of arteries to function properly.

There are two components in a blood pressure reading:

- Systolic pressure is the amount of force the heart uses on its initial contraction to move blood. It is the first number when referring to blood pressure and is the larger of the two numbers (the 120 in 120/80).
- Diastolic pressure is the measure of force when the contraction of the heart relaxes. It is the second number of the blood pressure measurement and the smaller of the two measurements (the 80 in 120/80).

What are the recommended blood pressure levels?

- The classifications in ( Figure 9.1 ) are for adults who are not taking blood pressure-lowering drugs and are not acutely ill. When a person's systolic and diastolic pressures fall into different categories, the higher category is used to classify the blood pressure status. Diagnosing high blood pressure is based on the average of two or more readings taken on different days.
- Blood pressures of 160/90 are seriously high.

> **What's the word...**
>
> **hypertension** High blood pressure.
>
> **systolic pressure** Higher blood pressure reading; measured when the heart contracts.
>
> **diastolic pressure** Lower blood pressure reading; measured when the heart relaxes between beats.

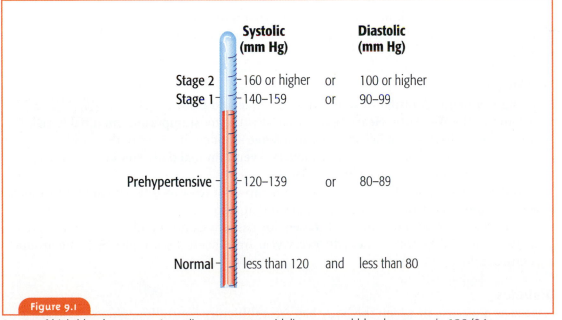

**Figure 9.1**

Stages of high blood pressure. According to current guidelines, normal blood pressure is 129/84 (systolic/diastolic) and high-normal is 139/89. High blood pressure (hypertension) is defined in four stages, with the risk of heart disease being greater the higher the blood pressure. Weight loss, exercise, not smoking, and stress reduction are recommended ways to control hypertension at earlier stages; drugs may also be necessary at later stages. (Adapted from the American Heart Association guidelines on blood pressure.)

**9**

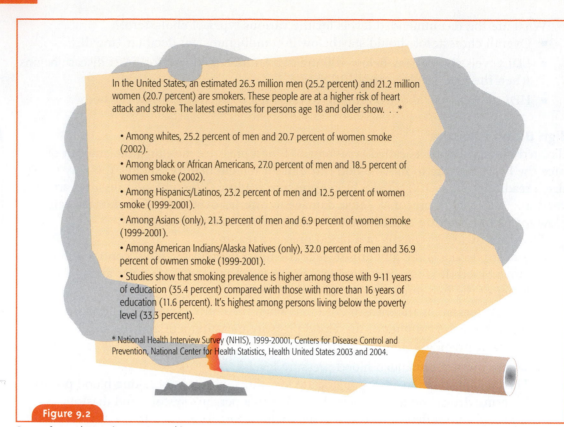

In the United States, an estimated 26.3 million men (25.2 percent) and 21.2 million women (20.7 percent) are smokers. These people are at a higher risk of heart attack and stroke. The latest estimates for persons age 18 and older show. . .*

- Among whites, 25.2 percent of men and 20.7 percent of women smoke (2002).
- Among black or African Americans, 27.0 percent of men and 18.5 percent of women smoke (2002).
- Among Hispanics/Latinos, 23.2 percent of men and 12.5 percent of women smoke (1999-2001).
- Among Asians (only), 21.3 percent of men and 6.9 percent of women smoke (1999-2001).
- Among American Indians/Alaska Natives (only), 32.0 percent of men and 36.9 percent of owmen smoke (1999-2001).
- Studies show that smoking prevalence is higher among those with 9-11 years of education (35.4 percent) compared with those with more than 16 years of education (11.6 percent). It's highest among persons living below the poverty level (33.3 percent).

* National Health Interview Survey (NHIS), 1999-20001, Centers for Disease Control and Prevention, National Center for Health Statistics, Health United States 2003 and 2004.

**Figure 9.2**

Some facts about cigarette smoking.

*Source:* Reproduced with permission. www.americanheart.org. © 2005, American Heart Association.

Individual blood pressures will vary from person to person. A physician should be consulted for dramatic increases or decreases from an individual's regular blood pressure measurement.

### Smoking

Smoking is a major contributor to the risk of stroke and heart attack (see **Figure 9.2**). According to the American Heart Association, it is the most important modifiable risk factor for heart disease. Studies indicate that some smokers have more than a five times greater risk for heart disease than nonsmokers; even minimal daily smoking produces a significantly greater risk (Kawachi et al. 1994).

Don't rationalize smoking. It's easy to come up with reasons to keep smoking—much easier than quitting. Don't let yourself fall into that trap!

Don't smoke around others. The Centers for Disease Control and Prevention (CDC) estimates that 35,000 nonsmokers die every year from heart disease just by being around cigarette smoke.

### Diabetes

**Diabetes** is a disease in which the body has great difficulty controlling glucose (sugar) levels. One form, type 1, begins early in life and requires regular shots of insulin. Type 2 diabetes shows similar symptoms as type 1 but can usually be controlled through lifestyle changes such as increased activity, diet management, and weight control. Most people

**What's the word. . .**

**diabetes** Disease characterized by the body's inability to manage insulin.

with diabetes exhibit other health problems, contributing to the likelihood of the development of heart disease:

- The increased glucose in the blood of diabetics can damage arteries, increasing the likelihood of atherosclerosis development. People with diabetes also have LDL that is more likely to stick to artery walls.

- Individuals with type 2 diabetes are 2.5 times more likely to suffer from heart disease than individuals without this condition (Nichols et al. 2004).

- According to the American Diabetes Association (ADA), people with diabetes are more likely to have low HDL levels and high triglyceride levels, both of which contribute to the increase in risk for heart disease (ADA 2004).

## What Can't Be Changed?

### Heredity

Some people have a genetic likelihood for the development of cardiovascular disease. If you have a first-degree relative (paternal grandparent, maternal grandparent, parent, sibling, or child) who developed heart disease early in life (age 55 in men, 65 in women), then you should screen aggressively for heart disease.

### Age

You can't stop the aging process—and when it comes to heart disease, age matters. The older we get, the more likely we are to have plaque buildup from cholesterol. Age makes it more likely that damage to arteries exists from the accumulation of lifestyle-related habits such as smoking, inactivity, and poor diet.

### Sex

Men are more likely to develop cardiovascular disease when we consider the risk for people in their younger years. Women, however, see a large increase in the incidence of heart disease after menopause. The changes in hormonal makeup—specifically, the reduction in production of estrogen—reduce the efficiency with which women can clean cholesterol out of their bodies.

## Current Studies

One of the most significant outcomes of current research has been the identification of disparities in the treatment of men and the treatment of women for cardiovascular disease. In the past, most of the research that sought to determine effective diagnosis and treatment of cardiovascular disease has been conducted on men. In turn, we've recently learned that women are less likely to receive drug therapy in the first 24 hours of hospital admission for heart-related illness and are less likely to undergo surgical procedures than men. Women are also more likely to die within 2 years of a heart attack than men (11% of women compared to 7% for men). The exact reasons for these differences are still being studied.

A study in the *New England Journal of Medicine* revealed that women younger than age 55 and minorities are more likely to be sent home from the physician's office when reporting shortness of breath as a symptom instead of chest pain. They are twice as likely to die from their heart problems, however, compared to white men.

Black women have been the least likely subgroup to receive clot-dissolving medication or to undergo angioplasty even when they meet the criteria for such a procedure. Black women are also less likely to be referred for cardiac catheterization than other women or men.

*What's the word. . .*

**cardiac catheterization** Passage of a thin, flexible tube into the heart to provide treatment for heart disease.

**9**

Other studies have focused on a variety of factors influencing heart disease:

- *Diabetes:* A study in the United Kingdom published in 2004 confirmed the relationship between blood-sugar levels and cardiovascular disease. The study followed more than 10,000 patients between 45 and 79 years old, some of whom were at risk for developing cardiovascular disease because of diabetes, by tracking their blood-sugar levels. Of the 806 participants who developed heart disease, 521 died. Those with higher blood-sugar levels at the start of the study were more likely to develop heart disease and die. Even those who did not have diabetes but had higher blood-sugar levels were more likely to develop cardiovascular disease and die.

- *Cholesterol:* A Texas study suggested that there may be a better predictor for cardiovascular disease risk than LDL cholesterol. While LDL cholesterol is the type of cholesterol that builds plaque on artery walls, LDL particles come in different sizes. The smaller, denser particles are of greater concern for development of heart disease. The Texas study measured the level of apoB (a smaller, denser form of cholesterol) and found it to be a better predictor of the development of heart disease in patients. The researchers also noted the test's convenience, as it does not require a fasting period as LDL testing does.

- *Stress:* Stress on the heart in the form of higher blood pressure or increased heart rate can be measured by looking for an increase in a stress protein called ST2. Increased levels of this protein in heart cells will most likely not serve as a measurable risk factor for heart attack or assist physicians in predicting a heart attack, but they could be used to predict recovery following a heart attack.

- *Nutrition:* Researchers at Boston University have suggested that black tea may help reduce the risk of heart attack in patients with atherosclerosis. The tea, which possesses antioxidants called flavonoids, helps arterial walls maintain their ability to prevent plaque buildup, keep inflammation down, and prevent blood clots from forming, all of which contribute to heart attack and stroke.

# Major Forms of Cardiovascular Disease

## Atherosclerosis

The form of cardiovascular disease of most concern in the United States is atherosclerosis. Atherosclerosis develops over time in a person who, for a reason such as smoking, has caused some damage to his or her arteries. Cholesterol and fatty deposits can then "catch" in the damaged area **Figure 9.3**. The sticky cholesterol builds on itself, forcing the flow of blood through an increasingly smaller area. Consider what happens when you place your thumb over the end of a garden hose. When it is unobstructed, the water runs smoothly out the hose end. If you block the flow, pressure builds up behind the blockage and the water must work harder to exit, causing it to spray. Likewise, when arteries are obstructed, the heart must work harder to force the blood through the restricted area. The result is increased blood pressure and a less efficient circulatory system.

## Angina Pectoris

Sharp pains in the chest, sometimes resembling a heart attack, are often the first sign of atherosclerosis. This warning from the body is called angina pectoris, and it indicates that the individual has plaque buildup in the arteries. The plaque has restricted the flow of blood. Recall that the blood carries oxygen throughout the body. If the heart does not receive enough oxygen, angina is the result. A person should see a doctor when this condition occurs to determine the significance of the blockage and develop a plan for reducing the amount of plaque built up in the arteries.

---

**What's the word...**

**apoB** A small, dense form of cholesterol.

**ST2** Stress-related protein that may be a predictor of how well an individual will recover from heart attack.

**atherosclerosis** Plaque buildup inside the arteries.

**cardiovascular disease** Series of diseases affecting the heart and blood vessels.

**angina pectoris** Chest pain caused by the early stages of cardiovascular disease.

**heart attack** Damage or death of all or part of the heart due to insufficient blood supply.

**myocardial infarction (MI)** Heart attack.

**angioplasty** Technique used to open arteries blocked by plaque buildup.

**plaque** Artery-blocking deposits impeding blood flow.

**stent** A mesh coil used to open blocked arteries.

**coronary bypass surgery** Procedure used to reroute blood flow around a damaged or blocked artery.

**ischemic stroke** Disruption of blood flow to the brain caused by blockage of an artery (clot).

**blood clot** Blockage that results from coagulation of blood.

## Heart Attack

If the heart continues to receive restricted amounts of blood as a result of arterial blockage, a heart attack can occur. Called a myocardial infarction (MI) in the medical community, a heart attack is often the first sign of the development of atherosclerosis. Approximately 500,000 people have heart attacks each year in the United States (AHA 2003).

Treating a heart attack is a complicated process. Time is of the essence when assisting a person having an MI. Within just a few minutes of the blood flow stoppage, heart muscle begins to die.

Treatment usually takes one of three forms:

- Angioplasty: The insertion of a small balloon into the blocked artery    Figure 9.4   . The balloon is inflated, compressing the plaque to the sides of the artery and reopening it for blood flow. The balloon is then deflated and removed.

- Stenting: A mesh coil inserted into the artery. The coil remains in the artery, moving the plaque aside and keeping the artery open for blood flow.

- Coronary bypass surgery: The removal of the damaged section of the artery and its rerouting with a new piece of artery taken from another area of the body. This procedure avoids the plaque-damaged section of artery, thereby restoring blood flow.

## Stroke

Whereas impeding blood flow to the heart causes a heart attack, impeding blood flow to the brain causes a stroke. The brain cannot survive without oxygen, and permanent damage can occur in very short periods of time without it—less than 5 minutes. During a stroke, blood flow to the brain can be disrupted in two primary ways:

- When blood flow is disrupted by the blockage of an artery, an ischemic stroke occurs. The blockage may consist of plaque or a blood clot formed from damage to an artery in another part of the body. The American Stroke Association states that eight out of nine strokes are caused by arterial blockage.

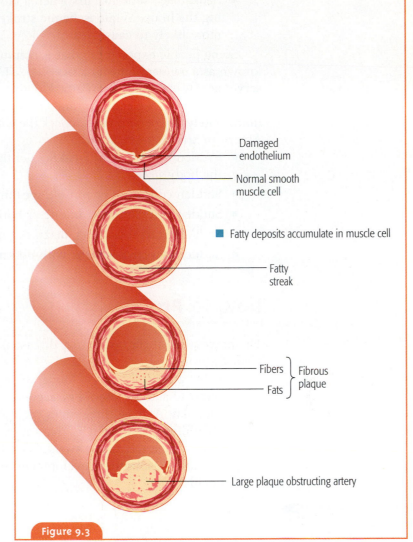

Damaged endothelium

Normal smooth muscle cell

Fatty deposits accumulate in muscle cell

Fatty streak

Fibers
Fats
} Fibrous plaque

Large plaque obstructing artery

**Figure 9.3**

Development of an atherosclerotic lesion (plaque) inside an artery. Plaque can eventually block blood flow, causing a heart attack or stroke. Many factors are suspected in the formation of a plaque, but none has been proven.

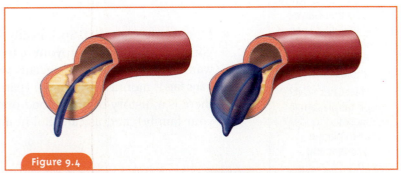

**Figure 9.4**

In balloon angioplasty, a thin tube containing a balloon is threaded through an artery until it reaches the area of plaque that is narrowing the vessel. The balloon is inflated, compressing the plaque against the artery wall and stretching the artery.

■ **Hemorrhagic stroke** occurs when a blood vessel bursts, preventing blood from reaching the brain. While ischemic strokes are more common, hemorrhagic strokes are more likely to cause death.

Some people experience what is commonly called a "mini-stroke," more formally known as a **transient ischemic attack (TIA)**. TIAs are warning signs, much as angina pectoris serves as a warning for heart attack. During a TIA, a blood clot remains in place only briefly, but sends a clear sign that trouble may lie ahead. A physician should be consulted immediately if a person experiences the warning signs of a stroke (as identified by the American Stroke Association):

■ Sudden numbness or weakness of the face, arm, or leg, especially on one side of the body

■ Sudden confusion or trouble speaking or understanding

■ Sudden trouble seeing in one or both eyes

■ Sudden trouble walking, dizziness, or loss of balance or coordination

■ Sudden, severe headache with no known cause

## How to Prevent It?

The prevention of cardiovascular disease is accomplished through:

■ Being physically active. Moderate levels of physical activity should be accomplished each day. At least three times each week, you should engage in activity that raises the heart rate enough to cause a sweat. See Chapter 3 on cardiorespiratory development for more details.

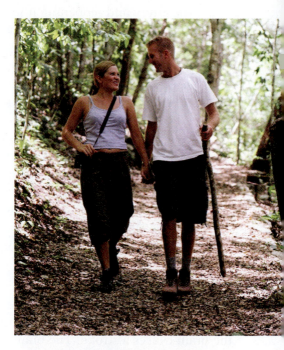

■ Monitoring your diet. Specifically, balance your calorie intake with your activity level, watch your fat intake (especially **saturated** and **trans fats**), monitor salt intake (particularly if there is a history of high blood pressure in your family), and use alcohol in moderation.

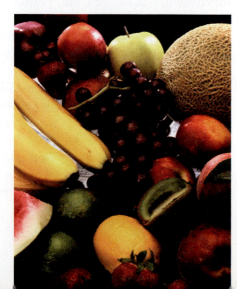

---

**What's the word...**

**hemorrhagic stroke**
Disruption of blood flow to the brain caused by leaking of a blood vessel.

**transient ischemic attack (TIA)** Warning sign of possible stroke.

**saturated fat** Form of fatty acid that has no available carbon bonds; promotes plaque development and high cholesterol.

**trans fat** Chemically derived fat present in hydrogenated foods; promotes plaque development and high cholesterol.

**chronic disease** Disease that takes many years to develop.

- Losing weight when necessary. Use Chapter 7 on weight management as your guide, be patient, and stick with it. The complete elimination of foods tends to make you want them even more, particularly if you eat them frequently, so use troublesome foods sparingly.

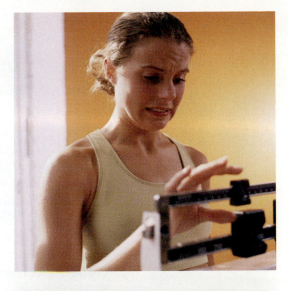

- Not smoking. If you do smoke, consider quitting now. Remember, cardiovascular disease is a chronic disease—it develops over time. What you do now can and will affect you later in life.

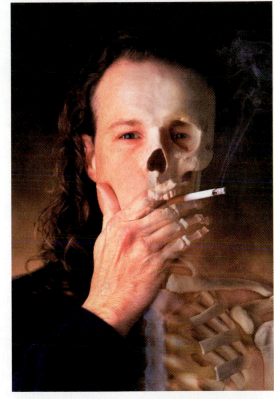

- Having your cholesterol and blood pressure checked by a health professional every few years, especially if you have a family history of heart disease or high blood pressure.

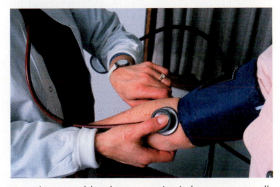

- Living life in a health-conscious fashion. You don't have to be a crusader against fun to have a healthy lifestyle. Be conscious of your choices, and try to make decisions based on what you've learned.

Knowing your blood pressure is vital to your overall health and well-being.

# Reflect ›››› Reinforce ›››› Reinvigorate

## Knowledge Check

*Answers in Appendix D*

1. Atherosclerosis is:

    A. A new method for cholesterol reduction
    B. The development of cholesterol buildup in arteries
    C. A procedure used to clean arteries
    D. A disorder caused by oxygen loss to the brain

2. Which of the following is a risk factor for developing heart disease?

    A. Participating in physical activity only occasionally
    B. Having a body mass index over 30
    C. Having a cholesterol level over 240 mg/dL
    D. All of the above

3. Which of the following is the level warranting a diagnosis of high blood pressure?

    A. 120/80
    B. 130/85
    C. 140/90
    D. 160/95

4. Which of the following is the upper limit for cholesterol before the risk of heart disease begins to increase?

    A. 180 mg/dL
    B. 200 mg/dL
    C. 240 mg/dL
    D. 275 mg/dL

5. At what age is an individual most likely to begin smoking?

    A. Younger than 18
    B. 20–25
    C. 25–44
    D. 44–65

6. Increasing metabolism and raising the level of high-density lipoproteins is a result of what behavior?

    A. Reducing calorie intake
    B. Being physically active
    C. Lowering blood pressure
    D. Losing weight

7. When blood flow to the brain is disrupted, a(n) _____ occurs.

    A. Heart attack
    B. Coma
    C. Angina
    D. Stroke

8. Approximately how many Americans suffer heart attacks each year?

   A. 100,000
   B. 250,000
   C. 500,000
   D. 1,000,000

9. Which of the following is *not* a method for treating heart attack?

   A. Stenting
   B. Coronary bypass surgery
   C. Angioplasty
   D. None of the above

10. Which of the following is the single greatest influence on lowering risk for development of cardiovascular disease?

   A. Reducing fat intake
   B. Lowering blood pressure
   C. Lowering resting heart rate
   D. Increasing physical activity level

## Modern Modifications

- Choose low-fat versions of foods you like to munch.
- Try walking when you can, and stay out of the elevator and off the escalator.
- Talk to your family about your health history.
- Get a physical examination.
- Make a personal contract.
- Quit smoking.

## Critical Thinking

Alfonse is a 27-year-old male. He is 5 feet 7 inches tall and weighs 235 pounds. He has had heart problems for several years and has shown signs of the development of type 2 diabetes. His doctors have repeatedly told him to lose weight, but have yet to offer a plan or suggest a location for Alfonse to visit for assistance. Alfonse would like to lose weight and become healthier, but has failed on diets many times, and has given up trying to lose the weight.

1. What stage of change is Alfonse in?
2. What methods would you suggest to move Alfonse to the next stage?
3. Where does the responsibility lie for Alfonse's failure to lose weight? Alfonse? His physician? Societal influences? A combination?
4. Based on your answers to questions 2 and 3, what is a reasonable next step for Alfonse to take?

## Going Above and Beyond

### Websites

American Diabetes Association
*www.diabetes.org*

American Heart Association
*www.americanheart.org*

American Stroke Association
*www.strokeassociation.org*

Centers for Disease Control and Prevention
*www.cdc.gov*

National Heart, Lung, and Blood Institute
*www.nhlbi.nih.gov*

## References and Suggested Readings

American Diabetes Association. Diabetes, cholesterol, and heart disease. http://www.diabetes.org/diabetes-cholesterol.jsp [accessed October 5, 2004].

American Heart Association (AHA). Heart disease and stroke statistics—2003 update. 2003.

——. Recent discoveries supported by the AHA. http://www.americanheart.org/presenter.jhtml?identifier=242 [accessed October 21, 2004].

Edlin G. and Golanty E. *Health and Wellness*, 8th ed. Sudbury, MA: Jones and Bartlett, 2004.

Kawachi I., Sparrow D., Vokonas P., and Weiss S. Symptoms of anxiety and risk of coronary heart disease: The normative aging study. *Circulation* 1994; 90:2225–2229.

Khaw T., Wareman N., Bingham S., Luben R., Welch A., and Day N. Association of hemoglobin A1c with cardiovascular disease and mortality in adults: The European prospective investigation into cancer in Norfolk. *Annals of Internal Medicine* 2004; 141:413–420.

McCormack Brown K., Thomas D. Q., and Kotecki J. E. *Physical Activity and Health*. Sudbury, MA: Jones and Bartlett, 2002.

Nichols G. A., Gullion C. M., Koro C. E., Ephross S. A., and Brown J. B. The incidence of congestive heart failure in type 2 diabetes. *Diabetes Care* 2004; 27:1879–1884.

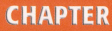
# Preventing Cancer

### Objectives

After reading this chapter, you should be able to:

- Describe the process by which cancer develops in the body.
- Identify the major forms of cancer.
- Explain the causes of and preventive measures related to cancer.

# Defining Cancer

**Cancer** is not a "single" disease. Rather, this term is used to describe a collection of diseases that share a set of common traits. Normally the body regulates how and when new cells are formed. Cancer cells, however, divide and grow in an uncontrolled fashion.

In cancer cells, the genes have been mutated, or changed. As a consequence, these cells have an abnormal shape and size. The irregular cells, which grow in an uncontrolled manner, may group together to form **tumors.**

Tumor development is accelerated by the presence of oncogenes. Oncogenes make proteins that are responsible for increasing the speed of cell growth.

Tumors may be either benign or malignant. **Benign** tumors grow slowly and tend to remain in or around their original location of development. **Malignant** tumors spread, invading tissues and organs in various places throughout the body. This spreading process is called metastasis ◗ **Figure 10.1** .

<aside>
### What's the word...

**cancer** A family of diseases characterized by rapid, uncontrolled growth of abnormal cells.

**tumor** A mass of cancer cells.

**benign** A noncancerous tumor that does not invade nearby cells.

**malignant** A cancerous tumor that invades other cells and inhibits their ability to function properly.
</aside>

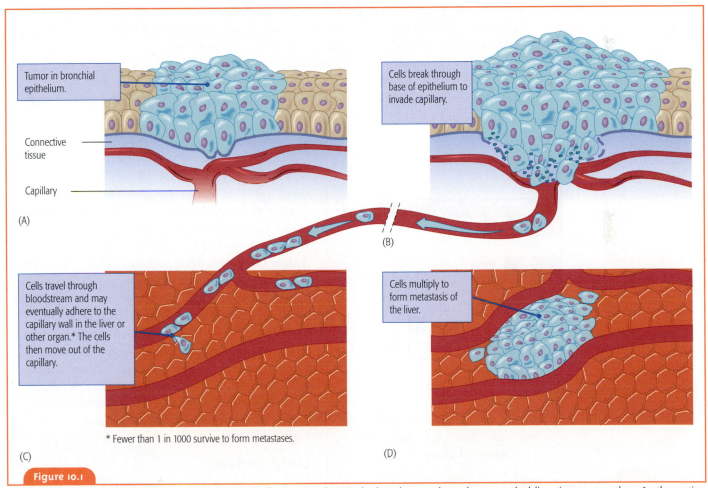

Tumor in bronchial epithelium.

Connective tissue

Capillary

(A)

Cells break through base of epithelium to invade capillary.

(B)

Cells travel through bloodstream and may eventually adhere to the capillary wall in the liver or other organ.* The cells then move out of the capillary.

Cells multiply to form metastasis of the liver.

* Fewer than 1 in 1000 survive to form metastases.

(C)                                                                 (D)

**Figure 10.1**

**How cancer cells multiply and spread.** Cancer cells secrete chemicals that destroy the substances holding tissues together. As these tissues break down, cancer cells move from their original site, enter the blood and lymph, and travel to other parts of the body.

**10**

## Susceptibility to Cancer

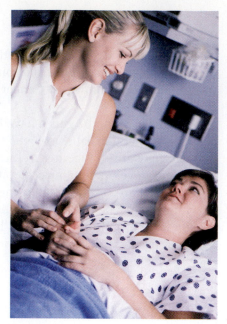

What makes a person susceptible to cancer? While a growing body of evidence indicates that a predisposition to some cancers may have a genetic link, the development of many cancers is directly related to individual lifestyle choices. Ask yourself the following questions to determine whether you are at risk for developing cancer:

1. Do I eat a minimum of five servings of fruit and vegetables every day?
2. Am I active for at least 30 minutes every day?
3. Am I within the healthy weight range for my height and age?
4. Do I use tobacco products of any kind?
5. When I am outside for a length of time, do I use sunscreen?
6. Do I not have a family history of cancer?

An important aspect in recovering from cancer is early detection. These questions will help you determine whether you are getting appropriate checkups:

1. Do I visit my physician for an annual checkup?
2. Women: If I am older than 40, do I have an annual mammogram?
3. Women: Do I conduct regular breast self-examinations?
4. Men: Do I conduct regular testicular examinations?
5. Men: If I am older than 50, do I have an annual prostate examination?

The more questions in either section to which you answered "no," the greater your risk for developing a form of cancer.

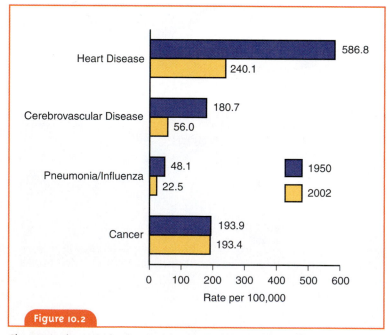

**Figure 10.2**

Change in the U.S. death rates* by cause, 1950 and 2002.
*Age-adjusted to 2000 U.S. standard population.
*Sources:* 1950 mortality data; CDC/NCHS, NVSS, Mortality Revised.
2002 mortality data: U.S. Mortality Public Use Data Tape, 2002, CDC/NCHS, 2004.

## Common Cancers

Cancer remains the second leading cause of death in the United States. In 2002, 557,000 deaths were cancer related, second only to the number of deaths caused by heart disease. In fact, since 1950, cancer is the only one of the major causes of death (heart disease, cancer, stroke, pneumonia/influenza) that has not seen a decrease in its death rate **Figure 10.2**. The American Cancer Society suggests that half of all men and one in three women will develop some form of cancer in their lifetime. Survival rates will vary depending on the type of cancer, the stage at which it is diagnosed, and the level of metastasis.

## Lung Cancer

- The most deadly cancer, it causes more deaths than any other cancer for both men and women.
- Most cases are directly related to smoking, which causes 87% of all lung cancers.

- **Death rates** are declining; incidence has leveled off. Because lung cancer takes many years to develop, today's relatively high death rate reflects the level of smoking in the 1960s and 1970s. As user rates decline, so will the long-term death rate from lung cancer in the future.

- Warning signs include chronic cough, wheezing, and excess saliva and mucus development.

- The best prevention method is to quit smoking.

- The overall 5-year survival rate after diagnosis is 15%.

## Breast Cancer

- Breast cancer is the most commonly diagnosed cancer in women, although men have seen a rapid increase in diagnosis in the last 10 years.

- A family history of breast cancer, aging, an early age of first menstrual cycle, and a previous personal diagnosis of breast cancer all increase the risk for developing breast cancer. Likewise, behavioral factors such as smoking, poor diet, and physical inactivity increase the level of risk.

- Breast cancer is the second leading cause of cancer death in women.

- Early detection of breast cancer can make a significant impact on the likelihood of successful treatment.

### Breast Self-Exam (BSE)

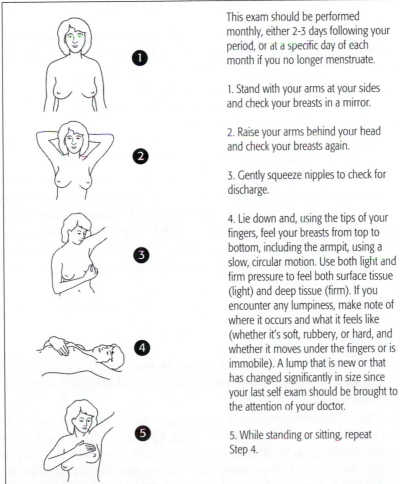

This exam should be performed monthly, either 2-3 days following your period, or at a specific day of each month if you no longer menstruate.

1. Stand with your arms at your sides and check your breasts in a mirror.

2. Raise your arms behind your head and check your breasts again.

3. Gently squeeze nipples to check for discharge.

4. Lie down and, using the tips of your fingers, feel your breasts from top to bottom, including the armpit, using a slow, circular motion. Use both light and firm pressure to feel both surface tissue (light) and deep tissue (firm). If you encounter any lumpiness, make note of where it occurs and what it feels like (whether it's soft, rubbery, or hard, and whether it moves under the fingers or is immobile). A lump that is new or that has changed significantly in size since your last self exam should be brought to the attention of your doctor.

5. While standing or sitting, repeat Step 4.

**Breast Self-Examination (BSE).** A monthly breast self-examination is recommended. Adapted from The National Cancer Institute.

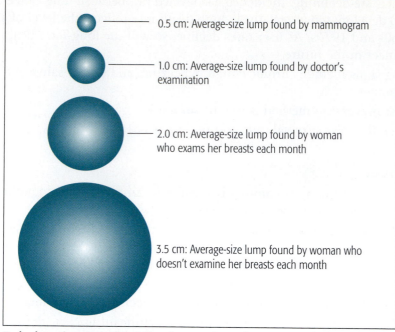

0.5 cm: Average-size lump found by mammogram

1.0 cm: Average-size lump found by doctor's examination

2.0 cm: Average-size lump found by woman who exams her breasts each month

3.5 cm: Average-size lump found by woman who doesn't examine her breasts each month

**Early detection saves lives!** The diagram above demonstrates the benefits of regular mammograms and self-exams. Reproduced with permission from St. Joseph Medical Center. http://www.osfstjoseph.org/cancered.html.

- The most prominent sign is the discovery of a lump in the breast through self-exam or **mammography**. Also, changes or distortions in the breast, discharge from the nipple, or discoloration of breast skin can be indicators.

- Estrogen appears to raise the risk level for breast cancer. Women receiving estrogen-based, **postmenopausal** hormone replacement therapy and women currently using estrogen-based fertility control methods have an increased risk for the development of breast cancer. The risk related to fertility control remains elevated as long as 10 years after discontinuation of the method.

- Adopting a lifestyle that includes physical activity, a moderate diet and weight, and not smoking appears to have a positive effect on risk of developing breast cancer. The American Cancer Society recommends having a mammogram every year or two after the age of 40. **Genetic testing** is currently available for those with a family history of breast cancer. While evidence is still emerging, researchers believe aspirin may have a protective effect for women with certain risk factors for the development of breast cancer.

- The 5-year survival rate for women diagnosed with breast cancer is 86%.

## Testicular Cancer

- Testicular cancer is the leading form of cancer in men between ages 15 and 35. It develops in the cells that help make sperm. There are about 7500 cases each year in the United States.

- The major risk factor associated with testicular cancer is having a testicle that has not (or has not *completely*) descended. In the fetus, testicles form in the abdomen and then drop into the **scrotum** as development progresses. For some men this descent does not occur or does not completely occur. Other risk factors include cancer in the other testicle, family history of testicular cancer, HIV infection, and race. White men are five times more likely than black men to develop testicular cancer.

## Testicular Self-Exam (TSE)

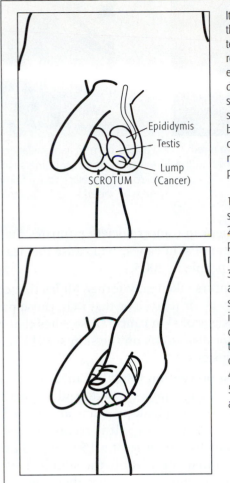

It is recommended that all men between the ages of 15 and 35 conduct monthly testicular self exams. The procedure is really quite simple, and routine self exams will make it easy to determine a difference in the nature of the testicles should a problem occur. The following steps are meant as a guide for self exam, but only a physician can make an actual cancer diagnosis. If you have any reason to be suspicious, see your physician immediately.

1. Visually examine the scrotum for swelling.
2. Examine each testicle individually by placing the testicle between the two middle fingers and thumb.
3. Gently roll the testicle between fingers and thumb. When in the habit of regular self exam, you will be able to determine if a new or unusual bump has developed on either testicle. Most testicular lumps are found on the sides of the testicle.
4. If you are unsure, consult a physician.
5. See the section on testicular cancer for additional warning signs of cancer.

**Testicular Self-Examination (TSE).** A regular testicular self-examination is recommended. Adapted from http://www.ontumor.com/testicular/selfexam.html.

- Early testicular cancer may or may not have associated symptoms. If symptoms are present you may notice a lump on or enlargement of a testicle, aching in the scrotum or abdomen, pain in the lower back, or infertility (rare).
- Most risk factors are not controllable. The best form of prevention is testicular self-exam.
- The 5-year survival rate is 95%.

## Skin Cancer

- Skin cancer is the most common cancer in the United States. More than 1 million new cases are diagnosed each year.
- There are three types of skin cancer: basal cell and squamous cell carcinomas (both easily curable) and malignant melanoma (much more serious).
- The greatest risk factor is exposure to ultraviolet (UV) rays from the sun. The unnatural form of UV rays produced by tanning machines is equally as dangerous. Having a light skin tone, a family history of skin cancer, repeated sunburns early in life, continued exposure to UV rays, and many moles or freckles make a person more susceptible to skin cancer.

**What's the word...**

**basal cell carcinoma** Form of skin cancer easily removed through surgery.

**squamous cell carcinoma** Cancer in the top layer of skin; highly curable when detected early.

**malignant melanoma** Dangerous form of skin cancer.

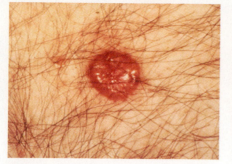

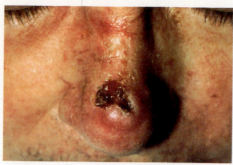

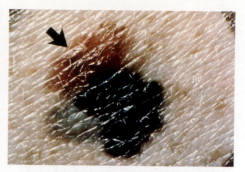

This basal cell carcinoma is on the cheek of a man. It is a raised lesion with central depressions that bleed and crust over.

Squamous cell carcinoma looks like a red rounded mass or a flat sore as shown in the photo.

Lesions of malignant melanoma are characterized by irregular borders with red, white, blue, or blue-black spots. Some portions may be raised.

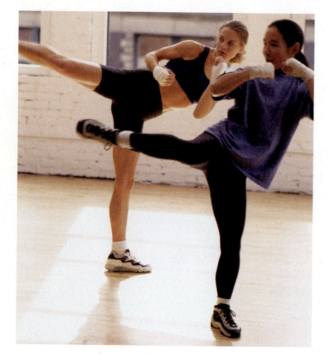

- The American Cancer Society estimates that the malignant form of skin cancer will cause the death of nearly 10,000 people in 2005.

- Skin cancers take many forms. Moles that change color, form, or texture or that itch, cause pain, or bleed can be signs of skin cancer. Also sores that won't heal and color distortions on the skin should be viewed as warning signs.

- The best prevention for skin cancer is primary prevention: using sunblock to defend against the sun's UV rays. All sunblock products are labeled with a sun protection factor (SPF). It is recommended that you use products with at least a 15 rating to protect your skin, and that you reapply the sunblock after swimming or engaging in activities that cause sweating. Check your body regularly and, if deemed necessary, see a dermatologist.

- The 5-year survival rate for malignant melanoma (the more dangerous form of skin cancer) is 89%.

## Prostate Cancer

- **Prostate** cancer is the second most commonly diagnosed form of cancer in men, behind skin cancer. It is one of the most successfully cured forms of cancer. However, because of the high volume of cases (nearly 200,000 each year), it is the second leading cancer-related killer. Prostate cancer is most commonly diagnosed after the age of 65, with a man's level of risk increasing quickly after age 50.

- Research has yet to clearly identify specific risk factors for this disease. Its specific causes are also unknown.

- Prostate cancer causes the death of more than 30,000 men annually in the United States.

- Symptoms include complications in urination, increased frequency in urination at night, pain in the lower pelvic region, blood in the urine, and sudden onset of impotence. However, these symptoms are found in other disorders of the prostate and are not specifically cancer related.

- Because a specific cause has yet to be identified for prostate cancer, prevention efforts focus on early identification of the problem. **Prostate-specific antigen (PSA)** testing and

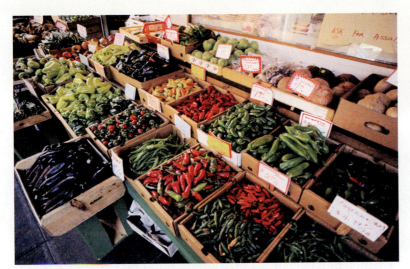

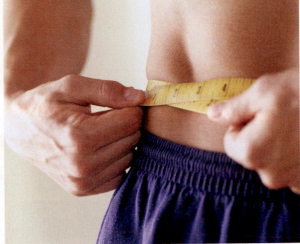

digital rectal examination (DRE) are used to identify prostate cancer. Other suspected but unconfirmed prevention ideas include maintaining a low-fat/high-fruit and -vegetable diet, increased intake of lycopene (an antioxidant found in tomato products), increased physical activity, and herbal remedies such as saw palmetto.

- When the disease is detected early and the cancer is localized, almost no deaths occur within 5 years of diagnosis.

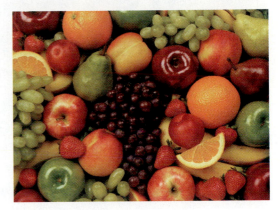

# Dietary Factors, Inactivity, and Obesity

The International Food Information Council reiterates what physicians and health professionals have been telling patients for some time: "Adopt a healthy lifestyle that includes getting regular physical activity, eating a balanced diet, and not smoking. A healthy lifestyle plays a major role in determining cancer risk." More specific or detailed information as to which foods help and which foods cause damage will vary from person to person because of the number and uniqueness of cancers. The organization does offer some general guidelines to increase your odds of remaining cancer free:

- Consume a diet rich in plant foods (whole grains, vegetables, fruit, beans) to help prevent colorectal, oral, and esophageal cancer.
- Diets high in animal products (red meat) have been associated with colon and prostate cancer, but other research attributes the relationship to other factors—primarily the fact that people who eat a great deal of red meat tend to eat less fruits and vegetables.
- Monitor your weight. Obesity is affected by diet, and eating more calories than you can burn through normal daily activity and added physical activity can increase your risk for certain cancers.

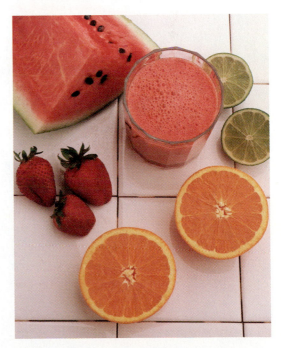

- Whole grains, vegetables, fruits, and beans contain fiber and **antioxidant** vitamins and minerals, which aid in the prevention of rectal and colon cancer.
- High-fat diets stimulate the production of estrogen, a hormone whose presence in larger volumes has been linked to breast cancer.

## Protecting Yourself

According to the American Cancer Society, one of the best defenses against cancer is regular screening. Use the acronym C.A.U.T.I.O.N. to raise your self-awareness of signs of possible cancer development:

**C**hange in bowel or bladder habits could be a sign of colorectal cancer.

**A** sore that does not heal on the skin or in the mouth could be a malignancy and should be checked by a doctor.

**U**nusual bleeding or discharge from the rectum, bladder, or vagina could mean colorectal, prostate, bladder, or cervical cancer.

**T**hickening of breast tissue or a new lump in the breast is a warning sign of breast cancer. A lump in the testes could mean testicular cancer.

**I**ndigestion or trouble swallowing could be cancer of the mouth, throat, esophagus, or stomach.

**O**bvious changes in moles or warts could mean skin cancer.

**N**agging cough or hoarseness that persists for 4 to 6 weeks could be a sign of lung or throat cancer.

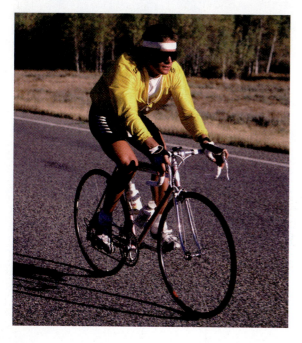

## Reflect ▸▸▸▸ Reinforce ▸▸▸▸ Reinvigorate

### Knowledge Check

*Answers in Appendix D*

1. Which of the following is *not* a quality of cancer cells?
   A. Uncontrolled growth
   B. Red and black color
   C. Mutated genes

2. It is recommended that women receive an annual mammogram after what age?
   A. 30
   B. 40
   C. 50

3. Men who are which of the following ages are most likely to develop testicular cancer?
   A. 25
   B. 40
   C. 55
   D. 65

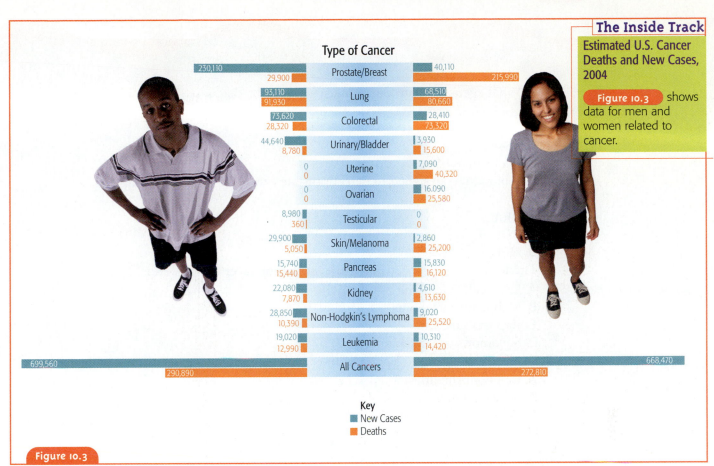

**The Inside Track**

Estimated U.S. Cancer Deaths and New Cases, 2004

**Figure 10.3** shows data for men and women related to cancer.

**Type of Cancer**

| Type of Cancer | Men New Cases | Men Deaths | Women New Cases | Women Deaths |
|---|---|---|---|---|
| Prostate/Breast | 230,110 | 29,900 | 40,110 | 215,990 |
| Lung | 93,110 | 91,930 | 68,510 | 80,660 |
| Colorectal | 73,620 | 28,320 | 28,410 | 73,320 |
| Urinary/Bladder | 44,640 | 8,780 | 3,930 | 15,600 |
| Uterine | 0 | 0 | 7,090 | 40,320 |
| Ovarian | 0 | 0 | 16.090 | 25,580 |
| Testicular | 8,980 | 360 | 0 | 0 |
| Skin/Melanoma | 29,900 | 5,050 | 2,860 | 25,200 |
| Pancreas | 15,740 | 15,440 | 15,830 | 16,120 |
| Kidney | 22,080 | 7,870 | 4,610 | 13,630 |
| Non-Hodgkin's Lymphoma | 28,850 | 10,390 | 9,020 | 25,520 |
| Leukemia | 19,020 | 12,990 | 10,310 | 14,420 |
| All Cancers | 699,560 | 290,890 | 668,470 | 272,810 |

**Key**
- ▇ New Cases
- ▇ Deaths

**Figure 10.3**

U.S. cancer incidence and mortality, 2004. *Source:* American Cancer Society, Surveillance Research, 2004.

4. Which type of cancer, when all variations are included, is the most diagnosed cancer in the United States?

   A. Breast
   B. Prostate
   C. Lung
   D. Skin

5. Which type of cancer causes the most deaths?

   A. Lung
   B. Breast
   C. Ovarian
   D. Colorectal

6. Tumor genes responsible for accelerating cell growth are called:

   A. Carcinogens
   B. Oncogenes
   C. Benign
   D. Metastasis

7. At what age is prostate cancer most likely to be diagnosed?
   A. Younger than 35
   B. 35–45
   C. 55–65
   D. Older than 65

8. The blood test designed to detect prostate cancer in men is called:
   A. DNA
   B. RRA
   C. PSA
   D. NFL

9. The form of skin cancer that forms in the top layer of the skin is:
   A. Basal cell carcinoma
   B. Malignant melanoma
   C. Kaposi's sarcoma
   D. Squamous cell carcinoma

10. Deaths related to _____ account for the largest percentage of cancer deaths.
    A. Cell abnormalities
    B. Genetic abnormalities
    C. Lifestyle factors
    D. Heredity

## Modern Modifications

- Eat a diet low in red meats, especially high-fat and processed meats.
- Eat a variety of fruits and vegetables daily.
- Women should perform monthly breast self-examinations.
- Men should perform monthly testicular self-examinations.
- Know the warning signs of cancer and see your health-care provider immediately if you detect any of them.
- Maintain a healthy weight.
- Women should consult their health-care providers regarding the use of oral contraceptives and estrogen replacement therapy with respect to cancer prevention and risk.
- Exercise most days of the week.
- Don't smoke cigarettes. If you can't quit, cut down.
- Avoid breathing environmental tobacco smoke.
- Don't chew tobacco products.
- Don't drink excessive amounts of alcoholic beverages.
- Avoid unnecessary exposure to ionizing radiation, such as X rays and ultraviolet light.
- Don't lie in the sun or in tanning beds.

## Critical Thinking

Abby is a 20-year-old college sophomore in her second year on the university softball team. She's been studying cancer in her health class and has been thinking about her diet, wondering if it might increase her risk for these diseases. Even if it does increase her risk, she is not confident in what to do about it. A typical day of eating for Abby consists of:

Breakfast: 2 eggs scrambled, 3 slices of bacon, 2 pieces of toast with butter

Lunch: Peanut butter sandwich, Big Grab bag of Doritos, milk

Dinner: Spaghetti with meat sauce, 4 bread sticks with butter and garlic, soda, pie slice

Snacks: Chocolate granola bar, 2 more sodas, hot wings with friends, "a couple" of beers

1. Is Abby getting the type of nutrition she needs to reduce her risk of cancers later in life? What makes you believe this?

2. What specific improvements would you suggest to Abby regarding her diet?

## Going Above and Beyond

### Websites

International Food Information Council

*www.ific.org*

American Cancer Society

*www.cancer.org*

Centers for Disease Control and Prevention

*ww.cdc.gov/cancer/nscpep/index.htm*

## References and Suggested Readings

Alters S. and Schiff W. *Essential Concepts for Healthy Living*, 3rd ed. Sudbury, MA: Jones and Bartlett, 2003.

American Cancer Society. Estimated new cancer cases and deaths by sex for all sites, US, 2004.

Centers for Disease Control and Prevention, National Center for Chronic Disease Prevention and Health Promotion. Colorectal cancer: The importance of prevention and early detection, 2004.

———. National Breast and Cervical Cancer Early Detection Program: Saving lives through screening, 2004.

———. Prostate cancer: The public health perspective, 2004.

———. Skin cancer: Preventing America's most common cancer, 2004.

DuBois R. N. Aspirin and breast cancer prevention: The estrogen connection. *Journal of the American Medical Association*, 2004; 291:20.

McCormack Brown K., Thomas D. Q., and Kotecki J. E. *Physical Activity and Health*. Sudbury, MA: Jones and Bartlett, 2002.

Melanoma and carcinoma skin cancer. http://www.melanoma-skin-cancer.com/warning-signs-of-skin-cancer.html [accessed December 1, 2004].

## Environmental Health

We live in a time when, if we're not paying attention, items in our everyday environment can cause us harm. Exposure to toxins outdoors, at work, or even in our own homes—not to mention our own personal choices—can lead to significant illness. How many of the items below need you look out for?

### Worksite/Industry

| Toxin | Source | Effects |
|---|---|---|
| Pesticides | Building supplies | Extended exposure in the workplace increases the risk for many cancers; widespread toxicity can create a condition known as "sick building syndrome" |
| Mercury | Chemicals | |
| Acids | Fireproofing | |
| Formaldehyde | Insulation | |
| Asbestos | Solvents | |
| | Metallurgy | |

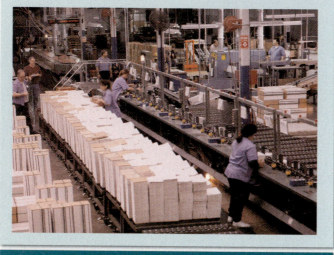

### Personal Behavior

| Toxin | Source | Effects |
|---|---|---|
| Tobacco | Personal behavior | Use, misuse and abuse of these items can lead to generally poor health, cancers, and death |
| Alcohol | | |
| Drugs | | |
| Diet | | |
| Activity | | |

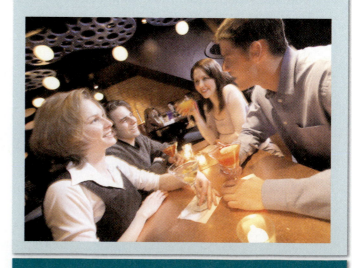

## Outdoors

| Toxin | Source | Effects |
| --- | --- | --- |
| Carbon dioxide | Vehicle exhaust | Increases breathing ailments, impacts hearing and vision, increases allergies, increases risk of birth defects and infertility |
| Methane | Fossil fuel burning | |
| Nitrogen oxides | Factory waste | |
| Carbon monoxide | Industrial waste | |
| Sulfur | Airplane pollution | |
| | Farming | |

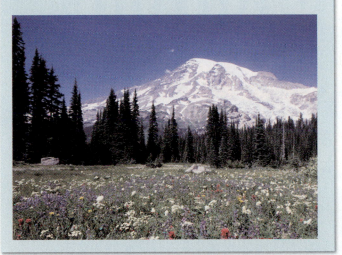

## Home

| Toxin | Source | Effects |
| --- | --- | --- |
| Radon | Insulation | Most poisons are ingested, but some are inhaled or absorbed through the skin; poisonous gases can come from dirt or old paint and insulation yet to be removed from the home |
| Asbestos | Thermometers | |
| Lead | Personal care items | |
| Mercury | Cleaning products | |
| Poisons | Paint | |
| | Mold | |
| | Noise | |
| | Medicines | |
| | Plants | |

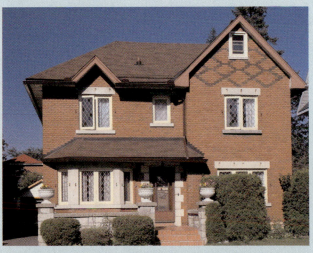

## CHAPTER 11

# Avoiding Addictive Behaviors

## Objectives

After reading this chapter, you should be able to:

- Distinguish between use, abuse, and addiction related to drug use, including alcohol and tobacco use.

- Describe the elements related to addiction.

- Describe the extent of alcohol, tobacco, and other drug use and abuse.

- List the various categories of drugs, and identify the types, functions, and effects of the specific drugs found within each category.

- Outline steps a person can take if he or she desires to stop smoking.

# Addictive Behavior

When you think about "addiction," what picture do you create in your mind's eye? A dark, dirty pub, with few people around, and a man passed out on the bar, half of his drink left in an unmoving hand while his head rests on the cherry wood? A deserted building in the inner city, with a group of people, shaking and nervous, huddled around a bag of drugs, a rubber hose, and a syringe? If those images resemble your first impressions, you are not alone. Those examples represent the most dramatic and visual forms addiction takes. However, the issue of addiction is much more prevalent, and hits much closer to home, than many of us would like to admit.

Drugs are any nonfood chemicals that can alter the way you think, act, feel, or process your environment. They can be legal (Tylenol, cough medicine, codeine, alcohol, caffeine, nicotine, aspirin) or illegal (marijuana, cocaine, Ecstasy, Rohypnol). They are found over the counter at the local store, in prescriptions from the physician, or on the street.

Addiction to a drug, regardless of its legality or availability, is a complex process. Many theories exist regarding the "cause" of addiction, but in reality trying to name just one item as the "cause" is futile. Addiction is a process influenced by genetics, personal behavior, personality, environment, social learning, personal history, and circumstance ( Table 11.1 ). Addiction shows no prejudice: It affects the poor and the rich, men and women, black and white, city and urban, and north, south, east, and west. Addiction does not care who you are; it affects what you do and how you think.

Addiction is also not limited to alcohol or other drug use. In addiction, the key is the pattern of behavior. This is why addiction can apply to gambling, sex, or two of the fastest growing addictions, cell phone and computer use.

Carlo DiClemente (2003) describes the conditions most commonly related to excessive exhibition of any behavior:

- Habitual patterns of intentional, craving-related behavior
- Behaviors that become excessive and produce serious consequences
- Problematic behaviors that continue over time
- Interrelationship of the physiological and psychological components of the behavior
- In all cases, addicted individuals who have difficulty ceasing the behavior

"Behaviors" and "consequences" are rather generic terms. When applied to addiction, they encompass a very particular set of characteristics:

- *Reward and reinforcement.* Physiologically, most addictive activities trigger the release of a chemical in the brain called dopamine. Dopamine is a pleasure drug, meaning that its presence in the brain makes you feel good. This sense of euphoria is why activities other than drug use can be addic-

**What's the word...**

**drug** Any nonfood substance that alters thought and/or behavior.

**addiction** Physiological and/or psychological need to perform a certain behavior.

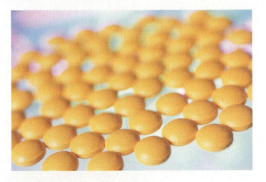

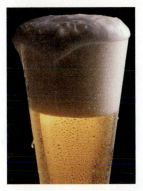

**Ask Yourself**
- How long can I go without using my cell phone or checking my e-mail?

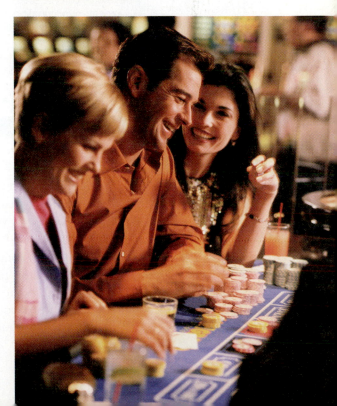

| Table 11.1 | Risk Factors for Addiction |
|---|---|

| Risk Factor | Leading to This Effect |
|---|---|
| **Biologically Based Factors** (genetic, neurological, biochemical, and so on) | |
| A less subjective feeling of intoxication | More use to achieve intoxication (warning signs of abuse absent) |
| Easier development of tolerance; liver enzymes adapt to increased use | Easier to reach the addictive level |
| Lack of resilience or fragility of higher (cerebral) brain functions | Easy deterioration of cerebral functioning, impaired judgment, and social deterioration |
| Difficulty in screening out unwanted or bothersome outside stimuli (low stimulus barrier) | Feeling overwhelmed or stressed |
| Tendency to amplify outside or internal stimuli (stimulus augmentation) | Feeling attacked or panicked; need to avoid emotion |
| Attention-deficit hyperactivity disorder and other learning disabilities | Failure, low self-esteem, or isolation |
| Biologically based mood disorders (depression and bipolar disorders) | Need to self-medicate against loss of control or pain of depression; inability to calm down when manic or to sleep when agitated |
| **Psychosocial/Developmental "Personality" Factors** | |
| Low self-esteem | Need to blot out pain, gravitate to outsider groups |
| Depression rooted in learned helplessness and passivity | Need to blot out pain; use of a stimulant as an anti-depressant |
| Conflicts | Anxiety and guilt |
| Repressed and unresolved grief and rage | Chronic depression, anxiety, or pain |
| Post-traumatic stress syndrome (as in veterans and abuse victims) | Nightmares or panic attacks |
| **Social and Cultural Environment** | |
| Availability of drugs | Easy frequent use |
| Chemical-abusing parental model | Sanction; no conflict over use |
| Abusive, neglectful parents; other dysfunctional family patterns | Pervasive sense of abandonment, distrust, and pain; difficulty in maintaining attachments |
| Group norms favoring heavy use and abuse | Reinforced, hidden abusive behavior that can progress without interference |
| Misperception of peer norms | Belief that most people use or favor use or think it's "cool" to use |
| Severe or chronic stressors, as from noise, poverty, racism, or occupational stress | Need to alleviate or escape from stress via chemical means |
| "Alienation" factors: isolation, emptiness | Painful sense of aloneness, normlessness, rootlessness, boredom, monotony, or hopelessness |
| Difficult migration/acculturation with social disorganization, gender/generation gaps, or loss of role | Stress without buffering support system |

*Source:* Hanson, G., Venturelli, P.J., Fleckenstein, A.E. (2004). *Drugs and Society,* 8th ed. Boston: Jones and Bartlett Publishers, p. 55.

---

*What's the word...*

**reinforcement** External support for a behavior.

tive. Socially, reward and **reinforcement** occur when the desired effect is accomplished. For instance, if you drink while believing that drinking makes you funny, and others tell you at a party, "Wow, you're really funny!" it reinforces your original belief and makes you more likely to drink the next time you desire to be funny.

- *Craving and compulsion.* Craving is related to the reward concept. The body, both physically and psychologically, adjusts quickly to the good feelings created by participating in the addictive activity. It seeks to replicate that sensation. As such, it creates a preoccupation with obtaining whatever the person is addicted to. Alcoholics think about when they'll have their next drink, sex addicts obsess about their next date, and computer addicts are preoccupied with the next chat room.

The preoccupation distracts the addict from living in the "here and now," and enjoying the present moment. Compulsion is a reflection of the increasing amount of time a user spends doing the activity.

- *Tolerance.* Tolerance refers to the body's adaptation to the addictive substance. The longer an individual is addicted to a substance, the more of that substance the body needs to achieve the original high or sense of euphoria. With some drugs, tolerance develops very quickly, and the need for using more of the drug to achieve the same effect happens rapidly.

- *Withdrawal.* Withdrawal is a key component of addiction, occurring when the addictive substance is taken away from the body. When an addict tries to quit, he or she may experience one or the entire set of symptoms: increased craving, nervousness, agitation, irritability, sweating, muscle twitching, insomnia, fever, rapid pulse, nausea, vomiting, and diarrhea.

> ## What's the word...
>
> **compulsion** An increase in the amount of time spent on an activity.
>
> **tolerance** The condition where more of a drug or activity is required to reproduce the initial sensation.
>
> **withdrawal** Symptoms related to the removal of a drug or activity.

## Relationship Addiction

The National Mental Health Association (NMHA) defines relationship addiction as "an emotional and behavioral condition that affects an individual's ability to have a healthy, mutually satisfying relationship." Those who battle with relationship addiction frequently enter into relationships with partners who are struggling with a chemical addiction on their own or significant conflict in their personal lives. Those with relationship addiction (also called co-dependency) feel an exaggerated sense of responsibility for the actions and behavior of their partner.

The NMHA fact sheet on co-dependency lists several other characteristics of relationship addiction:

- A tendency to "love" people whom the addict can pity and rescue
- A tendency to do more than his or her share, all of the time
- A tendency to become hurt when people don't recognize their efforts
- An unhealthy dependence on relationships
- A willingness to do anything to avoid the feeling of abandonment
- An extreme need for approval and recognition
- A sense of guilt when asserting oneself
- A compelling need to control others
- Lack of trust in oneself or others
- Difficulty identifying feelings
- Rigidity or difficulty adjusting to change
- Problems with intimacy and boundaries
- Chronic anger
- Lying and dishonesty

## Drug Addiction

To better define the relationship between personal choice or behavior, and drug use, we must consider the different effects that drug use can have on an individual. Not all people who use drugs are breaking the law, placing themselves at risk, or addicted—in fact, the vast majority are not. Taking this into consideration, the following definitions are often used to distinguish between the various types of use.

### Drug Use

- The appropriate use of a legal drug, for its appropriate purpose, in an appropriate amount
- Use of the drug is limited to the time of need

**11**

### Drug Misuse

- The temporary improper use of a legal drug
- May include use of a drug for a purpose other than which it was intended, or taken in the wrong dosage, frequency, or method of ingestion

### Drug Abuse

- The intentional use of any drug to the extent where daily living is adversely affected (negative social consequences)
- Can be related to medical or nonmedical use
- Even though the user recognizes negative effects, the behavior continues
- Emphasis shifts from the amount or frequency of use to the motive for use; attempting to alleviate stress, eliminate shyness, avoid conflict, or socially disconnect through use of a drug constitutes drug abuse

## Drug Effects on the Body

How a drug affects the body is influenced by many factors:

- *Drug pharmacology.* The chemical makeup of the drug will dictate many of the effects on the body.
- *Dosage.* The level of response to a drug is influenced by how much of the drug a person ingests (dosage). In general, the more drugs taken, the stronger the effect.
- *Time.* The longer a drug is in the body, the weaker the effect on the body.
- *Drug combinations.* Drug effects are multiplied or counteracted when combining them with other drugs. Drugs with similar pharmacology taken simultaneously will multiply the effect.
- *Method of use.* How the drug is ingested will influence the speed and impact of the drug's effect. Methods include injection, inhalation, absorption, and ingestion. The faster the drug reaches the bloodstream, and in turn the brain, the stronger the effect.

## Drug Categories

Drugs are classified into categories based on the effects they have on the body. Some have much greater addictive potential than others ( **Figure 11.1** ). What follows for each category is a list of applicable drugs, description of the effect, legitimate uses for the drugs (if any), and addictive qualities. ( **Table 11.2** ) summarizes these classifications, and ( **Table 11.3** ) highlights their potential for producing tolerance, dependence, and withdrawal.

### Central Nervous System (CNS) Depressants

CNS depressants include benzodiazepines (Xanax, Valium, Ativan, Halcion), sedatives (Phenobarbital, Quaaludes, Doriden), and alcohol. Medically, they are used to treat anxiety disorders, and for sedation and anesthesia in a clinical setting. There is no medical use for alcohol. Most CNS depressants have a moderate to high likelihood of dependence development, and all produce tolerance. Users may experience slurred speech, poor coordination, and disorientation. Common withdrawal symptoms include anxiety, insomnia, and delirium tremens.

---

**What's the word. . .**

**benzodiazepines** Central nervous system depressants used to reduce anxiety and induce sleep.

**sedatives** Sleep and anxiety reduction drugs with small margin of safety.

**insomnia** Inability to sleep.

**delirium tremens** DTs; withdrawal symptom characterized by uncontrollable shaking and hallucinations.

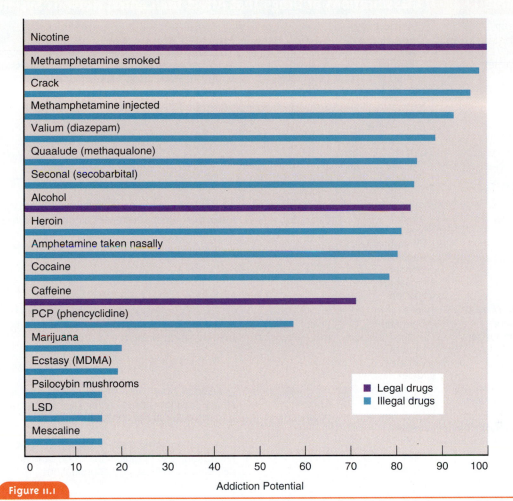

**Figure 11.1**

Addiction potential of various drugs. The chart shows health experts' ratings of the addiction potential of various drugs, with 100 being the highest addiction potential. Note that both legal and illegal drugs can be highly addictive. *Source:* Hanson, G., Venturelli, P.J. (2001). *Drugs and Society,* 6th ed. Boston: Jones and Bartlett Publishers, p. 95.

## Opioids (Narcotics)

Drugs in the opioid class include heroin, morphine, methadone, codeine, and opium. Medically, these drugs are painkillers, blocking the brain's ability to perceive pain. Narcotics are highly addictive, with tolerance to them developing rapidly. A user experiences a sense of euphoria, but may also experience a slowdown in breathing, drowsiness, and nausea. Withdrawal includes cold-like symptoms (runny nose, watery eyes), sleepiness, irritability, chills, sweating, nausea, and shaking.

## Cannabis

Drugs in this category include marijuana and hashish. The only medical use associated with these drugs is as antinausea agents for cancer patients (to counteract chemotherapy side effects). The intoxicating agent is tetrahydrocannabinol (THC). There is significant debate whether dependence is associated with cannabis products. One argument claims that, although no physical dependency develops, a psychological dependence is possible. No definitive consensus exists regarding the development of a tolerance level with this category of drugs. When they are taken at low doses, the user may experience euphoria, relaxation,

**What's the word...**

**opioids** Narcotics; used as pain relievers.

**euphoria** The effect associated with being "high."

**tetrahydrocannabinol (THC)** The active drug in marijuana.

## Table 11.2 — Classifications of Drugs That Affect the Central Nervous System

| Drug Classification | Common or Trade Name | Medical Uses | Effects of Average Dose |
|---|---|---|---|
| Opiates | Codeine<br>Darvon<br>Demerol<br>Fentanyl<br>Heroin<br>Methadone<br>Morphine<br>Opium<br>Oxycontin<br>Percodan<br>Vicodin | Analgesic (pain relief) | Blocks or eases pain; may cause drowsiness and euphoria; some users experience nausea or itching sensations |
| Sedatives | Amytal<br>Nembutal<br>Phenobarbital<br>Seconal<br>Doriden<br>Quaalude<br>Halcion | Sedation, tension relief | Relaxation, sleep; decreases alertness and muscle coordination |
| Minor tranquilizers | Dalmane<br>Equanil/Miltown<br>Librium<br>Valium<br>Xanax | Anxiety relief, muscle tension | Mild sedation; increased sense of well-being; may cause drowsiness and dizziness |
| Major tranquilizers (phenothiazines) | Mellaril<br>Thorazine<br>Prolixin | Control psychosis | Heavy sedation, anxiety relief; may cause confusion, muscle rigidity, convulsions |
| Alcohol | Beer<br>Wine<br>Liquor | None | Relaxation; loss of inhibition; mood swings; decreased alertness and coordination |
| Inhalants | Amyl nitrite<br>Butyl nitrite<br>Nitrous oxide | Muscle relaxant, anesthetic | Relaxation, euphoria; causes dizziness, headache, drowsiness |
| Stimulants | Benzedrine<br>Biphetamine<br>Desoxyn<br>Dexedrine<br>Methedrine<br>Preludin<br>Ritalin | Weight control; narcolepsy; fatigue and hyperactivity in children | Increased alertness and mood elevation; less fatigue and increased concentration; may cause insomnia, anxiety, headache, chills, and rise in blood pressure; organic brain damage after prolonged use |
| Cocaine | Cocaine hydrochloride | Local anesthetic, pain relief | Effects similar to stimulants |
| Cannabis | Marijuana<br>Hashish | Relief of glaucoma, asthma, nausea accompanying chemotherapy | Relaxation, euphoria, altered perception; may cause confusion, panic, hallucinations |
| Hallucinogens | LSD<br>PCP<br>Mescaline<br>Peyote<br>Psilocybin | None | Altered perceptions, visual and sensory distortion; mood swings |
| Nicotine | (In tobacco) | None | Altered heart rate; tremors; excitation |

**What's the word...**

**stimulants** Drugs used to increase activity in the central nervous system, causing increased energy and a sense of well-being.

**hallucinogens** Drugs that distort the senses and emotions, mimicking psychosis.

Source: Hanson, G., Venturelli, P.J., Fleckenstein, A.E. (2004). *Drugs and Society,* 8th ed. Boston: Jones and Bartlett Publishers.

| Table 11.3 | Tolerance, Dependence, and Withdrawal Properties of Common Drugs of Abuse |

| Drug | Tolerance | Psychological Dependence | Physical Dependence | Withdrawal Symptoms (Include Rebound Effects) |
|------|-----------|--------------------------|---------------------|-----------------------------------------------|
| Barbiturates | ++ | ++ | +++ | Restlessness, anxiety, vomiting, tremors, seizures |
| Alcohol | ++ | ++ | +++ | Cramps, delirium, vomiting, sweating, hallucinations, seizures |
| Benzodiazepines | + | ++ | ++ | Insomnia, restlessness, nausea, fatigue, twitching, seizures (rare) |
| Narcotics (heroin) | +++ | ++ | +++ | Vomiting, sweating, cramps, diarrhea, depression, irritability, gooseflesh |
| Cocaine, amphetamines | +* | +++ | ++ | Depression, anxiety, drug craving, need for sleep ("crash"), anhedonia |
| Nicotine | + | ++ | ++ | Highly variable; craving, irritability, headache, increased appetite, abnormal sleep |
| Caffeine | + | + | + | Anxiety, lethargy, headache, fatigue |
| Marijuana | + | + | + | Irritability, restlessness, decreased appetite, weight loss, abnormal sleep |
| LSD (lysergic acid diethylamide) | ++ | + | − | Minimal |
| PCP (phencyclidine) | + | + | + | Fear, tremors, some craving, problems with short-term memory |

+++ Intense   ++ Moderate   + Some   − Not significant
*Can sensitize.
*Source:* Hanson, G., Venturelli, P.J., Fleckenstein, A.E. (2004). *Drugs and Society,* 8th ed. Boston: Jones and Bartlett Publishers, p. 148.

disorientation, and hunger. Higher doses may trigger fatigue, hallucinations, lack of motivation, and paranoia. Withdrawal symptoms are minor, with some people experiencing insomnia and decreased appetite.

## Central Nervous System Stimulants

CNS stimulants include cocaine, caffeine, Ritalin, amphetamines, methamphetamine, and nicotine. Medically, these drugs are used as mild sedatives and for weight control, narcolepsy, and attention-deficit disorders. Nicotine has no medical value. A high degree of psychological and physical dependence is associated with these drugs, and tolerance to them does develop. Users may experience increased blood pressure and pulse, lack of appetite, excitation, increased concentration, and mood elevation/euphoria. Some users experience paranoia, hallucinations, and itching sensations in the skin (like something is crawling on them). Withdrawal from stimulants often results in long periods of sleep, depression and irritability, and lack of motivation.

## Hallucinogens

Hallucinogens include LSD, PCP, STP, MDMA (Ecstasy), mescaline, peyote, and Ketamine. There are no medical uses for hallucinogens. Levels of dependence are low or unknown for most hallucinogens, but tolerance

**The Inside Track**

**Side Effects of Marijuana Use**

Brain: THC changes the way your brain interprets information necessary for memory and learning, and destroys memory of behaviors that have already been learned.

Lungs: Tar and carbon monoxide levels are three to five times greater in marijuana users than in tobacco users. Also, respiratory problems such as cough, excessive phlegm, chronic bronchitis, and chest colds are common.

Learning and Social Behavior: Research supports the notion that skills related to attention, memory, and learning are impaired for people who smoke marijuana daily or almost daily. Student users have been shown to make more errors and to have problems processing and using information. Marijuana users have lower academic achievement than nonusers, are more likely to accept socially negative behavior such as skipping school and fighting, and have less satisfying relationships with their parents.

does develop. Users experience a distortion of perception under the influence of these drugs, as well as mood swings and hallucinations. Few withdrawal symptoms are reported with these drugs.

## Inhalants

Inhalants include butyl nitrite, amyl nitrite, and nitrous oxide. With rare exceptions, there are no medical uses for inhalant drugs. Dependence does not occur, and it is unknown whether tolerance develops. Users may experience brief (less than 30 minutes) euphoria, increased blood pressure and pulse, drowsiness, nausea, headache, and fainting and disorientation. Withdrawal symptoms include depression, loss of appetite, insomnia, and irritability.

# Alcohol

### The Current View

The National Youth Risk Behavior Survey is conducted every 2 years by the Centers for Disease Control and Prevention (CDC). In 2003, the CDC reported that by the time they reach the ninth grade, nearly 75% of adolescents have had at least one drink, and almost 30% report having had five or more drinks on one or more occasions during the previous month.

The National Institutes of Health report that among 12th graders, almost 30% reported drinking on three or more occasions per month. Approximately 30% of 12th graders engaged in heavy episodic drinking, now popularly termed binge drinking—that is, having at least five or more drinks on one occasion within the past 2 weeks—and it is estimated that 20% did so on more than one occasion (see **Figure 11.2**).

Most everyone knows and understands that the legal age to consume alcohol in the United States is 21. Most people also know and understand that this law is regularly broken, particularly on college campuses. One of the main reasons that this issue arises on college

*What's the word...*

**binge drinking** Having five or more drinks for men, or four or more drinks for women, in a single occasion.

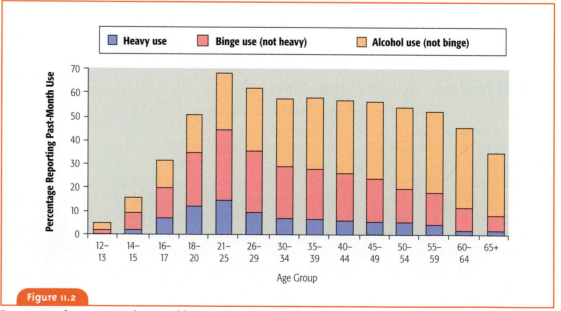

**Figure 11.2**

Percentage of persons aged 12 or older reporting past-month alcohol use, by level of use and age group, 2003. *Source:* Office of Applied Studies (OAS), Substance Abuse and Mental Health Services Administration (SAMHSA), The NHSDA Report: Alcohol Use. Rockville, MD: Substance Abuse and Mental Health Services Administration (SAMHSA), 2003. http://www.drugabusestatistics.samhsa.gov/.

campuses is that students come to the university environment anticipating that alcohol will have a positive influence on their college experience. This expectation makes it much easier to convince oneself to drink, even when a student knows it is against the law. It's considered the college norm—and besides, everyone does it, right? Well, actually, no. Almost one in five college students is an abstainer, meaning that he or she doesn't drink at all   Figure 11.4  . In addition, 70% of all alcohol consumed on campus is drunk by 20% of the students (NIAAA 2002).

According to the National Institute on Alcohol Abuse and Alcoholism (NIAAA), 40% of all college students report having been engaged in binge drinking (more than five drinks in an outing for a man, more than four drinks in an outing for a woman) at some point, but 20% reported having done so three or more times in the previous 2 weeks. These students are called frequent binge drinkers (or **heavy drinkers**), and they account for nearly 70% of all alcohol consumed on campus.

## The Intoxication Process

The intoxicating agent in alcohol is ethyl alcohol, also called grain alcohol or **ethanol**. Absorption of alcohol into the bloodstream happens in small amounts through the stomach, but primarily takes place in the small intestine. The bloodstream carries the alcohol throughout the body, to all major organs including the brain, heart, and liver.

The liver is responsible for processing out the alcohol, and it can do so at the rate of about one-half ounce per hour, or one drink per hour. As noted a "drink" is one 12-ounce beer, one 5- to 7-ounce glass of wine, or 1.5 ounces of 80–90 proof liquor   Figure 11.3  . You cannot speed up the rate at which the liver neutralizes alcohol: It is a constant. Taking a shower or drinking coffee merely gives you a wet, wide-awake drunk.

The **proof** of an alcoholic beverage is twice the percentage of alcohol in the beverage. Thus an 80 proof whiskey consists of 40% alcohol.

**Blood alcohol concentration (BAC)** is the measurement used to determine how much alcohol is in the bloodstream. In most states, the legal limit of intoxication for driving is 0.08 to 0.10, but impaired driving may begin with a BAC as low as 0.03   Table 11.4  .

Many things affect the BAC of a person. The presence of food in your stomach, the rate at which you drink, the amount you drink, and your body composition are the most significant factors. Fatty foods, such as milk and meat, will slow the body's ability to move alcohol into the small intestine, thereby slowing down the absorption process. Women, because they tend to have a larger percentage of body fat, will be more intoxi-

### What's the word. . .

**heavy drinkers** Individuals who consume five or more drinks on one occasion, five or more times in a 30-day period.

**ethanol** Grain alcohol; consumable form of alcohol in alcoholic beverages.

**proof** Two times the percentage of alcohol in an alcoholic beverage.

**blood alcohol concentration (BAC)** The concentration of alcohol found in the bloodstream; expressed as a percentage.

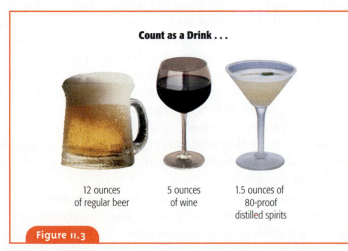

**Count as a Drink . . .**

| 12 ounces of regular beer | 5 ounces of wine | 1.5 ounces of 80-proof distilled spirits |

Figure 11.3

**Alcohol equivalents.** A can of beer, glass of wine, and a mixed drink have about the same amount of alcohol. So don't be fooled by the type of drink.

### Table 11.4    Blood Alcohol Concentration and Physical and Mental Behavior

| Blood Alcohol Concentration (%) | Physical and Mental Behavior |
|---|---|
| 0.01 | Clearing of the head. Slight tingling of mucous membranes. |
| 0.02 | Mild throbbing at the back of the head. A touch of dizziness. Personal appearance of no concern. Willing to talk. |
| 0.03 | Feeling of euphoria and superiority. ("Sure am glad I came to your party." "We will always be friends.") |
| 0.04 | Talking and laughing loudly. Movements a bit clumsy. Flippant remarks. ("You don't think I'm drunk, do you?") |
| 0.05 | Normal inhibitions almost eliminated. Many liberties taken. Talkative. Some loss of motor coordination. |
| 0.07 | Feeling of remoteness. Rapid pulse. Gross clumsiness. |
| 0.10 | Legally drunk in most states. Staggering, loud singing. Drowsiness. Rapid breathing. |
| 0.20 | Blackout level. Inability to recall events later. Easily angered. Shouting, groaning, weeping. |
| 0.30 and above | Stupor. Breathing reflex threatened. Deep anesthesia. Death is due to paralysis of the respiratory center and is generally preceded by 5 to 10 hours of stupor and coma. |

*Source:* Liska, K. *Drugs and the Human Body,* 6th ed. © 2000. Reprinted by permission of Pearson Education, Inc. Upper Saddle River, NJ.

cated than a man after consuming the same amount of alcohol. The best scenario, however, is not to place yourself in a position where you need to worry about such things.

There is only one well-recognized health "benefit" of alcohol consumption: drinking small amounts of red wine seems to reduce the risk of coronary heart disease. But is this single gain enough to balance the long list of alcohol-associated health and social problems? Moreover, Concord grape juice is more beneficial than wine for combating coronary heart disease and does not carry the potential dangers that alcohol does.

Why recommend a drug that we know leads to loss of control or alcohol addiction in about 10% of users? It makes little sense to recommend alcohol as a safeguard against coronary heart disease when there are so many much safer options already at hand. The NIAAA warns us that vulnerability to alcoholism and alcohol-related problems varies among individuals and cannot always be predicted before a person begins to drink.

If you choose to drink alcoholic beverages, follow the recommendations about their use from *The Dietary Guidelines for Americans, 2005:*

- Those who choose to drink alcoholic beverages should do so sensibly and in moderation—defined as a consumption of up to one drink per day for women and up to two drinks per day for men.

- Alcoholic beverages should not be consumed by some individuals, including those who cannot restrict their alcohol intake, women of childbearing age who may become pregnant, pregnant and lactating women, children and adolescents, individuals taking medications that can interact with alcohol, and those with specific medical conditions.

- Alcoholic beverages should be avoided by individuals engaging in activities that require attention, skill, or coordination, such as driving or operating machinery.

## The Problems

### Unintentional Injury

The Task Force on College Drinking, working through the NIAAA, reported in 2002 that alcohol consumption is linked to at least 1400 student deaths and 500,000 unintentional injuries annually. Motor vehicle crashes are the leading cause of death among youth ages 15 to 20, with the fatality rate among alcohol-involved drivers between 16 and 20 years old being more than twice the rate for alcohol-involved drivers 21 and older.

### Academic Failure

A direct relationship exists between the amount a student drinks and his or her academic achievement. More than 20% of college dropouts do so for alcohol-related reasons. One of every 14 college freshmen will not return for a second year of school because of an alcohol-related situation. Behaviors that affect academic performance include missing class, inattention while in class, failure to study, and poor performance on tests and projects.

### Sexual Issues

The initial sensation many people have while drinking is a reduction in inhibitions. While this may improve your ability to talk to a stranger, it increases the chances of you having sex when you normally would not. It also decreases the likelihood of you making wise decisions during sexual activity, such as wearing a condom, thereby increasing your chances for incurring an unwanted pregnancy or acquiring a sexually transmitted disease. It renders you less able to protect yourself in the event that someone makes an unwanted sexual approach. Approximately 3 in 10 female victims of acquaintance rape report being at least slightly intoxicated at the time of attack. Heavy drinking can also affect the body's ability to perform sexually.

### Suicide

The third leading cause of death among people between the ages of 14 and 25 is suicide. When alcohol becomes a part of the equation, conditions such as depression and stress may become more than a person can cope with.

### Cancer

Many cancers are directly related to the consumption of alcohol. Cancers of the pharynx, esophagus, colon, rectum, tongue, lungs, and liver are just a few of those associated with drinking.

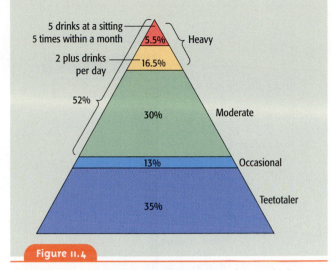

**Figure 11.4**

Throughout the U.S. adult population, 35% do not drink any alcoholic beverages whatsoever. *Source:* Hanson, G., Venturelli, P. J., Fleckenstein, A. E. (2004). *Drugs and Society*, 8th ed. Boston: Jones and Bartlett Publishers.

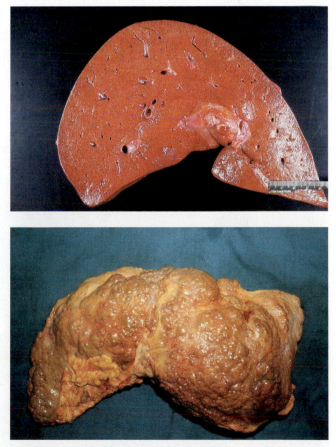

A normal liver (*top*) as it would be found in a healthy human body. An abnormal liver (*bottom*) that exhibits the effects of moderate to heavy alcohol consumption.

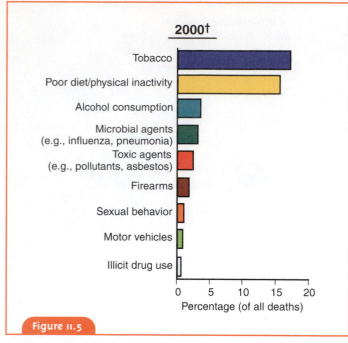

**2000†**

Tobacco
Poor diet/physical inactivity
Alcohol consumption
Microbial agents (e.g., influenza, pneumonia)
Toxic agents (e.g., pollutants, asbestos)
Firearms
Sexual behavior
Motor vehicles
Illicit drug use

Percentage (of all deaths)

**Figure 11.5**

Actual causes of death, United States, 2000.

*Source:* Mokad A., Marks J., Stroup D., and Gerberding J. Actual causes of death in the United States, 2000. *Journal of the American Medical Association,* March 10, 2004; 291:1238–1245.

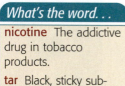

**What's the word. . .**

**nicotine** The addictive drug in tobacco products.

**tar** Black, sticky substance from tobacco smoke that builds up in the lungs and promotes cancer development.

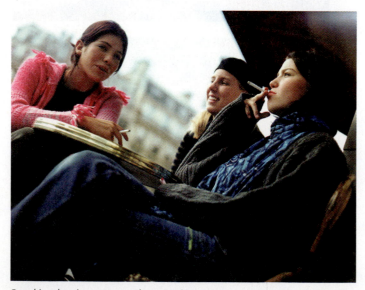

Smoking begins at an early age when peer acceptance is highly sought after.

# Tobacco

No single personal behavior has a more detrimental effect on society than tobacco use, particularly smoking. More than 60 million people in the United States were current smokers in 2001. The average number of deaths from 1995 to 1999 directly related to smoking was 442,000 **Figure 11.5**. That is almost 20% of all deaths in the United States. In addition, more than 8 million people in the United States have a major illness directly related to smoking.

In 1964, the U.S. Surgeon General released the first report establishing the relationship between smoking and lung cancer. In essence, we have known for more than 40 years that smoking causes a multitude of health problems and is the major reason for premature death in this country. So why do people still smoke? Some reasons include fitting into a desired group, perceived relaxation, and the stimulation received from use of tobacco. The most significant reason is nicotine addiction.

Nicotine is the addictive drug found in tobacco. Tobacco is the only source in which nicotine has ever been identified. It is found in all forms of tobacco, including cigarettes, cigars, and smokeless tobacco. There is no safe form of tobacco.

When compared to all other drugs, including crack cocaine, methamphetamine, and heroin, nicotine has the strongest addictive qualities of any drug. That means it is easier to get addicted to nicotine than any other drug.

The development of an addiction to nicotine starts immediately. For adolescents, addiction to nicotine is present when they smoke as few as two cigarettes per week. Among daily smokers, 75% say they started as teenagers **Figure 11.6**.

Because the adolescent brain is still developing, young teens are more susceptible to tobacco addiction than adults. In the 2003 Youth Risk Behavior Survey conducted by the CDC, more than half of all high school students said they had tried smoking at least once. One in five students was a current user, and one in 10 high school students was a frequent user (20 or more cigarettes in the past 30 days).

Addiction is merely the beginning of the problem for smokers. Smoking is a toxic behavior. More than 4000 chemicals are found in tobacco smoke, none of them good for you:

- Forty percent of smoke is in the form of tar. Tar is a sticky substance that lodges itself in the lungs as smoke is inhaled. A pack-a-day smoker will amass approximately 4 ounces of tar in his or her lungs each year. Tars are cancer causing.

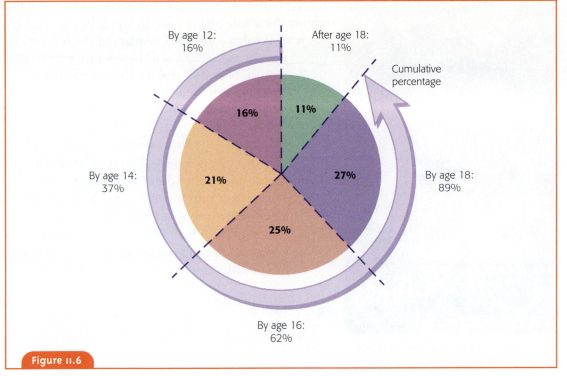

**Figure 11.6**

**Age at which adults say they started smoking.** Most smokers started this habit when they were in their teens or preteens.

*Source:* The National Household Survey on Drug Abuse, United States, 1991. Office on Smoking and Health, Centers for Disease Control and Prevention.

- **Carbon monoxide** is a poisonous gas found in cigarette smoke. Of all gases, it is one of the most prominent. Carbon monoxide binds to red blood cells, prohibiting oxygen from binding in the same place, and limiting the amount of oxygen the body can access.

- Smoking is the primary reason why heart disease is the number one killer in the United States. Because nicotine acts as a stimulant, smoking increases the smoker's heart rate and blood pressure, increasing the wear and tear on the heart over time. Smoking also promotes plaque buildup in arteries, called atherosclerosis. This buildup increases the risk for heart attack and stroke.

- Many cancers are related to smoking, including cancers of the lung, kidneys, esophagus, mouth, bladder, and stomach. Smoking causes more than 120,000 new cases of lung cancer each year, and approximately 30,000 cases of cancer in other areas of the body.

- **Chronic obstructive pulmonary disease (COPD)** is a term describing a group of diseases—most commonly chronic bronchitis and emphysema—that inhibit the body's ability to obtain and retain oxygen. Smoking damages the bronchi in the lungs. As a result, shortness of breath and a cough that produces a considerable amount of phlegm are common symptoms of these diseases. COPD kills about 80,000 people in the United States every year.

Smokeless tobacco is often seen as an alternative to smoking for tobacco users who do not wish to smoke. There are three common types of smokeless tobacco. **Snuff** (often called "spit" tobacco) is ground-up moist tobacco usually placed between the bottom lip and gum; this practice is also referred to as "dipping." **Chew** tobacco is shredded tobacco leaves placed between the cheek and gum; it is also referred to as "a wad." **Plug** tobacco is shredded tobacco leaves that are pressed into a hard block and

### What's the word...

**carbon monoxide** Most significant poisonous gas related to smoking.

**chronic obstructive pulmonary disease (COPD)** Family of breathing disorders most commonly contracted from smoking; includes emphysema and bronchitis.

**snuff** Ground-up moist tobacco placed between the bottom lip and gum.

**chew** Shredded tobacco leaves placed between the cheek and gum.

**plug** Shredded tobacco leaves that are pressed into a hard block.

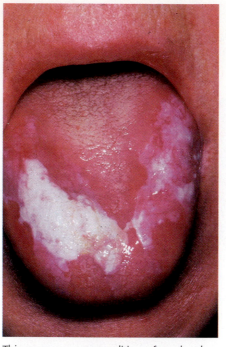

This precancerous condition often develops on the mucous membranes of the mouths of those who use smokeless tobacco products.

placed between the cheek and gum. None of these options is a safe alternative to smoking, however:

- Spit tobacco is used by placing the tobacco in the cheek, or between the lip and gum of the mouth. Nicotine and its associated chemicals are then absorbed through the mouth. Exposure to these chemicals increases one's risk for oral cancers, cancers of the pharynx and esophagus, and heart disease.

- One dip of smokeless tobacco, kept in the mouth for about 30 minutes, delivers the same amount of nicotine and chemicals as smoking two to four cigarettes.

- One tin (snuff like Skoal or Copenhagen comes in a round container) contains a lethal dose of nicotine, as much as 60 cigarettes.

## Reflect >>>> Reinforce >>>> Reinvigorate

### Knowledge Check

*Answers in Appendix D*

1. Behavior characterized by habitual patterns, craving, long-term persistence, and serious consequences is called:
   A. Co-dependence
   B. Addiction
   C. Abuse
   D. Reinforcement

2. Which chemical released in the brain is associated with feeling good?
   A. Cortisol
   B. Epinephrine
   C. Dopamine
   D. Norepinepherine

3. Needing more and more of a substance to produce a desired effect is called:
   A. Tolerance
   B. Reward
   C. Reinforcement
   D. Withdrawal

Youth are highly susceptible to use of tobacco, as they are more likely to be influenced when public figures are shown using the product. Youngsters seeing their favorite sports figure using chewing tobacco perceive that the behavior is acceptable ("My favorite baseball player wouldn't do anything that could harm him") and that chewing tobacco should happen during that activity. A dramatic increase in the amount of smoking shown on television and film also occurred during the 1990s.

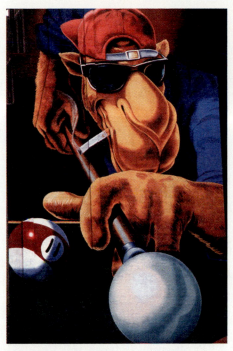

Cigarette advertisements such as this Joe Camel billboard are criticized because they appear to target preteens and teens.

4. Tom has a headache, and takes twice the amount of Tylenol described on the package to more quickly eliminate the pain. This is an example of:

   A. Drug use
   B. Drug misuse
   C. Drug abuse
   D. Addiction

5. The addictive element in marijuana is:

   A. NCC
   B. POT
   C. DNA
   D. THC

6. Which of the following has the least probability of producing addiction?

   A. Hallucinogens
   B. CNS depressants
   C. Opioids
   D. CNS stimulants

7. What percentage of high school students admit to binge drinking at least one time?

   A. 10%
   B. 30%
   C. 50%
   D. 75%

8. Which organ has the primary responsibility for cleansing the body of drugs and alcohol in the bloodstream?

    A. Heart
    B. Pancreas
    C. Lungs
    D. Liver

9. What poisonous gas is emitted from cigarettes, displacing oxygen in the lungs?

    A. Sulfur dioxide
    B. Helium
    C. Carbon dioxide
    D. Carbon monoxide

10. Bronchitis and emphysema are diseases in what family of breathing disorders?

    A. Asthma
    B. Pneumonia
    C. COPD
    D. Rheumatic fever

## Modern Modifications

### Quitting the Habit

The best decision you can make is not to smoke or use other forms of tobacco. If you have already begun, your best option is to quit. Here are some ideas on how to quit using tobacco:

- Commit to quitting. Tell everyone you know you're going to quit and ask them to support you.
- Pick a quit date and stick to it—no excuses.
- Throw away anything related to your tobacco use.
- Exercise. It will help with the stress you'll feel occasionally, and will also help with managing your weight.
- Calculate how much money you will save by not using tobacco.
- Try not to hang out in the places where you used to smoke or chew. Keep low-calorie snacks such as sugarless gum and candy, crunchy fruit and vegetables, and sunflower seeds (good for spitting, too) on hand to occupy your mouth when the urge to smoke or dip comes on.
- Plan to reward yourself frequently. Quitting may be one of the most difficult things you've tried, and you should explicitly recognize your efforts to quit.
- Plan for relapse. Most people do not quit successfully the first time they try. It may take a dozen attempts, but you must commit to regrouping, and trying over and over until you win the battle.

## Critical Thinking

1. You and some friends from campus have been at a local party for some time. When the group decides to leave, one friend intends to drive. You know that even a few drinks can impair a person's driving ability. Your friend has had several drinks and, you believe, should most likely not be behind the wheel of a car. No one else in the group says anything as the intoxicated person begins to enter their car. Would you

say anything to your friend? Would you stop him or her from driving? By any means necessary? Why or why not? What approach do you think might be successful?

2. What are your thoughts regarding the legalization of marijuana? Is there a legitimate public interest? Are the medical advantages significant enough to warrant legalization? Present evidence to support your stance.

## Going Above and Beyond

### Websites

American Cancer Society

*www.cancer.org*

National Institute on Alcohol Abuse and Alcoholism

*www.niaaa.nih.gov*

National Institute on Drug Abuse

*teens.drugabuse.gov*

National Institutes on Health

*www.nih.gov*

Youth Risk Behavior Surveillance Survey

*www.cdc.gov/yrbss*

### References and Suggested Readings

American Lung Association.  Facts about nicotine.

Centers for Disease Control and Prevention (CDC). Current trends in cigarette use. YRBSS, 2003.

———. Current trends in tobacco use. YRBSS, 2003.

———. Targeting tobacco use: The nation's leading cause of death. 2004.

DiClemente C. *Addiction and Change.* New York: Guilford Press, 2003.

Edlin G. and Golanty E. *Health and Wellness,* 8th ed. Sudbury, MA: Jones and  Bartlett, 2004.

Hanson G. R., Venturelli P. J., and Fleckenstein A. E. *Drugs and Society.* Sudbury, MA: Jones and Bartlett, 2004.

Johnston L. D., O'Malley P. M., and Bachman J. G. *Monitoring the  Future: National Survey Results on Drug Use, 1975–2001. Vol. II:  College Students and Adults Ages 19–40.* NIH Pub. No. 02–5107.  Bethesda, MD: NIDA, 2002.

McCormack Brown K., Thomas D. Q., and Kotecki J. E. (2002). *Physical Activity and Health.* Sudbury, MA: Jones and Bartlett, 2002.

National Center for Chronic Disease Prevention and Health Promotion. Women and tobacco fact sheet. May 2004.

———. Smokeless tobacco fact sheet. July 2004.

National Institute on Alcohol Abuse and Alcoholism (NIAAA), *Changing the Culture of Campus Drinking.* No. 58, October 2002.

———. *Underage Drinking: A Major Public Health Challenge.* No. 59, April 2003.

Saskatchewan Health. Facts you should know about smokeless (spit) tobacco. http://www.health.gov.sk.ca/rr_smokeless_tobacco.html [accessed January 5, 2005].

# Preventing Sexually Transmitted Infections

# Primary Sexually Transmitted Infections

Sex is everywhere you look—videos, music, films, books, television. Sex has become a centerpiece for marketing and publicity. It is a natural behavior, and it can be beautiful. But like any other behavior, it requires that an individual use his or her knowledge and skills to ensure that the experience is a positive one. If sexual activity is unplanned, impulsive, or undisciplined, it can have profound, and sometimes life-threatening, consequences.

Sexually transmitted infections (STIs) are diseases related to sexual behavior caused by the transfer of bacteria or viruses from one sexual partner to another. Often referred to as sexually transmitted diseases or sexually related diseases, 13 million new cases are reported every year at an annual cost of almost $10 billion. A single-cell microscopic organism that releases disease-causing toxins in the body causes a bacterial infection. Such STIs can be cured through the use of antibacterial medication. Viruses are the smallest pathogens, causing disease by entering cells and reproducing. Viruses cannot be cured. Once an individual has acquired a viral sexually transmitted disease, he or she has it for life.

Because sexual activity is happening at an earlier age and marriage is occurring later in life, people today are likely to have multiple sex partners. As a result, the incidence of STIs is on the rise. An increased sense of invincibility and youthful denial of the likelihood of infection help to make teens and college-aged students the most likely groups to have a STI. College students have indicated that, along with pregnancy and sexual violence, STIs and sexual activity consequences are their top concerns in relation to sexual behavior. **Table 12.1** summarizes the most common STIs.

## What's the word. . .

**sexually transmitted infections (STIs)** Infections and diseases transferred through intimate contact.

**bacteria** Microscopic organisms that cause disease.

**virus** Smallest of all disease-causing pathogens.

| Table 12.1 | Common Sexually Transmitted Infections | |
|---|---|---|
| **STI** | **Symptoms** | **Treatment** |
| AIDS | Flu-like symptoms followed by any of a number of diseases characteristic of immunodeficiency | New drugs may retard vital reproduction temporarily. Opportunistic infections can be treated to some degree. |
| Chlamydia | Usually occur within 3 weeks: infected men have a discharge from the penis and painful urination, women may have a vaginal discharge, but often are asymptomatic | Antibiotics |
| *Gardnerella vaginalis* | Yellow-green vaginal discharge with an unpleasant odor; painful urination; vaginal itching | Metronidazole |
| Genital warts | Usually occur within 1 to 3 months: small, dry growths on the genitals, anus, cervix, and possibly mouth | Podophyllin |
| Gonorrhea | Usually occur within 2 weeks: discharge from the penis, vagina, or anus; pain on urination or defecation or during sexual intercourse; pain and swelling in the pelvic region; genital and oral infections may be asymptomatic | Antibiotics |
| Hepatitis B | Low-grade fever, fatigue, headaches, loss of appetite, nausea, dark urine, jaundice | |
| Genital herpes | Usually occur within 2 weeks: painful blisters on site(s) of infection (genitals, anus, cervix); occasionally itching, painful urination, and fever | None; acyclovir relieves symptoms |
| Pubic lice | Usually occur within 5 weeks: intense itching in the genital region; lice may be visible in pubic hair; small white eggs may be visible on pubic hair | Gamma benzene hexachloride |
| Syphilis | Usually occur within 3 weeks: a chancre (painless sore) on the genitals, anus, or mouth; secondary stage—skin rash—if left untreated; tertiary stage includes diseases of several body organs | Antibiotics |
| *Trichomonas vaginalis* | Yellowish-green vaginal discharge with an unpleasant odor; vaginal itching; occasionally painful intercourse | Metronidazole |

*Source:* Edlin G., Golanty E., and McCormack Brown K. *Health and Wellness,* 6th ed., Boston: Jones and Bartlett, 1999:222.

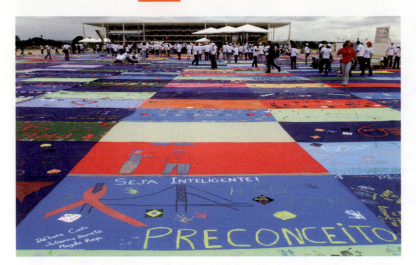

# HIV and AIDS

The human immunodeficiency virus (HIV) was first discovered and infection with it was first diagnosed as a new disease in 1981, although medical record reviews show the symptoms of HIV infection occurring well before then. The development of the virus is progressive, multiplying over the course over many years. During this time, the virus slowly causes the deterioration of the body's immune system. When the disease has progressed to a stage where the body becomes vulnerable to opportunistic infection, the disease is classified as acquired immunodeficiency syndrome

### What's the word...

**human immuno-deficiency virus (HIV)** The virus that causes AIDS.

**acquired immuno-deficiency syndrome (AIDS)** Late-stage development of HIV infection.

| Table 12.2 | HIV/AIDS Worldwide and in the United States | |
|---|---|---|
| | **World** | **United States** |
| Number living with HIV/AIDS | 37.8 million | 850,000–950,000 |
| Percent females/males | 50/50 | 20/80 |
| New cases annually | 4.8 million | 40,000 |
| New cases daily | 13,000 | 110 |
| Percent new cases less than 25 years old/more than 25 years old | 60/40 | 50/50 |
| Deaths from AIDS | 20 million | 500,000 |
| Cases by location | 70% sub-Saharan Africa<br>16% Asia/Pacific area<br>4% Europe<br>4% Latin America<br>3% North America<br>>1% Middle East<br>1% Caribbean<br><1% Australia | – |
| Method of infection in new cases: men | – | 60% homosexual sex<br>25% injection drug use<br>15% heterosexual sex |
| Race of infected person for new cases: men | – | 50% black<br>30% white<br>20% Hispanic<br><1% other |
| Method of infection in new cases: women | – | 75% heterosexual sex<br>25% injection drug use |
| Race of infected person for new cases: women | – | 64% black<br>18% white<br>18% Hispanic<br><1% other |

*Sources:* World Health Organization, 2002; National Institute of Allergy and Infectious Disease, 2004.

(AIDS). This deterioration eventually renders the body defenseless against all sorts of diseases.

Today, HIV is one of the top 10 causes of death among people aged 25 to 41. Nearly 1 million people in the United States are currently infected with HIV `Table 12.2`. More than 40,000 new cases of HIV in the United States were reported to the Centers for Disease Control and Prevention (CDC) in 2002. As `Figure 12.1` and `Figure 12.2` show, rates of infection are higher among men than among women in this country.

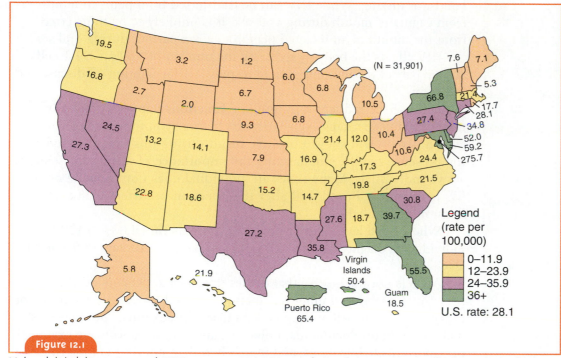

**Figure 12.1**

Male adult/adolescent annual AIDS rates per 100,000 population, for cases reported in 2001, United States. *Source:* Centers for Disease Control and Prevention. *HIV/AIDS Surveillance Report* 2001; 13:12.

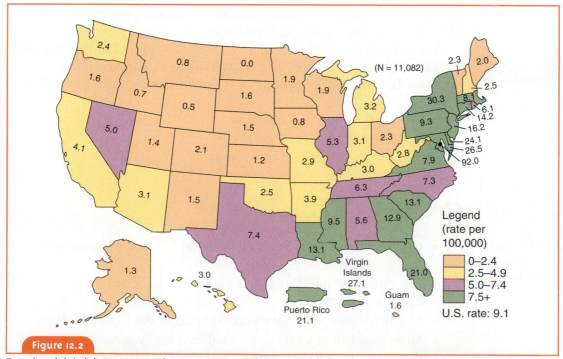

**Figure 12.2**

Female adult/adolescent annual AIDS rates per 100,000 population, for cases reported in 2001, United States. *Source:* Centers for Disease Control and Prevention. *HIV/AIDS Surveillance Report* 2001; 13:12.

## Opportunistic Infections

### Cancers
Kaposi's sarcoma
Primary lymphoma of the brain

### Protozoal and Helminthic
Cryptosporidiosis, intestinal (causing diarrhea for more than 1 month)
*Pneumocystis carinii* pneumonia
Strongyloidiasis (pneumonia, CNS infection, or disseminated infection)
Toxoplasmosis (pneumonia or CNS infection)

### Fungal Infections
Aspergillosis (CNS or disseminated infection)
Candidiasis (esophagitis)
Cryptococcosis (pulmonary, CNS, or disseminated infection)
Histoplasmosis (disseminated)

### Bacterial Infection
Atypical *Mycobacterium* species other than *M. tuberculosis* or *M. leprae* (disseminated infection)

### Viral Infection
Cytomegalovirus (pulmonary, gastrointestinal tract, or CNS infection)
Herpes simplex virus
　Chronic mucocutaneous ulcers persisting longer than 1 month
　Pulmonary, gastrointestinal tract, or disseminated infection
Progressive multifocal leukoencephalopathy (presumed papovavirus)

*Source:* www.AIDSMeds.com.

**What's the word. . .**

**intravenous drug use**
Drug use occurring by injecting the drug directly into the bloodstream using a needle and syringe.

**T cells** The immune system's primary defense system to fight disease.

**chlamydia** A bacterial infection caused by *Chlamydia trichomatis*.

HIV is transmitted in three ways: through sexual activity with an infected person, to a newborn child from exposure to infected blood of the mother or through breast-feeding, and through blood transfer caused by sharing needles during intravenous drug use. All methods of transfer (except breast-feeding) occur through the transfer of blood, semen, or vaginal fluids of an infected person to an uninfected person. HIV is not transferred through touch, casual contact, tears, or saliva. Thus you cannot obtain HIV by drinking from the glass of an infected person, shaking hands, or kissing. While HIV can be transferred from penis to mouth or from vagina to mouth during oral sex, it is unlikely to be transferred from the mouth of an infected person to a sex partner during oral sex.

HIV affects the body by reducing the number of T cells. CD4 T cells are the part of the immune system responsible for fighting off disease and infection.

Because the reduction in immune functions happens gradually, it may be many (perhaps even 10) years before symptoms occur. However, a person will show a positive result during this time if tested for the presence of HIV, emphasizing the importance of testing for sexually active individuals. Many times an individual does not know he or she has been infected until well after the infection occurred, making transmission more likely.

When T-cell levels drop below 200 (from an initial 800 to 1200), an individual is diagnosed with AIDS. It can take 7 to 10 years to reach this level.

AIDS is not the disease that causes the affected person's death. Because of its reduced immune function, the body is susceptible to opportunistic infections—that is, infections that take advantage of the body's inability to fight. Pneumonia, influenza, and certain cancers are examples of opportunistic infections, and more often than not they are the cause of death for persons with AIDS.

Testing is critical. HIV testing is conducted at local health departments, hospitals, private doctors' offices, and a variety of community sites. Look for testing at a place that also provides counseling so you can have any questions you might have answered.

You can call the CDC's National AIDS Hotline to find testing site locations throughout the country as well as to obtain additional information regarding HIV and AIDS. The service is provided 24 hours a day, 365 days a year at:

800-342-AIDS (800-342-2437)
800-AIDS-TTY (800-243-7889): TTY
800-344-SIDA (800-344-7432): Spanish

# Chlamydia

- **Chlamydia** is the most common bacterial STI in the United States **Figure 12.3**.
- It is caused by infection with *Chlamydia trichomatis* bacteria, invading cells and reproducing.
- Nearly 850,000 new cases were reported to the CDC in 2002.
- More than half of all those infected have no symptoms, increasing the opportunity for transmission to a new sex partner.

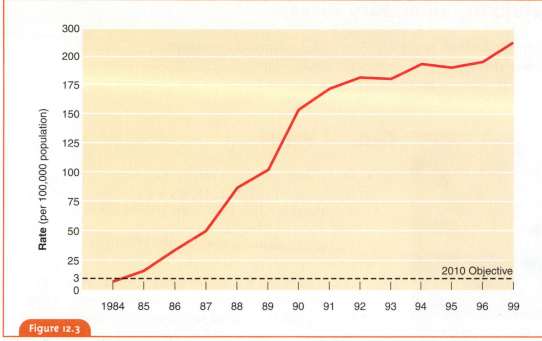

**Figure 12.3**

Chlamydia—reported rates: United States, 1984–1999.
*Source:* Division of STI Prevention. *Sexually transmitted disease surveillance, 1999.* U.S. Department of Health and Human Services, Public Health Service. Atlanta: Centers for Disease Control and Prevention (September 2000), 10.

- Those with symptoms experience urethritis, an inflammation of the urethra causing pain in urination or discharge from the penis or vagina.
- As a bacterial infection, once detected, chlamydia can be treated with antibiotics.
- Left untreated, chlamydia can develop into pelvic inflammatory disease (PID), which can lead to infertility.

## Gonorrhea

- Gonorrhea is a bacterial infection caused by *Niesseria gonorrhoeae*.
- It is often co-diagnosed with chlamydia.
- Approximately 700,000 new cases occurred in the United States in 2002.
- Frequently referred to as "clap" or "drip," gonorrhea infects the body by growing in the mucous membranes of the genital area.
- Symptoms, for those who have them, include painful urination and a pus-like, yellow discharge from the vagina or penis.
- As a bacterial infection, gonorrhea can be treated with antibiotics.
- Left untreated, it can cause sterility.
- Due to the widespread treatment of gonorrhea, some antibiotics have become ineffective, and the development of new treatment options is necessary.

**What's the word. . .**
**gonorrhea** A bacterial infection caused by *Niesseria gonorrhoeae.*

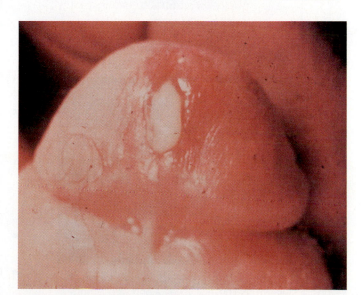

Gonorrheal discharge from the penis.

# Pelvic Inflammatory Disease

- **PID** develops as a result of untreated chlamydia or gonorrhea.
- It develops only in women and involves infection of the fallopian tubes and uterus.
- PID can lead to infertility if left untreated.

## Genital Warts

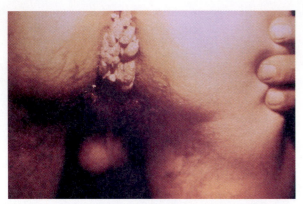

Genital warts in the anal area are caused by infection of the skin by papilloma viruses. Genital warts can be removed by a variety of treatments but sometimes recur.

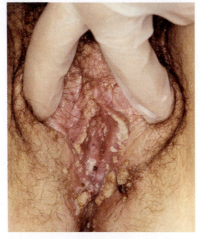

Genital warts on the vaginal area.

- **Genital warts** occur as a result of exposure to human papillomavirus (HPV). All warts—STIs and otherwise—are caused by HPV. More than 100 strains of HPV exist, only a few of which cause genital warts. Approximately 6.2 million people acquired HPV in 2002.
- Infection with HPV is most prevalent in college-aged (22 to 25 years) women. Because of their often high level of sexual risk taking—predominantly neglecting to use a condom during sexual activity—and a general lack of understanding of the likelihood and severity of acquiring HPV, as many as 60% of college women have or have had HPV.
- Genital warts appear as nonpainful, hard clusters of bumps on the penis of men, the vagina of women, and the anal region of both men and women. Bumps develop as a result of uncontrolled skin growth.
- The major concern of genital warts is their association with cervical cancer in women. Four strains of HPV are responsible for most of the cases of cervical cancer in the United States. All will be detected through a Pap smear, reinforcing the importance of annual testing for sexually active women.
- Genital warts are viral and cannot be treated with antibiotics. They are usually removed in one of three ways: freezing, application of a podophyllin-based cream, or burning through the use of an acid or laser technique.

## Genital Herpes

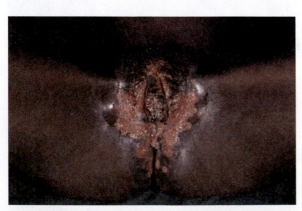

Symptoms of primary herpes genitalis include painful lesions, a sluggish feeling, and fever, along with lymph-node enlargement.

- **Genital herpes** is caused by the herpes simplex virus (HSV). Humans are susceptible to 4 of the approximately 70 viruses in the HSV family. Genital herpes is the sexually transmitted form of HSV. Humans are also susceptible to forms that cause chickenpox, shingles, and Epstein-Barr disease, and to cytomegalovirus, which can cause death in infants if acquired as a fetus.
- As a viral infection, genital herpes cannot be cured, although the frequency of outbreaks can be managed.
- Genital herpes appears as fluid-filled blisters or open sores most frequently found on or in the genitals (HSV-2), but can also appear in the mouth if transmitted

| Table 12.3 | STIs and Minorities |
|---|---|

Surveillance data show high rates of STIs for some minority racial or ethnic groups compared with rates for whites. Race and ethnicity in the United States are risk markers that correlate with other more fundamental determinants of health status such as poverty, access to high-quality health care, health-care–seeking behavior, illicit drug use, and residence in communities with high prevalence of STIs.

### Chlamydia

Chlamydia trends show consistently higher rates among women.

### Gonorrhea

In 2001, African Americans accounted for 75% of total cases of gonorrhea. The overall gonorrhea rates were 782.3 cases per 100,000 for African Americans and 74.2 for Hispanics compared to 29.4 for non-Hispanic whites.

In 2001, African American females 15 to 19 years old had a gonorrhea rate of 3495.2 cases per 100,000 population. African American men in this age group had a gonorrhea rate of 1794.1 per 100,000. These rates were on average 46 times higher than those of 15- to 19-year-old white adolescents. Among 20- to 24-year-olds, the gonorrhea rate among African Americans was almost 24 times that of whites.

### Syphilis

Since 1990, rates of primary and secondary syphilis have declined among all racial and ethnic groups. However, rates for African Americans and Hispanics continue to be higher than for non-Hispanic whites. In 2001, African Americans accounted for 62.5% of all cases of primary and secondary syphilis. Although the rate for African Americans declined from 12.2 cases per 100,000 population in 2000 to 11.0 per 100,000 in 2001, the rate was 15.7 times the non-Hispanic white rate of 0.7 per 100,000.

In 2001, the rate of congenital syphilis in African Americans was 37.8 per 100,000 live births and 20.1 in Hispanics compared to 1.8 in whites.

Reducing the prevalence of many of these STIs in minority populations will require a combination of strategies. Of course, education about prevention is important. Still, education will not have a significant effect in minority populations if it is not combined with strategies to reduce poverty, increase access to good-quality health care, decrease drug abuse and the sharing of drug "works," and create comprehensive sexuality education programs that start in schools at early ages and continue through community agencies into the adult years.

*Source:* Division of STI Prevention. *Sexually Transmitted Disease Surveillance, 2001.* U.S. Department of Health and Human Services, Public Health Service. Atlanta: CDC, September 2002.

**What's the word...**

**pelvic inflammatory disease (PID)** Complication in women caused by untreated chlamydia or gonorrhea.

**genital warts** One of many strains of human papillomavirus (HPV) transmitted through sexual contact, causing hard, round bumps on the skin surrounding the genitalia.

**genital herpes** Sexually transmitted disease caused by the herpes simplex virus.

through oral sexual contact (HSV-1). Symptoms subside after 2 or 3 weeks, but the virus remains in the body and symptoms may recur at any time.

■ It is estimated that in 2002 one in five American adults (approximately 45 million people older than age 12) had been infected with HSV. Each year, 500,000 people acquire the disease. The incidence rate must be estimated, as it is not mandatory for the medical profession to report cases of herpes to the CDC.

■ The most common medication used in reducing the number and severity of outbreaks is acyclovir.

■ Women with herpes are susceptible to cervical cancer and are encouraged to complete an annual Pap smear to check for cancerous cell development.

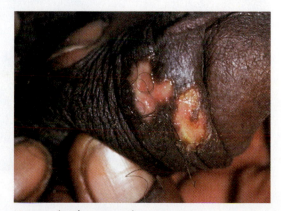

Herpes simplex on penis.

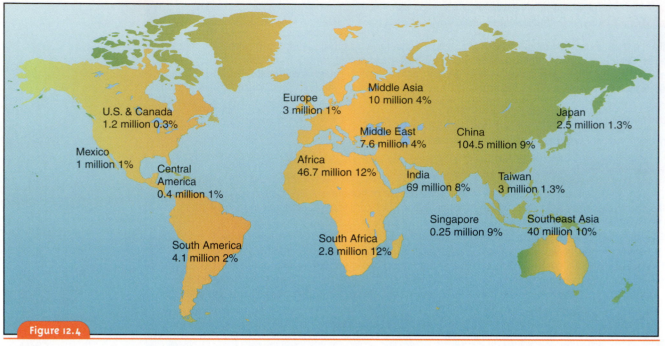

**Figure 12.4**

Hepatitis B infection worldwide. The number of people infected with hepatitis B virus in 1997 in the world and the percentage infected in each region. *Source:* World Health Organization, 1997.

**What's the word. . .**

**hepatitis B** One of a family of diseases that slowly destroy the functioning ability of the liver.

**syphilis** Sexually transmitted disease caused by spirochete bacteria.

**chancre** A predominantly painless open sore occurring in the early stages of syphilis.

# Hepatitis B

- There are currently seven known forms of **hepatitis** (A through G). Hepatitis B (see **Figure 12.4**) is the form most commonly transmitted through sexual contact, although it is also acquired through other blood transfer methods such as needle sharing in drug use, sweat, saliva, and breast milk.
- Hepatitis slowly destroys the ability of the liver to function properly. A transplant is often necessary after a person has had the disease for many years.
- A vaccine for this disease does exist.

# Syphilis

- **Syphilis** is a bacterial infection, meaning that it can be treated with antibiotics. Penicillin has long been the most effective treatment for syphilis.
- Approximately 32,000 new cases were reported in 2002, although the number of cases of syphilis seems to vary more than the numbers of cases of other STIs from year to year.
- Early symptoms are generally mild and can be missed. The first sign is usually a **chancre**, an open sore that does not cause pain and is located on or around the genitals, anus, or mouth. It may appear between 1 and 3 months after the initial infection is acquired.

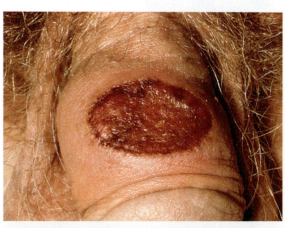

The first physical sign of a syphilis infection is an open lesion called a chancre.

■ When left untreated or undetected, syphilis can turn into a body-wide rash. In later stages it can affect the heart and nervous system and, while it may take years to develop, can eventually cause death.

# Prevention of Sexually Transmitted Infections

You can protect yourself from STIs. Educating yourself is the first step. Understanding the likelihood of contracting STIs will help you to make wise decisions regarding your sexual activity.

Self-assessment is absolutely necessary to keep yourself aware of possible behaviors or risk factors that may increase your chance of being infected with an STI. Answer the following questions regarding your sexual behavior to take an initial look at your possible risks:

1. Are you sexually active (including vaginal, oral, or anal sexual activity)?
2. Are you sexually active with several partners?
3. Have you been sexually active while under the influence of alcohol or other drugs?
4. When you are sexually active, do you rarely or never use a barrier-type contraceptive?
5. Have you used a needle to inject drugs?
6. Do you rarely or never ask about the sexual history of the individuals with whom you choose to be sexually active?

Answering "yes" to any of these questions indicates that you have an increased risk for the acquisition of an STI. Answering several questions with a "yes" indicates a need to expand your knowledge regarding the risks involved with being sexually active.

Practicing safer sex is essential to safeguarding against an STI. This includes practicing safer sex. **Abstinence**, a complete refrain from sexual activity, is the only sure method to stay STI free. If you choose to be sexually active, there are many ways to diminish your personal risk. See **Table 12.4** for some of these strategies.

> **What's the word . . .**
>
> **abstinence** Complete refrain from sexual activity.

| Table 12.4 | Eliminating or Reducing Your Risk of HIV Infection and Other STIs |
|---|---|
| **How to Eliminate Your Risk** | **How to Reduce Your Risk** |
| • Abstain from sex.<br><br>If that is not an option:<br>• Do not have sex with HIV-infected individuals or those infected with any STI.<br>• Engage in sex only in a monogamous relationship in which it is certain that neither partner is infected.<br>• Abstain from using drugs. | • Reduce your number of sexual partners.<br>• Avoid having sex with high-risk partners.<br>• Avoid having sex with people you do not know well.<br>• Avoid having sex while under the influence of drugs, including alcohol.<br>• Use a new latex condom during each act of sexual intercourse.<br>• Never share needles or syringes. |

*Note:* People in certain professions, such as health care workers and police officers, have additional risks of infection due to the nature of their work. Such risks are not eliminated by these practices. These people can become infected with hepatitis B virus or HIV if their blood mixes with the blood or bodily secretions of an infected person.

## Reflect >>>> Reinforce >>>> Reinvigorate

### Knowledge Check

*Answers in Appendix D.*

1. The virus that causes AIDS is called:

   A. HSV
   B. HPV
   C. HIV
   D. PID

2. An individual believing that he or she can never contract a sexually transmitted disease is in which stage of change?

   A. Precontemplation
   B. Contemplation
   C. Action
   D. Maintenance

3. The most common sexually transmitted infection is:

   A. Syphilis
   B. Genital warts
   C. Chlamydia
   D. HIV

4. Which of the following STIs has no cure?

   A. Chlamydia
   B. Gonorrhea
   C. Syphilis
   D. Herpes

5. Which of the following increases the likelihood of contracting an STI?

   A. Poor communication skills
   B. Failure to use a condom every time there is sexual intercourse
   C. Denying one's likelihood of obtaining an STI
   D. All of the above

6. Which of the following develops as a complication from an undetected STI?

   A. Pelvic inflammatory disease
   B. Herpes
   C. HIV
   D. Genital warts

7. A disease that takes advantage of the body's weakened immune system is called a(n):

   A. Sexually transmitted disease
   B. Biological intruder
   C. Opportunistic infection
   D. Viral disease

8. An open sore that usually appears as a result of exposure to syphilis is called a:

   A. Sarcoma
   B. Chancre
   C. T-cell abnormality
   D. Blot

9. Refraining from sexual intercourse is called:
   A. Deterrence
   B. Suspension
   C. Abstinence
   D. Asceticism

10. The type of sexually transmitted infection that slowly destroys the liver's ability to function properly is called:
   A. Syphilis
   B. Herpes
   C. Chlamydia
   D. Hepatitis B

## Modern Modifications

- Develop a comfort level for discussing sex. Like any other skill, the more you practice communicating about sexual activity, the more naturally it will come over time. In this instance, what you don't know can and will hurt you.
- Always use a condom during sexual activity.
- Because so many STIs have no visible symptoms, make a point of being tested regularly if you are sexually active.
- Sexually active women should visit their physician for a Pap smear every year.
- Don't believe that "it won't happen to you." Every person who has an STI said the same thing.
- Don't make decisions regarding your sexual activity while under the influence of alcohol or other drugs. If you are in a social situation and are concerned you'll make a poor decision, ask a friend to help you get home safely.
- Try to remember that there are alternatives to intimacy: Vaginal or oral sex are not your only options.

## Going Above and Beyond

### Websites

American Social Health Association
*www.ashastd.org*

National Center for Health Statistics
*www.cdc.gov/nchs/fastats/Default.htm*

Facts about Sexually Transmitted Diseases
*www.womenshealth.about.com/cs/stds/a/sextrandisfacts.htm*

American International AIDS Foundation
*www.aids.com*

Communication in Sexual Behavior
*www.couns.msu.edu/self-help/behavior.htm*

National HIV Testing Resources
*www.hivtest.org*

## References and Suggested Readings

Alters S. and Schiff W. *Essential Concepts for Healthy Living,* 3rd ed. Sudbury, MA: Jones and Bartlett, 2003.

Bernard A. and Prince A. HIV testing practices and attitudes of college students. *American Journal of Health Studies* 1998; 14:84.

Centers for Disease Control and Prevention (CDC). National HIV testing resources. www.hivtest.org (accessed March 22, 2005).

Edlin G. and Golanty E. *Health and Wellness,* 8th ed. Sudbury, MA: Jones and Bartlett, 2004.

Greenberg J. S., Bruess C. E., and Haffner D. W. *Exploring the Dimensions of Sexual Activity.* Sudbury, MA: Jones and Bartlett, 2004.

*HIV/AIDS Statistics: Facts and Figures.* Bethesda, MD: Office of Communications and Public Liaison, National Institute of Allergy and Infectious Disease, National Institutes of Health, 2004.

Ingledue K., Cottrell R., and Bernard A. College women's knowledge, perceptions, and preventative behaviors regarding human papillomavirus and cervical cancer. *American Journal of Health Studies* 2004; 19:28.

Luquis R. R., Garcia E., and Ashford D. A qualitative assessment of college students' perceptions of health behaviors. *American Journal of Health Studies* 2003; 18:156.

McCormack Brown K., Thomas D. Q., and Kotecki J. E. *Physical Activity and Health.* Sudbury, MA: Jones and Bartlett, 2002.

World Health Organization (WHO). *Report on the Global HIV/AIDS Epidemic.* 2002: 190–201.

## Critical Thinking

Herpes is a sexually transmitted disease that lasts a lifetime; however, herpes can be managed with medication. Explain, in detail, how you would go about telling your new partner that you have herpes.

## Relationships

Relationships don't just happen; they must be built. They require a commitment and effort, every day, often when you don't feel like giving to your partner or working through conflict.

### Why the House?

- Foundation: Issues such as money, commitment, sex, and personal values are items that relationships must work on bringing balance to the relationship.
- When the foundation is strong, the house stands tall. When the foundation is weak, the house may fall.
- Just because one aspect of the relationship may be weaker than the others, it is the accumulation of strength from all the pillars that keeps the house standing. Working on the weaker aspects doesn't diminish the other pillars, but it does strengthen the entire foundation.
- Each room in the house represents a skill necessary to maintain the foundation.

## Rooms

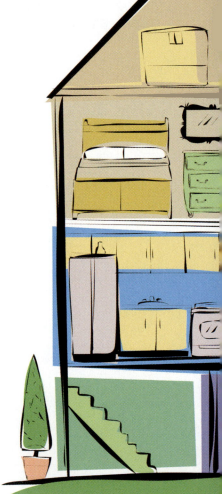

Foundation: Values, Career, Money, Faith, Health, Sex, Children, Activities, Friends, Education, Commitment, Time

### 1 Communication

- The largest room in the house.
- When at its best, feelings are recognized and shared, respect is created, and agreements can be made.
- When at its worst, feelings are ignored and resentment develops. Eventually, one partner may feel as though he or she has no value.
- Includes taking responsibility for your feelings (not blaming another for how you feel), proposing constructive solutions to issues, effective listening, and using appropriate nonverbal communication.

### 2 Conflict Resolution

- All relationships have conflict.
- Members of successful relationships understand how to work through feelings of anger and frustration without causing physical or emotional damage to their partners.
- Be clear about the issue you wish to discuss.
- Address only one issue at a time.
- Agree with each other that the discussion will be civil, even when there is disagreement.
- Propose a resolution to the issue.
- Reconnect at a later date to make sure the agreement is working.

## 3 Respect

- A key to gaining the trust of your partner is to show respect when conflict is present.
- Conflict and disagreement are inevitable. It's how you handle the inevitable that determines the quality of the relationship.
- Show your partner you understand how he or she feels. Then try to determine what might have happened to generate the misunderstanding.
- Remember that feelings are genuine, even when they are in opposition with yours. You cannot dictate how another person will feel; you can only try to help that person understand your side of the story.
- Belittling, demeaning, or failing to acknowledge another's feelings (for example, "Oh, that's just ridiculous!") will only grow resentment in the relationship.

## 4 Intimacy

- Intimacy is the ability to relate emotions in the relationship, to effectively tell your partner how you feel. When we can honestly tell someone how we feel and what we need, without blaming or accusing, we open the door to communication.
- It has nothing to do with sex.
- Relationships with well-developed intimacy feature a bond between partners beyond the physical limitations of the sexual component of the relationship.

## 5 Love

- Love is the combination of the set of emotions involving intimacy, respect, and commitment to a long-term future.
- It is the result of a mutual attempt by both partners in the relationship to address the needs of their partner, often before one's own needs are considered.
- A person in love does not have the desire to be with someone other than his or her partner.
- Love is a reflection of a sense of obligation to another.

# Responsible Decision Making

## Objectives

After reading this chapter, you should be able to:

- Describe a lifetime fitness program.
- Evaluate a health/fitness club for reliability.
- Recognize myths and false claims about exercise nostrums.
- Assess exercise equipment before purchasing.
- List precautions to take when using hydrotherapy equipment or facilities.
- Evaluate Internet information.
- Identify exercise misinformation and quackery.

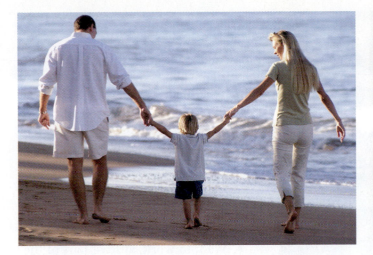
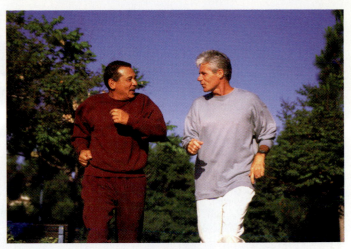

## Childhood to Old Age

If you expect to become a parent, bear this in mind: A physically active life begins in childhood. You will do your children no favors if you allow them to watch television or play computer games most of the time. Encourage children to balance those activities with sports, games, or other physical activity that they enjoy. Also, remember that as a parent you are a model for your child. Take time to do activities with your children to encourage them to spend time exercising.

Continue to exercise as you age. You'll have a healthier heart and fitter body. Exercise can reduce blood pressure, make your joints more flexible, and increase muscular strength and endurance. Not only your body benefits: You will improve your mood and your cognitive functions as well.

Keeping your balance as you age is a major issue. Falls that a young person bounces back from can incapacitate or be fatal for older people. Falls in old age are usually the result of poor balance, and keeping fit improves balance.

Even if you did not start early, you can start late. Light to moderate exercise will improve your health at any age—for example, mall-walking, dancing, t'ai chi, or fitness classes designed for older people.

### What's the word...

**endurance** Ability to work out for a period of time without fatigue.

**mall-walking** Walking a circuit around the lobby floors of an enclosed shopping mall in the morning, often before the stores open.

**t'ai chi** Thirteenth-century Chinese exercise routine involving graceful dance-like movements.

## College Students

Now is the time to make exercise a permanent part of your life. Most colleges try to make it convenient for you. Did you know the following?

- Your college or university probably offers a variety of fitness and sports courses and intramural athletic programs.
- College gyms and athletic fields usually have times designated for recreational student use and have some of the best trainers and equipment.

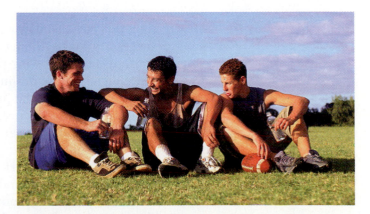

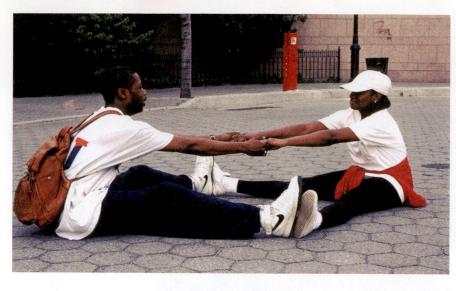

## After College

It may take a bit more initiative, especially if your job is desk-bound, but you will be healthier if you create a personal program of physical activity and exercise after college.

Choose activities you like; you are more likely to stick with them throughout your life.

There are some simple ways to make a difference in your daily physical activity:

- Walk to work, at least part of the way.
- Use the stairs, not the elevator.
- Walk during lunchtime.
- Ride a bicycle.

To be more serious about it, you can exercise at home, join a fitness club, or use the exercise facilities in your office building.

If you like to exercise at home, you can buy barbells and hand weights for **resistance training**, and for aerobic exercise, use a rowing machine, stationary bike, treadmill, stair climber, or cross-country ski machine. A great way to decide whether these are the best pieces of equipment to purchase for home use is to try them out at a fitness club before buying them.

If you like the social aspects of belonging to a fitness club or find it more motivating, by all means join one, but look before you leap.

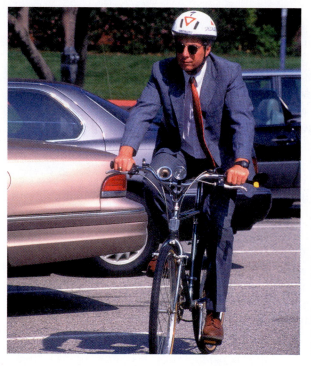

> **What's the word...**
> **resistance training**
> Building muscle by working against the resistance of weights.

## Steps in Decision Making

After reading this book, and especially this chapter, you should realize that many decisions are necessary for beginning and maintaining a healthy lifestyle. To make good decisions, you can use the following procedure. This procedure applies to any of life's decisions, not merely those dealing with a healthy lifestyle:

1. **Identify and clarify the problem.** You must recognize that a problem exists. Some may simply be annoyances, while others are big issues.
2. **Gather information.** Learn more about the problem situation. Look for possible causes and solutions.
3. **Evaluate the evidence.** How accurate is the information? Is it fact or opinion?
4. **Consider alternatives and implications.** Draw conclusions, then weigh the advantages and disadvantages of each alternative.
5. **Choose and implement the best alternative.**

## Tipping Point

### Selecting a Fitness Professional Who Is Right for You

- Is the fitness professional's workspace convenient to your workplace or home, or is training available in your home?
- Are new clients provided with a pre-exercise screening for health risk factors, and is a fitness program designed specifically for their needs?
- Does the fitness professional offer the expertise, programs, and services you need to achieve your fitness goals?

## How to Choose a Fitness Facility

Gyms offer a great number of resources and allow you access to expensive equipment and a variety of fitness classes. But be wary of a high-pressure sales pitch. Once you walk into a gym with one of its promotional fliers, the sales staff will do everything in their power to persuade you to join that day. Take some steps to find out if this is the best gym for you and then take some time to assess whether you can afford the membership.

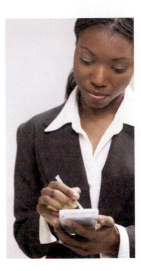

- Find out how much it costs: Can you afford it? Never join a gym the first time you go. Ask to try out the club for a period of time before signing up. Then you can assess whether you will make the effort to go before making the financial investment. Membership frequently requires a year-long commitment.
- Check equipment quality and general cleanliness. Check out the changing rooms and showers.
- Interview the club's trainers. Ask for their credentials and names of clients you can call.
- Ask them to describe a plan they might recommend for you.
- Ask how long the club has been in business.

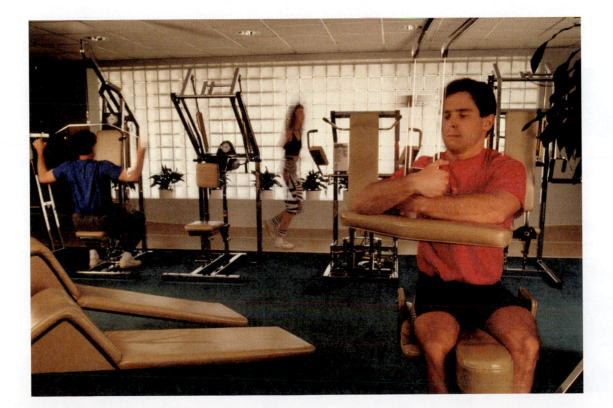

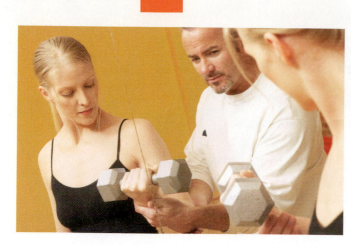

- Check references. Talk to current clients, the Better Business Bureau, and the consumer protection department of the local district attorney's office to see if there are any complaints against the club.
- Again, do not sign a contract on the spot. Double-check what the monthly fees are and ask what the initial joining fee is. Ask if fees exist for special programs, pool time, or court time.
- How do you end membership at the gym? Do you need to show proof of moving from the area? Do you have to pay a penalty for leaving before the contract ends?
- Check with your health insurance company. Often many insurance companies reinburse some or all of the cost of a gym membership.
- How far is the gym from your house and work? If it is too far out of the way, will you go often enough to make joining the gym a cost-effective decision?
- Does the fitness professional have **CPR** certification, the appropriate educational background, and fitness certification from nationally recognized organizations? Is the fitness professional accredited?
- Does the fitness professional abide by recognized regulations, standards, or guidelines accepted for personalized training in the fitness industry, and if so, what are they?

## Precautions When Using Hydrotherapy Equipment

One of the benefits of a health club membership can be using the sauna, steam bath, whirlpool, or hot tub. They do not do anything to make you more fit, but they can make you feel better. However, there are some precautions to keep in mind:

- Make sure the equipment is kept clean, and that a hot tub/whirlpool is chlorinated and has the right **pH**.
- Make sure the temperature is not hotter than 100 °F for a whirlpool/hot tub, 120 °F for a steam bath, or 190 °F for a sauna.
- Shower with soap before and after using the facilities.
- Don't stay in longer than 10 to 15 minutes.
- Stay hydrated: Drink water before or during use.
- Be careful about overheating yourself:
  - Wait an hour after eating.
  - Cool down after exercising.
  - Don't drink alcohol beforehand.
  - Don't exercise while you are in the hot tub or sauna.
  - Get out immediately if you get a headache or feel dizzy, hot, chilled, or nauseated.

**What's the word...**

**CPR (cardiopulmonary resuscitation)** Clearing air passages to the lungs, giving mouth-to-mouth respiration, and massaging the heart to restore normal breathing after cardiac arrest.

**pH** Condition of a solution represented by a number on a scale of acidity to alkalinity.

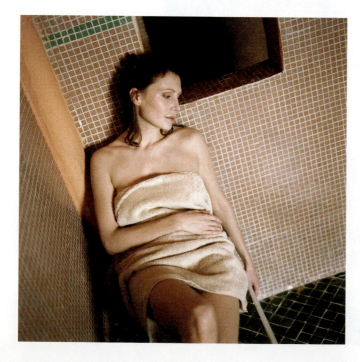

- Don't wear makeup, skin lotion, or jewelry.
- Don't go in by yourself.
- If you have any health problems or are on medication, check first with your doctor.
- Do not submerse you entire body if you have a heart condition or may be pregnant. The hot temperature may be harmful to the fetus.

# Purchasing Exercise Equipment

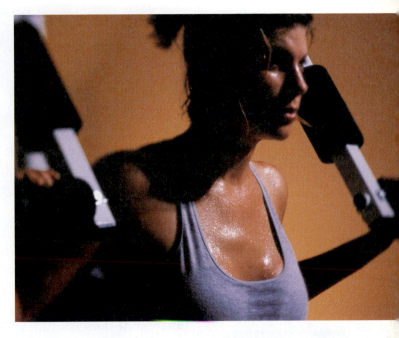

After checking the advertised claims for exercise equipment, consider these questions before buying:

- Most important, will the equipment help you achieve your desired goal—build strength, improve endurance, and so on?
- Will you use the equipment? Most home exercise equipment goes unused.
- Do you have room for it?
- Will you have to disassemble the equipment to store it?
- Is it so noisy it will bother your neighbors?
- Check out consumer and fitness magazines that rate exercise equipment.
- Test equipment at a local gym or retailer to find one that feels comfortable to you.
- What's the best deal? Shop around.
- Get details on warranties, guarantees, and return policies. Try to buy from a seller who offers a 30-day money-back guarantee.
- Check out the seller's customer service and support.

You may get a great deal from a secondhand store, consignment shop, yard sale, or the classified ads, but be aware:

- Items bought secondhand usually cannot be returned and don't carry the warranties of new equipment.
- Ask about total costs before buying. The ad may quote a low price, but not include shipping and handling fees, sales tax, and delivery and set-up fees.

# Exercise Myths or Misconceptions

Misconceptions exist about what is exercise fact and what is exercise fiction. Here are some common exercise-related fallacies:

- Passive muscle stimulators expend energy from the electrical outlet in the wall, not from your cells. The energy expended to bring about fat loss must be from within your body.
- Taking a pill to bring about instant changes in fitness is an illusion. Fitness takes time and effort. The body systems (muscular, cardiovascular, and skeletal) become stronger in response to regular physical activity.
- Cellulite is not something a health gadget or cream can eliminate. Rapid gain or loss of body fat causes the dimpled look associated with the term *cellulite*.
- Shake, rattle, or roll your fat—it won't disappear. The *only* way to reduce body fat is to use more energy than you consume in calories.

*What's the word. . .*

**cellulite** Adipose tissue surrounded by stretched connective tissue.

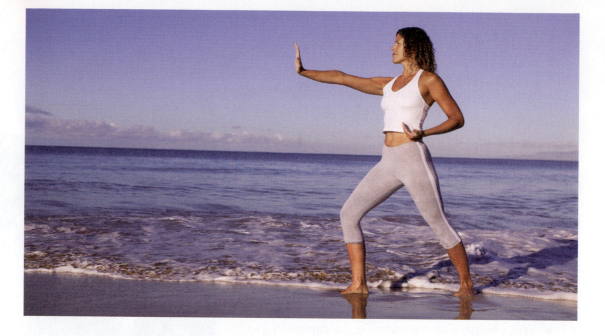

- Wearing rubberized suits, extra layers of clothing, or working out in a hot environment loses water, not fat. It takes a great deal of heat to melt fat. Such heat would melt the rest of you as well.

- If spot reduction worked, everyone who chewed gum or talked a lot would have a narrow face.

- Exercise does not turn fat cells into muscle cells, nor does inactivity turn muscle cells into fat. They are different types of cells. Eat too much and be inactive, and you will enlarge (hypertrophy) the fat cells in your body and shrink (atrophy) the muscle cells. Eat right and exercise to do the reverse.

- Rubbing lotions on the skin to lose fat, firm up muscles, or remove lactic acid does not work. Resistance training firms up muscles.

- Eating extra protein to build stronger muscles doesn't work. Eat more protein than your body uses and the extra will be stored by your body as fat. Increased muscle size comes through resistance training.

- Losing inches is not necessarily loss of fat. It can also be loss of water or lean muscle tissue.

- Exercise is only tiring momentarily. It then makes you feel more energetic as you become more fit.

- In women, resistance training mainly increases muscle strength, not size.

- Drinking liquids during exercise does not cause cramping. Cool water or other appropriate drinks (not soda) should be consumed before, during, and after exercising to replace lost fluids.

## Evaluating the Quality of Internet Information Sources

You can find information on just about everything on the Internet. Of course, not all Internet sites are created equal. Some present research and information, some are trying to sell a product, and some are flat-out misinformation. Here are some suggestions on how to decide whether the information you find is quality and reputable:

1. **Check for the creator of the site.** It is important to be able to identify whom the authors or creators of the site are. The author should include his or her credentials

to demonstrate his or her training and expertise in the subject matter. If this information is missing, be cautious.

2. **Check the URL.** Website addresses that end with .edu are material from an educational or research institution. Those ending in .gov are government sources. Those ending with .com or .biz are commercial sites generally intended to sell a product. Because the content of websites is not monitored for accuracy, you may be reading inaccurate, biased, misleading, partial, or false information. This is much more likely to occur on commercial sites than on any other type of website. In addition, if the URL includes a personal name, the site may simply be an individual creating a forum for his or her personal opinion.

3. **Check for advertising.** Websites often accept advertising to help pay the cost of maintaining the site. If the products being advertised are the same as or related to the nature of the information you seek, be cautious. You'd hate to rely on information that has been biased so as not to offend or upset an advertiser. When that happens, you can be certain the information you are viewing is misleading.

4. **Look for accuracy.** Be on the lookout for sites that integrate personal opinions, testimonials, or leading statements about the material you are searching for. Do not assume the first site you visit has accurate information. Gather information from several sites on the same topic and look for common themes. Sites that go into greater depth with their information (as opposed to stating one "fact" and then presenting opinion afterward) are more likely to be accurate. Always back up data from Internet sources with other forms of information to make your data gathering more comprehensive and, in turn, more accurate.

5. **Look for timeliness.** Websites should always contain "updated on" dates to indicate when the information was created. If these dates are missing, you should find additional sources to support the materials' timeliness. Some websites are created but then never updated, and there is no systematic removal of old sites from the Internet. In addition, many sites contain links to other websites or other information. If many of the links are no longer available or contain outdated material, exercise caution regarding what you find. Make certain you find supporting materials from other sources.

# Identifying Fitness Misinformation and Quackery

Some advertisers claim—without evidence—that their fitness products offer a quick, easy way to shape up, keep fit, and lose weight. There is no such thing as a no-work, no-sweat way to a healthy, fit body. To get the benefit, you have to do the work. Watch for these and other warning signs:

- If the claim sounds too good to be true, it probably is.
- If a product really worked, you would see it in headlines, not just in ads.
- The ads claim the product treats a wide range of ailments.
- The information given is unclear, vague, and highly emotional.
- Changes are promised to be quick, dramatic, or miraculous.
- Results are promised to be easy, effortless, guaranteed, or permanent.

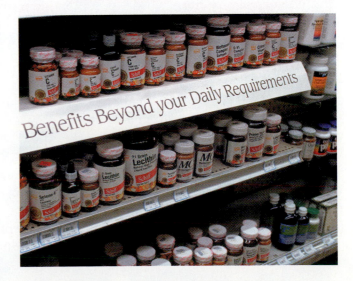

- The ads claim relief from conditions for which there are few treatments and no cures.
- The promoter blames problems on a buildup of toxins in the body.
- Ads declare the medical community to be against the discovery.
- The ads rely on a guru, testimonials, case histories, and before-and-after photos.
- Products are sold door-to-door, in fliers, through pop-up ads, or by mail order and television advertisements.
- The promoter uses high-pressure sales tactics, one-time-only deals, recruitment for a pyramid sales organization, or demands for large advance payments or long-term contracts.

## Choosing Supplements

The next time you watch a TV commercial or see a flyer for a quick weight-loss program, take a moment to consider it. What is being said to you? Who is saying it? In today's day and age we find that to be healthy consumers we need to be educated consumers. The next time you see one of these ads, take a minute to answer the following questions:

- What claim is being made on behalf of this product?
- Who is making this claim? Is it an outside source or the company that makes the product?
- Is everything a testimony about how miraculous the product is?
- Does the ad list any studies that have been done to demonstrate the product's effectiveness?
- If yes, is this a credible source?
- Does it seem like a miracle cure or solution?
- How does it make you feel that ineffective or dangerous products may be marketed without any sound research?

## Reflect ▸▸▸▸ Reinforce ▸▸▸▸ Reinvigorate
### Knowledge Check
*Answers in Appendix D*

1. If you don't begin exercising when you are young, you will never get any benefit from it.
    A. True
    B. False
2. Perhaps the most important question to ask yourself when purchasing a piece of exercise equipment is:
    A. Do I have room for it?
    B. Will I use the equipment?
    C. Will the equipment help me achieve my goals (e.g., build strength)?

## For centuries, doctors in the Orient have known about the wonders of herbal medicines— nature's botanical cures for human ailments.

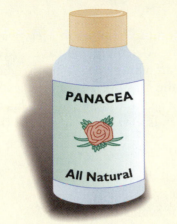

PANACEA

All Natural

### Finally, American scientists are recognizing the healthful benefits of these herbs.

**SwayCon Pharmaceuticals** has developed a capsule that contains everything you need to reduce suffering, enhance health, and regain youthful vigor.

A team of medical experts from three major medical schools in the United States have clinical proof that the ingredients of Panacea are effective! Panacea contains a chemical-free mixture of natural enzymes and exotic herbs that

- relieve up to 80% more arthritis pain than aspirin;
- lower blood pressure by up to 20%;
- lower cholesterol by up to 45%;
- reduce lung cancer risk by as much as 50%, even in smokers;
- and reduce the risk of heart attack by 75%.*

### Other remarkable findings

Taking Panacea for a few months can improve intelligence. R.P., a college student at a large East Coast university reports, **"**At the beginning of the fall semester, I started taking three capsules of Panacea a day. My G.P.A. went from a 1.8 to a 3.4! Panacea has helped me get all A's!"

Reports are coming into our offices that Panacea acts as a sexual stimulant, increasing potency. S.D., a computer programmer in St. Louis, writes, "Thanks for saving my marriage. Before taking Panacea, my husband complained about my lack of interest in sex. One of my friends told me that Panacea can help. Just a few days after taking the capsules, our marriage turned into a perpetual honeymoon."

**Panacea is only available in fine health food stores. Order a three-month supply now, while supplies last**

\* These statements have not been evaluated by the FDA.

> "Clinical proof" is a red flag. The medical experts, the medical schools, or journals where the research has been published are not identified. Objective testing could show the product is neither safe nor effective. The ad should cite the specific effects of the product, including negative ones.

> "Chemical-free" is a red flag; herbs, other plants, indeed all matter is chemical. Furthermore, scientific studies should be cited to provide evidence for these value claims. These statements are not verifiable facts.

> A testimonial from an individual is not scientific evidence. This student's G.P.A. my have risen for a variety of reasons. Studies conducted to show that a treatment is useful in particular ways should contain at least 30 subjects.

> No scientific evidence is cited that a daily Panacea pill prevents serious illness. Additionally, this statement attacks conventional medical practitioners by implying that they are interested only in making money, which suggests that physicians can't be trusted.

This ad is merely a collection of value claims that are not supported by scientific research. The ad further attempts to encourage the reader to purchase the product by suggesting that it is better (and less expensive) than conventional therapies. It claims to relieve a wide range of health conditions. The red-flag phrases and testimonials rather than scientific evidence, the lack of details concerning the medical experts' credentials, and the lack of caution about the hazards of using the product all suggest the ad is an unreliable source of health-related information. *Source:* Alters S. and Schiff W. *Essential Concepts for Healthy Living,* 3rd ed. Sudbury, MA: Jones and Bartlett, 2003:13.

3. What should you look for in using a hot tub?

A. Its cleanliness

B. It has 12, not 6, jets

C. The bubbler signals you when to get out

4. Phil is a 55-year-old overweight salesman with high blood pressure. What course of action do you recommend to help him reach his 56th birthday?

A. He should immediately join a gym and start vigorous daily workouts.

B. He should check with his doctor about starting a program of gradually increasing daily physical activity coupled with a better diet.

C. He should cut down a bit on the martinis at lunch.

D. He doesn't need to change anything so long as he feels okay.

5. Sales of health and fitness club memberships are at an all-time high. What should you do in selecting a health/fitness club for your workouts?

   A. Ask questions (e.g., What are the trainers' credentials?).
   B. Check out the social amenities the club offers.
   C. Look around to see if everyone in the club looks fit.
   D. You should do all of the above.

6. Your mother has Alzheimer's disease. You want to help her in every way possible. In a magazine you read this advertisement: "Cure Alzheimer's Disease!!! My husband has Alzheimer's. On September 2, 1998, he began taking one teaspoon a day of Emu's Liver Oil. Now (in just 22 days) he mows the grass, cleans out the garage, weeds the flower beds, and we take our morning walk again. It hasn't helped his memory much yet, but he is more like himself!!!" What sends a warning signal that this product and its claims may not be valid?

   A. The ad appeared in a magazine.
   B. An unsupported testimonial is used to sell the product.
   C. Emus do not develop Alzheimer's disease.

7. Which of the following is not a criterion for evaluating websites?

   A. Sites should show the date they were last updated.
   B. Site authors should explain their credentials.
   C. Sites should have several links to related products.
   D. Sites should be cross-referenced with other materials.

8. Which of the following product statements would support a product's safety?

   A. "These statements have not been evaluated by the FDA."
   B. "A 7-year study conducted at State University shows the product's effectiveness."
   C. "Our product is 'chemical free'."
   D. "This product was the best thing I've ever done for my health!"

## Modern Modifications

- Look through your local community education or college intramurals programs for a new activity or sport class that you would like to try.
- Aerobic classes or sports not your style? Learn a new type of dance instead.
- Take a walk during your lunch break.
- Ride a bike or walk to work or class if you live a reasonable distance away.
- Check any supplements or home exercise equipment that you have at home using the guidelines provided in this chapter.

## Critical Thinking

Identify three websites addressing the same health issue (e.g., Alzheimer's disease, colon cancer). Using the criteria set out in this chapter, discuss the quality of each site, specifically citing the items that make each a strong or weak example of a website.

## Going Above and Beyond

### Websites

American Dietetics Association
*http://www.eatright.org*

American Medical Association, Health Insight
*http://www.ama-assn.org*

Center for Science in the Public Interest
*http://www.cspinet.org*

Food and Drug Administration
*http://www.fda.gov*

Healthfinder
*http://www.healthfinder.gov*

Mayo Clinic
*http://www.mayohealth.org*

National Council Against Health Fraud
*http://www.ncahf.org*

National Council for Reliable Health Information
*http://www.ncahf.org*

Office of Dietary Supplements
*http://dietarysupplements.info.nih.gov*

Quackwatch
*http://quackwatch.com*

### References and Suggested Readings

Angell M. and Kassirer J. P. Alternative medicine: The risks of untested and unregulated remedies. *New England Journal of Medicine* 1998; 339:839.

Armsey T. D. and Gree G. A. Nutrition supplements: Science vs. hype. *Physician and Sports Medicine* 1997; 25:76.

Kuntzleman C. T. and Wilkerson R. A primer to recommending home aerobic equipment. *American College of Sports Medicine Health and Fitness Journal* 1997; 1:24.

The mainstreaming of alternative medicine. *Consumer Reports* 2000; 65:17–25.

Stamford B. Choosing and using exercise equipment. *Physician and Sports Medicine* 1997; 25:107–108.

## Health Procedure Timeline

With all of the health issues discussed in this text, not to mention what you see and hear every day, it can be confusing to figure out just when to have yourself examined by a doctor. **Table TO5.1** identifies the most common examinations, as well as who should have them done, and how often.

No schedule or list, however, can take the place of routine communication with your physician. Keep your doctor "in the loop" about your self care efforts to make sure you are on the right track!

## Table TO5.1 | Health Procedures

| Procedure | Males | Females | Age | Conditions |
|---|---|---|---|---|
| Blood pressure | X | X | Over age 18 | Every year |
| Blood Sugar | X | X | Over age 18 | Annually if at high risk: obese and over age 40, family history |
| Breast exam | | X | Under age 40<br>Over age 40 | Every 3 years<br>Annually |
| Breast self-exam | | X | Over age 18 | Same date every month |
| Cholesterol | X | X | Men over age 35<br><br>Women over age 45 | Cholesterol <200, every 5 years, age 35–65<br>Cholesterol <200, every 5 years, age 45–65<br>Total cholesterol >200, annually |
| Colorectal exam (sigmoidoscopy) | X | X | Over age 50 | Every 5 years until age 80 |
| Colonoscopy | X | X | Over age 65 | Every 10 years unless there are strong family histories of colon cancer |
| Dental exam | X | X | | Annually |
| Hearing and vision | X | X | Over age 50 | Annually |
| Influenza | X | X | Over age 50 | Annual vaccination |
| Mammography | | X | Under age 40<br>Age 40–50<br>Age 50–65<br>Over age 65 | Not recommended<br>Every 1–2 years, based on history<br>Annually<br>Every 1–2 years until age 75 |
| Medical oral exam (tobacco users) | X | X | Over age 18 and tobacco user | Every 1–2 years |
| Pap and pelvic exam | | X | Under age 40 | Every 3 years (if three consecutive years have returned normal); After age 65, if pap exam is negative for 3 years in a row, exam can be performed every 1-3 years |
| Physical exam | X | X | Age 18–40<br>Age 40–50<br>Over age 50 | Occasionally<br>Every 2 years<br>Annually |
| Pneumonia | X | X | Over age 65 | Single dose |
| Rectal and prostate exam | X | X | Men over age 40<br>Women over age 65 | Prostate annually for men only<br>Rectal annually for both genders |
| Skin self-exam | X | X | Over age 18 | Monthly |
| Testicular self-exam | X | | Over age 18 | Monthly |
| Tetanus booster | X | X | Over age 18 | Every 10 years |

# Dietary Guidelines for Americans 2005*

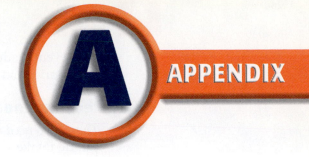

The *Dietary Guidelines for Americans* provides science-based advice to promote health and to reduce risk for major chronic diseases through diet and physical activity. Major causes of morbidity and mortality in the United States are related to poor diet and a sedentary lifestyle. Some specific diseases linked to poor diet and physical inactivity include cardio-vascular disease, type 2 diabetes, hypertension, osteoporosis, and certain cancers. Furthermore, poor diet and physical inactivity, resulting in an energy imbalance (more calories consumed than expended), are the most important factors contributing to the increase in overweight and obesity in this country. Combined with physical activity, following a diet that does not provide excess calories according to the recommendations in this document should enhance the health of most individuals.

## Adequate Nutrients within Calorie Needs

### Key Recommendations

- Consume a variety of nutrient-dense foods and beverages within and among the basic food groups while choosing foods that limit the intake of saturated and trans fats, cholesterol, added sugars, salt, and alcohol.
- Meet recommended intakes within energy needs by adopting a balanced eating pattern, such as the USDA Food Guide or the DASH Eating Plan.

### Key Recommendations for Specific Population Groups

- *People over age 50.* Consume vitamin $B_{12}$ in its crystalline form (i.e., fortified foods or supplements).
- *Women of childbearing age who may become pregnant.* Eat foods high in heme-iron and/or consume iron-rich plant foods or iron-fortified foods with an enhancer of iron absorption, such as vitamin C–rich foods.
- *Women of childbearing age who may become pregnant and those in the first trimester of pregnancy.* Consume adequate synthetic folic acid daily (from fortified foods or supplements) in addition to food forms of folate from a varied diet.
- *Older adults, people with dark skin, and people exposed to insufficient ultraviolet band radiation (i.e., sunlight).* Consume extra vitamin D from vitamin D–fortified foods and/or supplements.

## Weight Management

### Key Recommendations

- To maintain body weight in a healthy range, balance calories from foods and beverages with calories expended.

*From Department of Health and Human Services (DHHS) and U.S. Department of Agriculture (USDA), *Dietary Guidelines for Americans 2005*, joint statement released on January 12, 2005. http://www.healthierus.gov/dietaryguidelines/.

- To prevent gradual weight gain over time, make small decreases in food and beverage calories and increase physical activity.

### Key Recommendations for Specific Population Groups

- *Those who need to lose weight.* Aim for a slow, steady weight loss by decreasing caloric intake while maintaining an adequate nutrient intake and increasing physical activity.
- *Overweight children.* Reduce the rate of body weight gain while allowing growth and development. Consult a health care provider before placing a child on a weight-reduction diet.
- *Pregnant women.* Ensure appropriate weight gain as specified by a health care provider.
- *Breast-feeding women.* Moderate weight reduction is safe and does not compromise weight gain of the nursing infant.
- *Overweight adults and overweight children with chronic diseases and/or on medication.* Consult a health care provider about weight-loss strategies prior to starting a weight-reduction program to ensure appropriate management of other health conditions.

## Physical Activity

### Key Recommendations

- Engage in regular physical activity and reduce sedentary activities to promote health, psychological well-being, and a healthy body weight.
  - To reduce the risk of chronic disease in adulthood: Engage in at least 30 minutes of moderate-intensity physical activity, above usual activity, at work or home on most days of the week.
  - For most people, greater health benefits can be obtained by engaging in physical activity of more vigorous intensity or longer duration.
  - To help manage body weight and prevent gradual, unhealthy body weight gain in adulthood: Engage in approximately 60 minutes of moderate- to vigorous-intensity activity on most days of the week while not exceeding caloric intake requirements.
  - To sustain weight loss in adulthood: Participate in at least 60 to 90 minutes of daily moderate-intensity physical activity while not exceeding caloric intake requirements. Some people may need to consult with a health care provider before participating in this level of activity.
- Achieve physical fitness by including cardiovascular conditioning, stretching exercises for flexibility, and resistance exercises or calisthenics for muscle strength and endurance.

### Key Recommendations for Specific Population Groups

- *Children and adolescents.* Engage in at least 60 minutes of physical activity on most—preferably all—days of the week.
- *Pregnant women.* In the absence of medical or obstetric complications, incorporate 30 minutes or more of moderate-intensity physical activity on most—if not all—days of the week. Avoid activities with a high risk of falling or abdominal trauma.

- *Breast-feeding women.* Be aware that neither acute nor regular exercise adversely affects the mother's ability to successfully breast-feed.
- *Older adults.* Participate in regular physical activity to reduce functional declines associated with aging and to achieve the other benefits of physical activity identified for all adults.

# Food Groups to Encourage

## Key Recommendations

- Consume a sufficient amount of fruits and vegetables while staying within energy needs. Two cups of fruit and $2\frac{1}{2}$ cups of vegetables per day are recommended for a reference 2000-calorie intake, with higher or lower amounts depending on the calorie level.
- Choose a variety of fruits and vegetables each day. In particular, select from all five vegetable subgroups (dark green, orange, legumes, starchy vegetables, and other vegetables) several times a week.
- Consume 3 or more ounce-equivalents of whole-grain products per day, with the rest of the recommended grains coming from enriched or whole-grain products. In general, at least half the grains should come from whole grains.
- Consume 3 cups per day of fat-free or low-fat milk or equivalent milk products.

## Key Recommendations for Specific Population Groups

- *Children and adolescents.* Consume whole-grain products often; at least half the grains should be whole grains. Children 2 to 8 years should consume 2 cups per day of fat-free or low-fat milk or equivalent milk products. Children 9 years of age and older should consume 3 cups per day of fat-free or low-fat milk or equivalent milk products.

# Fats

## Key Recommendations

- Consume less than 10% of calories from saturated fatty acids and less than 300 mg/day of cholesterol, and keep trans fatty acid consumption as low as possible.
- Keep total fat intake between 20% and 35% of calories, with most fats coming from sources of polyunsaturated and monounsaturated fatty acids, such as fish, nuts, and vegetable oils.
- When selecting and preparing meat, poultry, dry beans, and milk or milk products, make choices that are lean, low fat, or fat free.
- Limit intake of fats and oils high in saturated and/or trans fatty acids, and choose products low in such fats and oils.

## Key Recommendations for Specific Population Groups

- *Children and adolescents.* Keep total fat intake between 30% and 35% of calories for children 2 to 3 years of age and between 25% and 35% of calories for children and adolescents 4 to 18 years of age, with most fats coming from sources of polyunsaturated and monounsaturated fatty acids, such as fish, nuts, and vegetable oils.

# Carbohydrates

### Key Recommendations

- Choose fiber-rich fruits, vegetables, and whole grains often.
- Choose and prepare foods and beverages with little added sugars or caloric sweeteners, such as amounts suggested by the USDA Food Guide and the DASH Eating Plan.
- Reduce the incidence of dental caries by practicing good oral hygiene and consuming sugar- and starch-containing foods and beverages less frequently.

# Sodium and Potassium

### Key Recommendations

- Consume less than 2300 mg (approximately 1 teaspoon of salt) of sodium per day.
- Choose and prepare foods with little salt. At the same time, consume potassium-rich foods, such as fruits and vegetables.

### Key Recommendations for Specific Population Groups

- *Individuals with hypertension, blacks, and middle-aged and older adults.* Aim to consume no more than 1500 mg of sodium per day, and meet the potassium recommendation (4700 mg/day) with food.

# Alcoholic Beverages

### Key Recommendations

- Those who choose to drink alcoholic beverages should do so sensibly and in moderation—defined as the consumption of up to one drink per day for women and up to two drinks per day for men.
- Alcoholic beverages should not be consumed by some individuals, including those who cannot restrict their alcohol intake, women of childbearing age who may become pregnant, pregnant and lactating women, children and adolescents, individuals taking medications that can interact with alcohol, and those with specific medical conditions.
- Alcoholic beverages should be avoided by individuals engaging in activities that require attention, skill, or coordination, such as driving or operating machinery.

# Food Safety

### Key Recommendations

To avoid microbial foodborne illness:
- Clean hands, food contact surfaces, and fruits and vegetables. Meat and poultry should not be washed or rinsed.
- Separate raw, cooked, and ready-to-eat foods while shopping, preparing, or storing foods.
- Cook foods to a safe temperature to kill microorganisms.

- Chill (refrigerate) perishable food promptly and defrost foods properly.
- Avoid raw (unpasteurized) milk or any products made from unpasteurized milk, raw or partially cooked eggs or foods containing raw eggs, raw or undercooked meat and poultry, unpasteurized juices, and raw sprouts.

## Key Recommendations for Specific Population Groups

- *Infants and young children, pregnant women, older adults, and those who are immunocompromised.* Do not eat or drink raw (unpasteurized) milk or any products made from unpasteurized milk, raw or partially cooked eggs or foods containing raw eggs, raw or undercooked meat and poultry, raw or undercooked fish or shellfish, unpasteurized juices, and raw sprouts.
- *Pregnant women, older adults, and those who are immunocompromised:* Only eat certain deli meats and frankfurters that have been reheated to steaming hot.

| Table 1 | Percentage Contributed by Each Energy System to Overall Energy Needs of Various Activities | | |
|---|---|---|---|
| Physical Activity | Immediate System (%) | Anaerobic System (%) | Aerobic System (%) |
| Running: 100 meters | 98 | 2 | — |
| Running: 3 miles | 10 | 20 | 70 |
| Marathon | — | 5 | 95 |
| Swimming: 50 meters | 98 | 2 | — |
| Swimming: 400 meters | 20 | 40 | 40 |
| Swimming: 1500 meters | 10 | 20 | 70 |

# Nutrition and Health for Canadians*

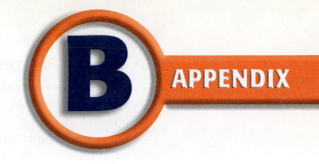

## Canadian Guidelines for Nutrition

For the past 60 years, the government has worked to promote healthy and nutritious eating habits in Canadians. In 1987, Health and Welfare Canada began a major review of the system for guiding Canadians on their food choices. To perform the review, the government appointed two advisory committees—the Scientific Review Committee and the Communications and Implementation Committee.

After examining research evidence available on nutrition and public health, the Scientific Review Committee issued a report in 1990 called Nutrition Recommendations. The report included both updated Recommended Nutrient Intakes (RNI) and a scientific description of a healthy dietary pattern that would deliver adequate nutrients for health and reduce the risk of nutrition-related chronic diseases.

Meanwhile, the Communications and Implementation Committee translated these scientific findings into understandable guidelines and outlined implementation strategies in a report called *Action Towards Healthy Eating: Technical Report* (1990). This report suggested that Canada develop a "total diet approach" toward healthy eating. A total diet approach would give consumers a better idea of eating patterns associated with reducing the risk of developing chronic diseases.

In 1990, the government issued *Nutrition Recommendations: A Call for Action*, a summary report produced jointly by the Scientific Review Committee and the Communications and Implementation Committee.

## A Revised Food Guide

In accordance with the recommendations of its two advisory groups, the Health Department undertook to revise *Canada's Food Guide*. In 1992, the agency launched *Canada's Food Guide to Healthy Eating* and an explanatory document called *Using the Food Guide*. This promotes dietary diversity, reduction of total fat intake, and an active lifestyle. It also offers consumers a pattern for establishing healthy eating habits in their daily selection of foods.

Moreover, the guide introduced a number of new concepts. A range of servings from the four food groups accommodates the wide range of energy needs for different ages, body sizes, activity levels, genders, and conditions such as pregnancy and nursing. The wide range of servings in grain products, vegetables, and fruits is designed to give consumers a better idea of the type of diet that would help reduce the risk of developing nutrition-related chronic diseases.

The guide also introduced a category of "other" foods such as sweets, fats such as butter, and drinks such as coffee that, though part of the diets of many Canadians, would traditionally not have been mentioned in a food guide. The guide recommends moderation in the consumption of these foods and acknowledges their role, along with the wide range of servings in grains, vegetables, and fruits, as a "total diet approach" to healthy eating.

*Adapted with permission from Insel P., Turner R. E., and Ross D. *Nutrition*, 2nd ed. Sudbury, MA: Jones and Bartlett, 2004.

**B**

### A Work in Progress

Some groups and organizations challenged specific aspects of the government's Nutrition Recommendations. In a typically Canadian twist, the government responded to challengers by including them in the development process. When the Canadian Pediatric Society, for example, queried the dietary recommendations on fat consumption in children, the Society was invited to join Health Canada in researching the issue. The result was *Nutrition Recommendations Update: Dietary Fat and Children* (1993), which adjusted the recommendation of appropriate levels of dietary fat for growing children. In 1995, Health Canada issued *Canada's Food Guide to Healthy Eating: Focus on Preschoolers* as a background paper for educators and communicators.

Health Canada also has positioned nutrition in a broader health context, which includes physical activity and a positive outlook on life. One result of this comprehensive approach was the *Vitality Leaders Kit* (1994), intended to help community leaders promote healthy eating, active living, and positive self- and body-image in an integrated way.

# Canada's *Food Guide to Healthy Eating*

Scientists have known for some time that adequate nutrition is essential for proper growth and development. More recently, healthy eating has been accepted as a significant factor in reducing the risk of developing nutrition-related problems, including heart disease, cancer, obesity, hypertension (high blood pressure), osteoporosis, anemia, dental decay, and some bowel disorders.

## Healthy Eating in Canada

The Food Guide is based on nutrition and food science. A key reference is *Nutrition Recommendations: The Report of the Scientific Review Committee*, published in 1990 by Health Canada. This report contains a review of nutrition research conducted by a committee of scientists and provides recommendations describing the desired characteristics of the Canadian diet. The Nutrition Recommendations, which are reviewed regularly, act as the foundation for all nutrition and healthy eating programs in the country.

## *Canada's Guidelines for Healthy Eating*

A committee of experts in communications and program planning worked with the committee of scientists and prepared the report *Action Towards Healthy Eating*. They adapted the Nutrition Recommendations into a more user-friendly set of statements called *Canada's Guidelines for Healthy Eating*. These guidelines promote healthy eating in a general way:

- Enjoy a variety of foods.
- Emphasize cereals, breads, other grain products, vegetables, and fruit.
- Choose lower-fat dairy products, leaner meats, and foods prepared with little or no fat.
- Achieve and maintain a healthy body weight by enjoying regular physical activity and healthy eating.
- Limit salt, alcohol, and caffeine.

## *Canada's Food Guide to Healthy Eating*

*Canada's Food Guide to Healthy Eating* takes *Canada's Guidelines for Healthy Eating* one step further and provides consumers with more detailed information for establishing healthy eating habits through the daily selection of food ( **Figure B.1** ). The Food Guide is a basic nutrition education tool used:

- To help plan healthy meals for individuals or groups; and
- To evaluate a person's eating habits in a general way but not to assess nutritional status.

The Food Guide meets the nutritional needs of all Canadians 4 years of age and over and has been designed specifically for the general public with a reading level of grade 7. It is not appropriate for those under the age of 4 because the number of servings and the serving sizes are too large for toddlers and preschoolers.

### Food Guide Materials

- *Canada's Food Guide to Healthy Eating*: a tear sheet for consumers.
- *Using the Food Guide*: a booklet for consumers that explains the basic concepts of the tear sheet more fully.
- *Food Guide Facts: Background for Educators and Communicators*: fact sheets that provide background information for nutrition professionals, health educators, home economists, fitness leaders, and others involved in promoting healthy eating.
- *Canada's Food Guide to Healthy Eating*: tear sheet, consumer booklet, and the fact sheets for educators and communicators are available from provincial or local health departments or from Publications, Health Canada, Ottawa, Ontario K1A 0K9, tel. (613) 954-5995.

# Canada's Physical Activity Guide to Healthy Active Living

High levels of physical inactivity are a serious threat to public health in Canada. Nearly two thirds of Canadians are not active enough to achieve optimal health benefits. These Canadians are at risk for heart disease, obesity, high blood pressure, adult-onset diabetes, osteoporosis, stroke, depression, and colon cancer. Although physical activity levels increased during the 1980s and early 1990s, the progress has stalled. Health Canada estimates that physical inactivity results in at least 21,000 premature deaths annually.

*Canada's Physical Activity Guide to Healthy Active Living*, produced by a joint effort of Health Canada and the Canadian Society for Exercise Physiology, provides the first set of Canadian guidelines for physical activity ( **Figure B.2** ). It provides information to help Canadians understand how to achieve health benefits by being physically active. The guide complements the popular *Canada's Food Guide to Healthy Eating* and provides concrete examples of how to incorporate physical activity into daily life.

Designed for adults, the guide recommends 60 minutes of physical activity every day to stay healthy or improve your health. As a person progresses to more intense activity, he or she can cut down to 30 minutes, 4 days a week. The guide also suggests Canadians can add up their activities in periods of at least 10 minutes each, starting slowly and building up.

Federal, provincial, and territorial governments are working to reduce the number of inactive Canadians. *Canada's Physical Activity Guide to Healthy Active Living* is a major step toward building the knowledge and awareness necessary for all Canadians to become more active. The healthy active living series now also includes *Physical Activity Guide to Healthy Active Living for Older Adults, Physical Activity Guide for Youth, Physical Activity Guide for Children*, and *Active Living at Work*.

*Text continued on p. 260.*

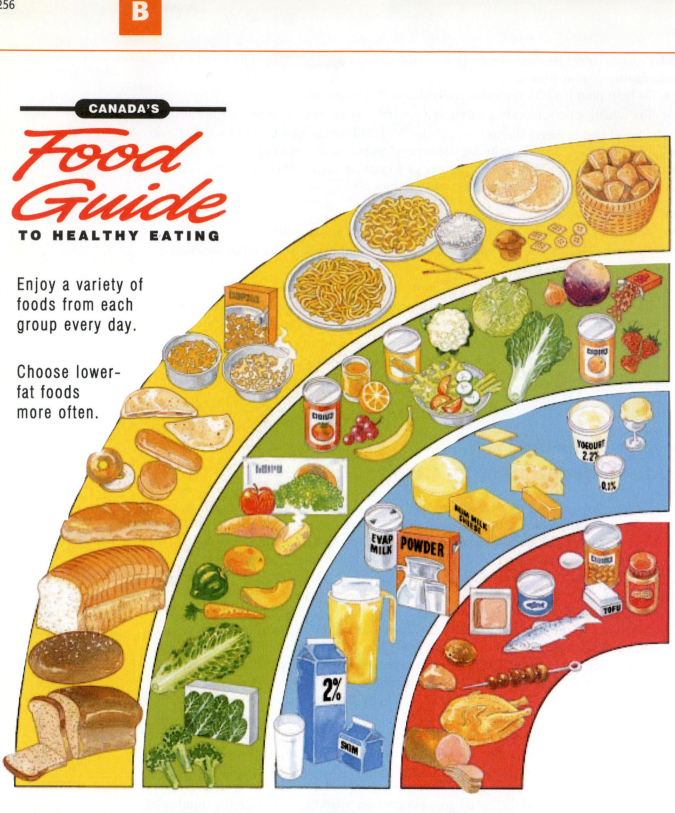

## CANADA'S

# Food Guide

## TO HEALTHY EATING

Enjoy a variety of foods from each group every day.

Choose lower-fat foods more often.

**Grain Products**
Choose whole grain and enriched products more often

**Vegetables & Fruit**
Choose dark green and orange vegetables and orange fruit more often.

**Milk Products**
Choose lower-fat milk products more often

**Meat & Alternatives**
Choose leaner meats, poultry and fish, as well as dried peas, beans and lentils more often

**Figure B.1**

*Canada's Food Guide. Source:* © Minister of Public Works and Government Services Canada, 1997.

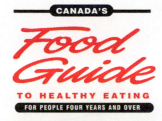

## Different People Need Different Amounts of Food

The amount of food you need every day from the 4 groups and other foods depends on your age, body size, activity level, whether you are male or female and if you are pregnant or breast-feeding. That's why the Food Guide gives a lower and higher number of servings for each food group. For example, young children can choose the number of servings, while male teenagers can go to the higher number. Most other people can choose servings somewhere in between.

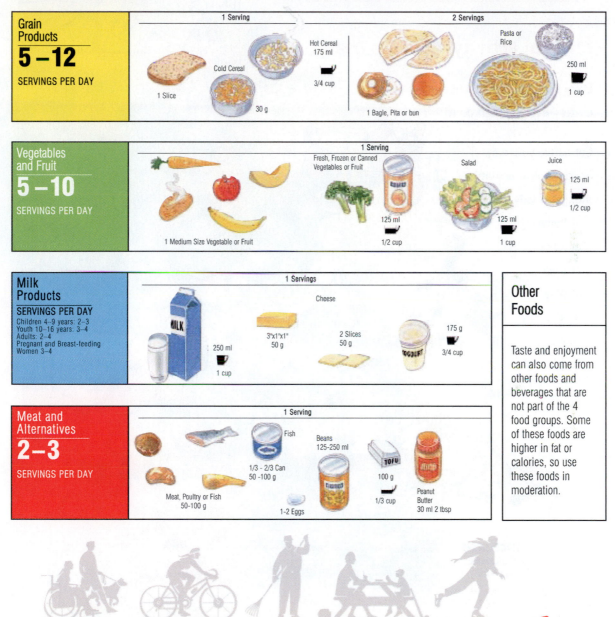

Enjoy eating well, being active and feeling good about yourself. That's *VITALITÉ*

©Minister of Supply and Services Canada 1992 Cat. No. H39-252/1992E No changes permitted. Reprint permission not required.
ISBN 0-662-19648-1

**B**

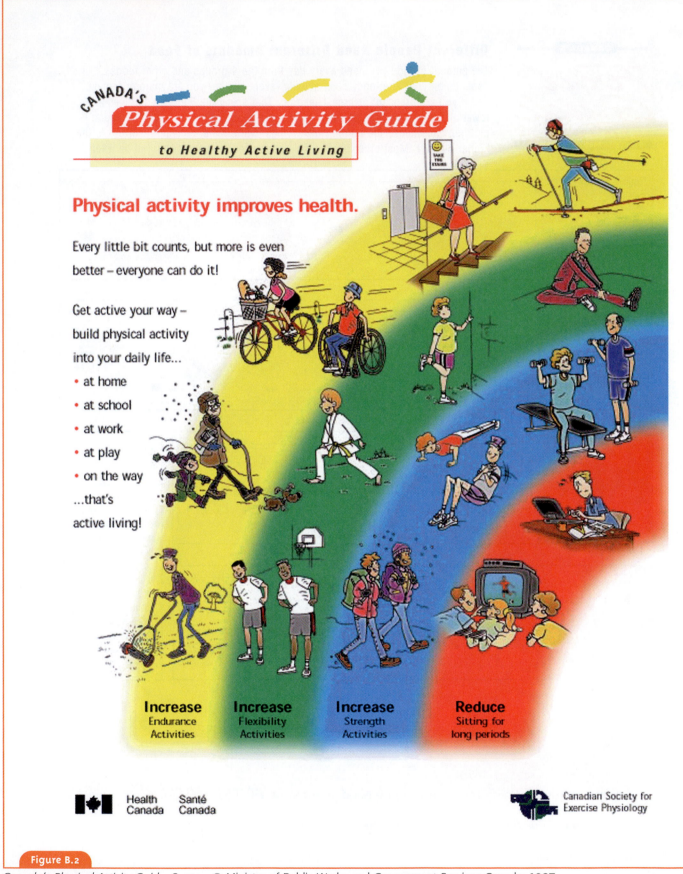

Figure B.2

*Canada's Physical Activity Guide. Source:* © Minister of Public Works and Government Services Canada, 1997.

**Choose a variety of activities from these three groups:**

### Endurance

*4-7 days a week*
Continuous activities for your heart, lungs and circulatory system.

### Flexibility

*4-7 days a week*
Gentle reaching, bending and stretching activities to keep your muscles relaxed and joints mobile.

### Strength

*2-4 days a week*
Activities against resistance to strengthen muscles and bones and improve posture.

Starting slowly is very safe for most people. Not sure? Consult your health professional.

For a copy of the *Guide Handbook* and more information: **1-888-334-9769**, or **www.paguide.com**

Eating well is also important. Follow *Canada's Food Guide to Healthy Eating* to make wise food choices.

# Get Active Your Way, Every Day—For Life!

Scientists say accumulate 60 minutes of physical activity every day to stay healthy or improve your health.  As you progress to moderate activities you can cut down to 30 minutes, 4 days a week. Add-up your activities in periods of at least 10 minutes each. Start slowly… and build up.

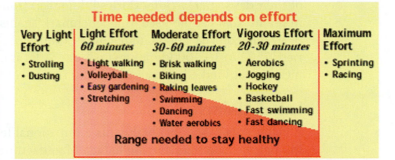

### Time needed depends on effort

| Very Light Effort | Light Effort *60 minutes* | Moderate Effort *30-60 minutes* | Vigorous Effort *20-30 minutes* | Maximum Effort |
|---|---|---|---|---|
| • Strolling<br>• Dusting | • Light walking<br>• Volleyball<br>• Easy gardening<br>• Stretching | • Brisk walking<br>• Biking<br>• Raking leaves<br>• Swimming<br>• Dancing<br>• Water aerobics | • Aerobics<br>• Jogging<br>• Hockey<br>• Basketball<br>• Fast swimming<br>• Fast dancing | • Sprinting<br>• Racing |

**Range needed to stay healthy**

## You Can Do It – Getting started is easier than you think

Physical activity doesn't have to be very hard.  Build physical activities into your daily routine.

- Walk whenever you can – get off the bus early, use the stairs instead of the elevator.
- Reduce inactivity for long periods, like watching TV.
- Get up from the couch and stretch and bend for a few minutes every hour.
- Play actively with your kids.
- Choose to walk, wheel or cycle for short trips.

- Start with a 10 minute walk – gradually increase the time.
- Find out about walking and cycling paths nearby and use them.
- Observe a physical activity class to see if you want to try it.
- Try one class to start – you don't have to make a long-term commitment.
- Do the activities you are doing now, more often.

## Benefits of regular activity:

- better health
- improved fitness
- better posture and balance
- better self-esteem
- weight control
- stronger muscles and bones
- feeling more energetic
- relaxation and reduced stress
- continued independent living in later life

## Health risks of inactivity:

- premature death
- heart disease
- obesity
- high blood pressure
- adult-onset diabetes
- osteoporosis
- stroke
- depression
- colon cancer

*Physical Activity Guide*

# Nutrition Labeling for Canadians

The nutrition label is one of the most useful tools in selecting foods for healthy eating. The Food Guide outlines a pattern of healthy eating; the nutrition label supports the Food Guide by helping consumers to choose foods according to healthy eating messages.

Consumers can use labels to compare products and make choices on the basis of nutrient content. For example, consumers can choose a lower-fat product based on the fat content given on the labels **Figure B.3** and **Figure B.4**.

Consumers also can use label information to evaluate products in relation to healthy eating. For instance, the Nutrition Recommendations advise Canadians to get 30% or less of their day's energy (kilocalories/kilojoules) from fat. This translates into a range of fat, in grams, that can be used as a benchmark against which individual foods and meals can be evaluated. The Food Guide covers a range of energy needs from 1800 to 3200 kilocalories (7500 to 13,400 kilojoules) per day. A fat intake of 30% or less of a day's calories means a fat intake between 60 and 105 grams of fat.

## Label Claims

A claim on a food label highlights a nutritional feature of a product. It is known to influence consumers' buying habits. Manufacturers often position label claims in a bold, banner format on the front panel of a package or on the side panel along with the nutrition label. Since a label claim must be backed up by detailed facts relating to the claim, the consumer should look for the nutrition label for more information.

## Nutrient Content Claims

A nutrient content claim describes the amount of a nutrient in a food. A food whose label carries the claim "high fiber" must contain 4 grams or more fiber per reference amount and serving of stated size. A "sodium-free" food must contain less than 5 mg of sodium per reference amount and serving of stated size.

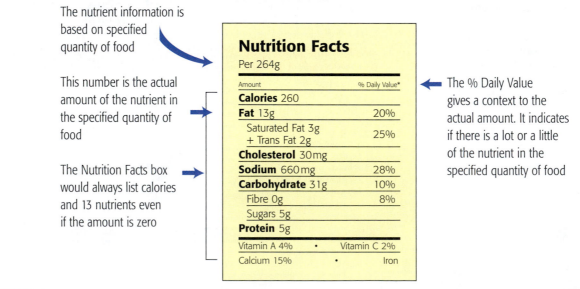

### The Nutrition Facts Box

The Nutrition Facts box allows consumers to make informed choices.

The nutrient information is based on specified quantity of food

This number is the actual amount of the nutrient in the specified quantity of food

The Nutrition Facts box would always list calories and 13 nutrients even if the amount is zero

**Nutrition Facts**
Per 264g

| Amount | % Daily Value* |
|---|---|
| **Calories** 260 | |
| **Fat** 13g | 20% |
| Saturated Fat 3g + Trans Fat 2g | 25% |
| **Cholesterol** 30mg | |
| **Sodium** 660mg | 28% |
| **Carbohydrate** 31g | 10% |
| Fibre 0g | 8% |
| Sugars 5g | |
| **Protein** 5g | |
| Vitamin A 4% • Vitamin C 2% | |
| Calcium 15% • Iron | |

The % Daily Value gives a context to the actual amount. It indicates if there is a lot or a little of the nutrient in the specified quantity of food

**Figure B.3**

How to read a food label.

**INGREDIENTS:** Fructose Syrup (from Grapes, Corn, and Pears), Oat Bran, Maltodextrin (Complex Carbohydrate), Modified Milk Ingredients (Milk Protein with Lactose removed), Brown Rice, Almond Butter, Natural Berry Flavours, Carmine, Citric Acid. **VITAMINS AND MINERALS:** Dicalcium phosphate, Potassium bicarbonate, Ascorbic acid, Magnesium carbonate, Alpha tocopherol (vit. E), Zinc gluconate, Ferrous fumarate, Salt, Potassium iodide, Beta carotene (vit. A), Copper gluconate, Manganese sulfate, Calcium pantothenate, Pyridoxine hydrochloride (vit. $B_6$), Riboflavin (vit. $B_2$), Niacin, Thiamin hydrochloride (vit. $B_1$), Cholecalciferol (vit. D), Folic acid, Biotin, Cyanocobalamin (vit. $B_{12}$).

**INGRÉDIENTS:** Sirop de fructose (de Raisin, de Maïs, et de Poire), Son d'avione, Maltodextrine (glucide complexe), Substances latières modifées (protéines du lait, lactose enlevé), Riz brun, Beurre d'amande, Arômes naturels de baie, Carmin, Acide citrique. **VITAMINES ET MINERAUX:** Phosphate bicalcique, Bicarbonate de potassium, Acide ascorbique, Carbonate de magnésium, Alpha tocophérol (vit. E), Gluconate de zinc, Fumarate ferreux, Sel, Iodure de potassium, Bêta-carotène (vit. A), Gluconate de cuivre, Sulfate de manganèse, Pantothénate de calcium, Chlorhydrate de pyridoxine (vit. $B_6$), Riboflavine (vit. $B_2$), Niacine, Chlorhydrate de thiamine (vit. $B_1$), Cholécalciférol (vit. D), Acide folique, Biotine, Cyanocobalamine (vit. $B_{12}$).

**Ingredients List** must be included by law and must list all of the ingredients used in the product. Ingredients are listed in the order of the amount used. The amount is based on the weight of an ingredient rather than its volume.

**Figure B.4**

Ingredients list.

## Diet-Related Health Claims

Optional health claims highlight the characteristics of a diet that reduces the chance of developing a disease such as cancer or heart disease. They also tell how the food fits into the diet.

### Characteristic of the Diet:

Low in sodium and high in potassium
Adequate in calcium and vitamin D
Low in saturated and trans fats
Rich in fruit and vegetables
Sugar alcohols (such as sorbitol)

### Reduced Risk of:

High blood pressure
Osteoporosis
Heart disease
Some types of cancer
Tooth decay

New nutrition labeling regulations were published on January 1, 2003. For the latest information, visit the Nutrition Labeling area of the Health Canada website at http://www.hc-sc.gc.ca/hpfb-dgpsa/onpp-bppn/labelling-etiquetage/index_e.html.

## Food Choice System

The CDA Food Choice System is a method of meal planning created by the Canadian Diabetes Association to make it easier for people with diabetes to eat the right amount of food for their insulin supply. This system is based on two concepts: Most foods are eaten by people with diabetes in measured amounts, and foods within each of the system's seven food groups can be interchanged.

The CDA Food Choice System started with the nutritional principles in *Canada's Food Guide to Healthy Eating* and modified them to meet the special needs of people with dia-

**B**

betes. People with diabetes must eat a certain amount of carbohydrate, protein, and fat at each meal to control the amount of glucose (sugar) that enters the blood after a meal. The CDA Food Choice System helps them select the proper type and amount of food to manage their diabetes.

The Food Choice System classifies foods into seven food groups according to the food's carbohydrate, protein, and fat content. The Food Choice Values tell a person with diabetes what group a food belongs to and how much of that food is interchangeable with another food in the same food group. The Food Choice Values, therefore, help someone with diabetes eat a balance of foods in the right amounts.

In the Food Choice System, the seven food groups and their symbols are:

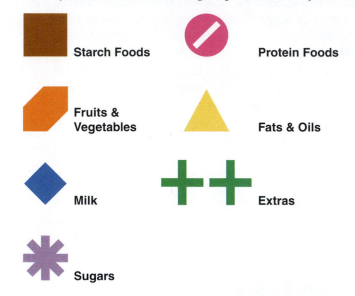

Because food groups in CDA's Food Choice Systems may be confused with the food groups in *Canada's Food Guide to Healthy Eating*, the government does not permit them to be listed by name on food labels. The federal government regulation states that only the assigned quantity, the Food Choice "Symbol," and the word "Choice" can be published on a label.

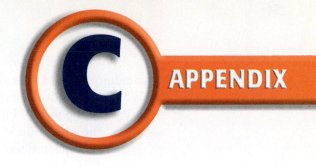

# Injury Care and Prevention

## Exercise-Related Injuries

Most exercise-related injuries do not threaten life, nor are they severe. However, exercise-related injuries demand that you make a decision about the proper care for an injury.

This section helps in such decision making with its decision table (If…, then…) format. Decision tables not only help identify what may be wrong (the "If" column), but also help determine what action to take (the "Then" column).

This appendix does not cover life-threatening conditions requiring rescue breathing and CPR, nor many other injuries and conditions that a quality first-aid course may cover. For a quality first-aid course, go to the American Academy of Orthopaedic Surgeons/American College of Emergency Physicians Emergency Care and Safety Institute website—http://www.safetycampus.org—to locate a training center near you. Many colleges and universities use the AAOS/ACEP first-aid, CPR, and AED (automated external defibrillator) program.

## How to Examine for an Injury

See Table C.1 .

Signs of an exercise-related injury may include:

- Loss of use. "Guarding" occurs when movement produces pain; the person refuses to use the injured part.
- A grating sensation (crepitus) can be felt, and sometimes even heard, when the ends of a broken bone rub together.

| Table C.1 | How to Examine for an Injury |
|---|---|
| **What to Do** | **How to Do It** |
| Determine the location of the problem. | Ask yourself or the injured person "What's wrong?" or "Where do you hurt?" |
| Find out if an injury exists. | Look and feel the area for one or more of the following signs of injury: deformity, open wounds, tenderness, and swelling. The mnemonic "D-O-T-S" helps in remembering the signs of an injury:<br>• **D**eformities occur when bones are broken, causing an abnormal shape. Deformity might not be obvious. Compare the injured part with the uninjured part on the other side of the body.<br>• **O**pen wounds break the skin and there is bleeding.<br>• **T**enderness (pain) means sensitive when touched or pressed. It is commonly found only at the injury site. The person usually will be able to point to the site of the pain.<br>• **S**welling is the body's response to injury that makes the area larger than usual. It appears later and is due to fluid from inflammation and/or bleeding. |

For extremity (arms and legs) injuries, check blood flow and nerves. Use the mnemonic CSM (circulation, sensation, movement) as a way of remembering what to do.

- **Circulation:** For an arm injury, feel for the radial pulse (located on the thumb side of the wrist). For a leg injury, feel for the posterior tibial pulse (located between the inside ankle bone and the Achilles tendon). An arm or leg without a pulse requires immediate surgical care.
- **Sensation:** Lightly touch or squeeze one of the victim's fingers or toes and ask the victim what he or she feels. Loss of sensation is an early sign of nerve damage.
- **Movement:** Inability to move develops later. Check for nerve damage by asking the victim to wiggle his or her fingers or toes. If the fingers or toes are injured, do not have the victim try to move them.

A quick nerve and circulatory check is very important. The tissues of the arms and legs cannot survive for more than 3 hours without a continuous blood supply. If you note any disruption in the nerve and blood supply, seek immediate medical care.

## RICE Procedures

RICE is the acronym—rest, ice, compression, and elevation—for the treatment of all bone, joint, and muscle injuries. The steps taken in the first 48 to 72 hours after such an injury can help to relieve, and even prevent, aches and pains.

Treat all extremity bone, joint, and muscle injuries with the RICE procedures. In addition to RICE, fractures and dislocations should be stabilized against movement.

### R: Rest

Injuries heal faster if rested. Rest means to stay off the injured part and avoid moving it. Using any part of the body increases the blood circulation to that area, which can cause more swelling of an injured part.

### I: Ice

An ice pack should be applied to the injured area for 20 to 30 minutes every 2 or 3 hours during the first 24 to 48 hours. Skin treated with cold passes through four stages: cold, burning, aching, and numbness. When the skin becomes numb, usually in 20 to 30 minutes, remove the ice pack. After removing the ice pack, compress the injured part with an elastic bandage and keep it elevated (the "C" and "E" of RICE).

Cold constricts the blood vessels to and in the injured area, which helps reduce the swelling and inflammation. Cold should be applied as soon as possible after the injury— healing time often is directly related to the amount of swelling that occurs. Heat has the opposite effect when applied to fresh injuries: It increases circulation to the area and greatly increases both the swelling and the pain.

Put crushed ice (or cubes) into a double plastic bag or commercial ice bag. Place the ice pack directly on the skin and then use an elastic bandage to hold the ice pack in place. Ice bags can conform to the body's contours.

### C: Compression

Compressing the injured area may squeeze some fluid and debris out of the injury site. Compression limits the ability of the skin and of other tissues to expand and reduces internal bleeding. Apply an elastic bandage to the injured area, especially the foot, ankle, knee, thigh, hand, or elbow. Fill the hollow areas with padding, such as a sock or washcloth, before applying the elastic bandage.

Start the elastic bandage several inches below the injury and wrap in an upward, overlapping spiral with an even, slightly tight pressure. Pale skin, pain, numbness, and tingling are signs that the bandage is too tight. If any of these appear, immediately remove the elastic bandage. Rewrap later when the symptoms disappear.

For a bruise or strain, place a pad between the injury and the elastic bandage.

### E: Elevation

Elevating the injured area, in combination with ice and compression, limits circulation to an area, helps limit internal bleeding, and minimizes swelling.

# Returning to Physical Activity After an Injury

Returning to physical activity is generally permissible once an injury is fully healed. Fully healed means:

- No pain
- No swelling
- No limping, favoring, or instability

Full rehabilitation means:

- Return of full range of motion and flexibility
- Muscle strength and endurance in the affected extremity (arm or leg) equal to that of the unaffected extremity
- Resumption of pre-injury endurance levels
- Good balance and coordination

Sometimes, clearance to return to exercising should come from a physician (e.g., after surgery).

# Definitions

- **Contusions:** Bruising of tissue.
- **Strains:** Muscles are stretched or torn.
- **Sprains:** Tearing or stretching of the joints that causes mild to severe damage to the ligaments and joint capsules.
- **Dislocations:** Bones are displaced from their normal joint alignment, out of their sockets, or out of their normal positions.
- **Tendonitis:** Inflammation of a tendon from overuse.

# Specific Injuries

## Foot

Foot injuries are common among exercisers because of the foot's role in bearing weight. Careless treatment can have consequences that may include lifelong disability Table C.2 .

## Ankle

Most ankle injuries are sprains. About 85% of sprains involve the ankle's outside (lateral) ligaments and are caused by having the foot turned or twisted inward. If not treated properly, a sprained ankle becomes chronically susceptible for future injuries. See Table C.3 for symptoms and treatment.

## Lower Leg

The two bones of the lower leg are the tibia ("shin bone") and fibula. Most shin injuries are "shin splints," which are strains from overuse. Occasionally, a bone is fractured from overuse. See Table C.4 .

**C**

| Table C.2 | Determining and Treating Foot Injuries |
|---|---|
| **If...** | **Then...** |
| Pain is at top of the heel (over Achilles tendon)<br>Pain is aggravated by activity—worse at beginning of activity and improved with warm-up | Suspect **Achilles tendonitis:**<br>• Apply ice to decrease inflammation and pain.<br>• Use an anti-inflammatory for 7 to 10 days.<br>• Reduce or stop activity until no more pain occurs while either walking or resting.<br>• Elevate heel with a heel cup or pads in the shoe.<br>• Calf muscles should be stretched after warm-up and cool-down. |
| Pain is at back of the heel<br>Injury resembles Achilles tendonitis | Suspect **retrocalcaneal bursitis**:<br>Treat the same as for Achilles tendonitis. |
| Pain, often disabling, is at bottom of the heel | Suspect **plantar fasciitis** ("heel spur"):<br>• Apply ice for 20–30 minutes after activity and 3–4 times daily.<br>• Use a heel cup in the shoe.<br>• Reduce or stop activity.<br>• Use an anti-inflammatory for 7 to 10 days. |
| Pain is in fifth metatarsal bone, possibly with swelling | Suspect **fracture** (Jones fracture):<br>• Apply ice.<br>• Stop activity.<br>• Seek medical care. |
| Pain is on ball of foot between second and third toes | Suspect **Morton's neuroma:**<br>• Wear wider, softer shoes.<br>• If there is no improvement, surgery may be required. |
| Pain is on ball of foot at the big toe | Suspect **seasmoiditis or a stress fracture:**<br>• Apply ice for 20–30 minutes, 3–4 times daily.<br>• Rest.<br>• Use an anti-inflammatory for 7 to 10 days.<br>• If pain persists, seek medical care. |
| Area on skin has a "hot spot" (not very painful, red area) from rubbing | Suspect a **blister:**<br>• Cool the hot spot with an ice pack.<br>AND/OR<br>• Tape several layers of moleskin, which are cut into a "doughnut shape" to fit around the blister.<br>OR<br>• Apply duct tape tightly over the painful area. |
| Blister is broken and fluid is seeping out | • Leave the "roof" on for protection.<br>• Clean with soap and water.<br>• Tape several layers of moleskin, cut into a "doughnut shape" to fit around the blister.<br>• Apply an antibiotic ointment in the hole over the blister.<br>• Cover with an uncut gauze pad and tape in place. |
| Blister on foot is very painful, affects walking, and is not broken | • Drain the blister by puncturing the roof with several holes.<br>• Leave the "roof" on for protection.<br>• Clean with soap and water.<br>• Tape several layers of moleskin, cut into a "doughnut shape" to fit around the blister.<br>• Apply an antibiotic ointment in the hole over the blister.<br>• Place gauze pad over the moleskin and tape in place. |

| Table C.3 | Determining and Treating Ankle Injuries (Ottawa Ankle Rules) |
|---|---|
| **If…** | **Then…** |
| Ankle is able to bear weight<br>He/she is able to take four steps immediately after the injury and an hour later<br>No tenderness or pain is felt when you push on the ankle knob bone | Suspect **ankle sprain:**<br>• Use RICE procedures.<br>• For the compression part of RICE, apply an elastic bandage over any soft pliable material (e.g., sock or T-shirt) placed in a "U" shape around the ankle knob with the curved part down.<br>• Use an anti-inflammatory.<br>• If pain and swelling do not decrease within 48 hours, seek medical care. |
| Ankle is unable to bear weight<br>He/she is unable to take four steps immediately after the injury and an hour later<br>Tenderness and pain is felt when you push on the ankle knob bone | Suspect **ankle fracture:**<br>• Use RICE procedures.<br>• For the compression part of RICE, apply an elastic bandage over any soft pliable material (e.g., sock or T-shirt) placed in a "U" shape around the ankle knob with the curved part down.<br>• Use an anti-inflammatory.<br>• Stabilize ankle against movement.<br>• Seek medical care. |

| Table C.4 | Determining and Treating Lower Leg Injuries |
|---|---|
| **If…** | **Then…** |
| Shin aches during activity, but:<br>• Ache subsides significantly after activity stops<br>• Ache is result of increase in workout routine (e.g., running longer, jogging on hills)<br>• Shin is tender when pressed | Suspect **shin splints:**<br>• Apply ice before activity and for 30 minutes after activity.<br>• Stop activity until pain free.<br>• Use an anti-inflammatory. |
| Leg receives direct hit that produces: deformity, open wound, tenderness, and/or swelling | Suspect **fracture or bruise:**<br>• Use RICE procedures.<br>• Use an anti-inflammatory.<br>• Control any bleeding.<br>If fracture is suspected:<br>• Stabilize leg against movement.<br>• Seek medical care. |
| He/she feels a pop or sudden, sharp, burning pain in calf muscle while running or jumping | Suspect a **muscle strain** (tear, pull):<br>• Use RICE procedures.<br>• Use an anti-inflammatory. |
| He/she feels a pop while running or jumping causing pain just above the heel<br>Leg is tender when pressed<br>He/she is unable to bear weight on injured leg<br>He/she has difficulty with controlling foot (flops around) | Suspect a **torn Achilles tendon:**<br>• Use RICE procedures.<br>• Use an anti-inflammatory.<br>• Seek medical care. |
| A muscle (most often the calf muscle) goes into an uncontrolled spasm and contraction, resulting in severe pain and restriction or loss of movement | Suspect a **muscle cramp:**<br>• Gently stretch the affected muscle, or<br>• Relax the muscle by applying pressure to it.<br>• Apply ice to the muscle.<br>• Drink lightly salted cool water (dissolve $\frac{1}{4}$ teaspoon salt in a quart of water). Do not give salt tablets. |

C

## Knee

Knee injuries are among the most serious joint injuries Table C.5 . Their severity is difficult to determine; thus you should seek medical care.

## Thigh

The thigh consists of a single bone, the femur, which is surrounded and protected by heavy muscle. The muscle group on the front of the thigh is the "quadriceps." Most thigh injuries are from direct hits. As with other leg muscles, a quadriceps strain can happen. See Table C.6 .

| Table C.5 | Determining and Treating Knee Injuries |
|---|---|
| **If...** | **Then...** |
| Immediate swelling occurs after injury<br>Knee locks<br>Knee gives way<br>Pain occurs below kneecap<br>Pain occurs under the kneecap when climbing stairs | Suspect **knee injury** (acute and/or chronic):<br>• Use RICE procedures.<br>• Stabilize knee against movement.<br>• Use an anti-inflammatory.<br>• Seek medical care. |
| Examining for an acute injury (not overuse type of injury):<br>**Pittsburgh Knee Rules:**<br>Any blunt trauma or fall type injury and one of the following present:<br>• Age younger than 12 years or over 50 years<br>• Inability to walk four weight-bearing steps<br>OR<br>**Ottawa Knee Rules:**<br>• Age over 55 years<br>• Tenderness at the patella (kneecap)<br>• Tenderness at head of fibula (bony knob on outside of knee)<br>• Inability to flex knee to 90° angle<br>• Inability to bear weight and take four steps immediately after injury and later | Suspect serious **knee injury:**<br>• Use RICE procedures.<br>• Stabilize knee against movement.<br>• Use an anti-inflammatory.<br>• Seek medical care. |
| Deformity obvious, with the kneecap (patella) on the outside (lateral side) of the knee. Compare it with the other kneecap. | Suspect a **dislocated kneecap:**<br>• Apply ice.<br>• Stabilize against movement.<br>• Seek medical care. |

| Table C.6 | Determining and Treating Thigh Injuries |
|---|---|
| **If...** | **Then...** |
| Pain at front of thigh | Suspect a **bruise:**<br>• Use RICE procedures.<br>• Use an anti-inflammatory. |
| Pain at back of thigh | Suspect a **muscle strain** (pulled hamstring):<br>• Use RICE procedures.<br>• Use an anti-inflammatory. |

## Hip

See **Table C.7** for information on how to determine and treat hip injuries.

## Finger

Most finger injuries are not severe. In rare cases a finger can dislocate, producing a grotesque deformity that requires immediate medical care. See **Table C.8**.

## Elbow

More often than not, elbow injuries are nagging nuisances. Occasionally an elbow will be more seriously injured. Rarely will an elbow dislocate. See **Table C.9**.

## Shoulder

Shoulder injuries can range from mild to those that pose medical emergencies **Table C.10**. A dislocated shoulder usually occurs during contact sports and requires immediate medical care. A shoulder dislocation can be confused with a shoulder separation. The key difference is that in separation the shoulder joint and upper arm remain mobile. In dislocation, the mobility is lost.

| Table C.7 | Determining and Treating Hip Injuries |
|---|---|
| **If…** | **Then…** |
| Pain is in groin | Suspect **muscle strain:**<br>• Use RICE procedures.<br>• Use an anti-inflammatory. |
| Pain is on upper hip | Suspect **hip pointer:**<br>• Use RICE procedures.<br>• Use an anti-inflammatory. |
| Pain is on outer thigh to knee | Suspect **muscle strain or bursitis:**<br>• Use RICE procedures.<br>• Use an anti-inflammatory. |

| Table C.8 | Determining and Treating Finger Injuries |
|---|---|
| **If…** | **Then…** |
| Deformed<br>Tender/painful<br>Swollen | Suspect a possible **fracture and/or dislocation:**<br>• Test for a finger fracture:<br>  – If possible, straighten the fingers and place them flat on a hard surface.<br>  – Tap the tip of the injured finger toward the hand. Pain lower down in the finger or into the hand can indicate a fracture.<br>• Do **not** try to realign a dislocation.<br>• Apply ice.<br>• Stablize finger against movement by "buddy" taping for support.<br>Or<br>• Keeping hand and fingers in cupping shape as though holding a baseball with extra padding in the palm, secure the hand, fingers, and arm to a rigid board or folded newspapers.<br>• Seek medical care. |

**C**

## Table C.9 — Determining and Treating Elbow Injuries

| If… | Then… |
|---|---|
| Severe elbow pain after fall on arm | Suspect **dislocation or fracture:**<br>• Apply ice.<br>• Give an anti-inflammatory.<br>• Stabilize against movement.<br>• Seek medical care. |
| Elbow pain on inside (medial) | Suspect **"little league, golf, or racquetball" elbow:**<br>• Use RICE procedures.<br>• Give an anti-inflammatory.<br>• Seek medical care if pain persists. |
| Elbow pain on outside (lateral) | Suspect **"tennis" elbow:**<br>• Use RICE procedures.<br>• Give an anti-inflammatory.<br>• Seek medical care if pain persists. |
| Elbow with:<br>• Tenderness/pain<br>• Swelling | Suspect a **bruise:**<br>• Use RICE procedures.<br>• Seek medical care if tingling and/or weakness continue for 24 hours (can be serious because of possible nerve injury). |

## Table C.10 — Determining and Treating Shoulder Injuries

| If… | Then… |
|---|---|
| Pain is on top of shoulder after a fall or being hit | Suspect a **separation:**<br>• Apply ice.<br>• Use an anti-inflammatory.<br>• Seek medical care. |
| Extreme pain is at front of shoulder after a fall<br>Victim holds upper arm away from the body, supported by the uninjured arm<br>Arm cannot be brought across the chest to touch the opposite shoulder<br>Victim describes a history of previous dislocations | Suspect a **dislocation:**<br>• Apply ice.<br>• Stabilize shoulder against movement and immediately seek medical care. |
| Burning pain is felt down arm after twisting neck | Suspect a **"stinger":**<br>• Apply ice.<br>• Use an anti-inflammatory.<br>• Seek medical care. |
| Arm goes limp | Suspect a **subluxation:**<br>• Apply ice.<br>• Use an anti-inflammatory.<br>• Seek medical care. |
| Pain is felt when raising arm | Suspect a **rotor cuff:**<br>• Apply ice.<br>• Use an anti-inflammatory.<br>• Seek medical care. |

## Muscle

See [ Table C.11 ] for information on how to determine and treat muscle injuries.

## Chest

See [ Table C.12 ] for symptoms and treatment of chest injuries.

## Breathing Difficulty

See [ Table C.13 ] for information on how to determine and treat breathing difficulty.

| Table C.11 | Determining and Treating Muscle Injuries |
|---|---|
| **If…** | **Then…** |
| Muscle pain occurs 12 to 72+ hours after physical activity | Suspect **delayed-onset muscle soreness:**<br>• Apply ice (some experts suggest heat).<br>• Warm up.<br>• Stretch the muscle.<br>• Do not use nonsteroidal medications (e.g., ibuprofen, aspirin). |

| Table C.12 | Determining and Treating Chest Injuries |
|---|---|
| **If…** | **Then…** |
| Sudden, severe central chest pain:<br>• Can occur at rest<br>• Worse when exerting<br>• Pain is crushing, vice-like<br>• May radiate up to the jaws or down the left arm<br>Nausea<br>Breathlessness<br>Sweating<br>Blueness of lips | Suspect a **heart attack:**<br>1. Give one aspirin to chew (not any other analgesic, only aspirin).<br>2. Seek medical care immediately—usually by calling 9-1-1.<br>3. Monitor for possible cardiac arrest requiring CPR.<br>4. Help victim into least painful position—usually sitting with legs bent at the knees.<br>5. Ask if he or she is taking a medication known as nitroglycerin; if so, help person take it. |
| No chest pain, but:<br>• Sudden general tiredness<br>• Breathlessness as a new symptom<br>• Sudden worsening of existing breathlessness | Suspect a **silent heart attack:**<br>• Treat as you would a heart attack. |

| Table C.13 | Determining and Treating Breathing Difficulty |
|---|---|
| **If…** | **Then…** |
| Coughing<br>Wheezing, especially when breathing out<br>Chest feels "tight"<br>Sweating, breathless, rapid pulse<br>Neck muscles strain in an attempt to increase breathing<br>As attack worsens, blue lips, tiredness, drowsiness<br>Confusion, coma<br>Poor response to usual medication | Suspect **asthma** (asthma can be induced during exercise):<br>1. Place victim in a comfortable, upright position to help breathing.<br>2. Help victim use medicines (inhaler and/or pills).<br>3. Give plenty of fluids.<br>4. Seek medical care if:<br>• No improvement within 2 hours after using medications.<br>• There are repeated attacks.<br>• Attack is severe and prolonged. |

C

# How Heat Affects the Body

Human bodies dissipate heat by varying the rate and depth of blood circulation, by losing water through the skin and sweat glands, and—when blood is heated above 98.6 °F—by panting. The heart begins to pump more blood, blood vessels dilate to accommodate the increased flow, and the bundles of tiny capillaries threading through the upper layers of skin are put into operation. The body's blood is circulated closer to the skin's surface, and excess heat drains off into the cooler atmosphere. At the same time, water diffuses through the skin as perspiration. The skin handles about 90% of the body's heat dissipating function.

Sweating, on its own, does nothing to cool the body, unless the water is removed by evaporation—and high relative humidity retards evaporation. The evaporation process works this way: The heat energy required to evaporate sweat is extracted from the body, thereby cooling it. Under conditions of high temperature (above 90 °F) and high relative humidity, the body is doing everything it can to maintain an internal temperature of 98.6 °F. The heart is pumping a torrent of blood through dilated circulatory vessels; the sweat glands are pouring liquid—including essential dissolved chemicals, like sodium and chloride—onto the surface of the skin.

## Too Much Heat

Heat disorders generally occur from a reduction or collapse of the body's ability to shed heat by circulatory changes and sweating, or a chemical (salt) imbalance caused by too much sweating. When heat gain exceeds the level the body can remove, or when the body cannot compensate for fluids and salt lost through perspiration, the temperature of the body's inner core begins to rise and heat-related illness may develop.

Heat illnesses include a range of disorders ( Table C.14 ). Some of them are common, but only heatstroke is life threatening. Untreated heatstroke victims always die.

Ranging in severity, heat disorders share one common feature: The individual has been overexposed or has overexercised for his or her age and physical condition in the existing thermal environment.

Studies indicate that, other factors being equal, the severity of heat disorders tends to increase with age—heat cramps in a 17-year-old may be heat exhaustion in a 40-year-old, and heatstroke in a person over age 60.

Acclimatization concerns adjusting the sweat–salt concentration, among other things. The idea is to lose enough water to regulate body temperature, with the least possible chemical disturbance.

The heat index (or apparent temperature) is how the heat and humidity in the air combine to make us feel ( Figure C.1 ). Higher humidity plus higher temperatures often combine to make us feel a perceived temperature that is higher than the actual air temperature. The old saying, "It's not the heat, it's the humidity," holds true.

The National Weather Service is using a new "mean heat index" to alert people to the dangers of heat waves. The index, which went into use in May 2002, measures how hot a person will feel over a full day.

The idea is the same as the traditional heat index, which shows how hot a particular combination of heat and humidity feels. This index has usually been used to show the danger during the hottest part of the day.

The mean heat index averages the heat index from the hottest and coolest parts of a day.

## Table C.14 | Determining and Treating Heat-Related Illnesses

| If... | Then... |
|---|---|
| Skin is extremely hot when touched—usually dry, but may be moist<br>Altered mental status, ranging from slight confusion, agitation, and disorientation to unresponsiveness | Suspect **heatstroke:**<br>Heatstoke is life threatening and must be treated immediately.<br>1. Move victim to a cool place. Monitor ABCs.<br>2. Remove clothing down to victim's underwear.<br>3. Keep victim's head and shoulders slightly raised.<br>4. Quickly cool the victim:<br>• Spray the victim with water and vigorously fan. This method does not work well in high humidity.<br>• If ice is available, place ice packs into the armpits, sides of the neck, and groin.<br>5. Stop cooling when mental status improves or if shivering occurs.<br>6. Evacuate to medical care ASAP. Continue cooling during evacuation. |
| Sweating<br>Thirsty<br>Fatigued<br>Flu-like symptoms—headache, nausea<br>Shortness of breath<br>Rapid pulse<br>Differences from heatstroke:<br>• No altered mental status<br>• Skin is not hot, but clammy | Suspect **heat exhaustion:**<br>Uncontrolled heat exhaustion can evolve into heatstroke.<br>1. Move victim to a cool place.<br>2. Have the victim remove excess clothing.<br>3. Have the victim drink cool fluids.<br>4. For more severe cases, give lightly salted cool water (dissolve ¼ teaspoon salt in a quart of water). Do not give salt tablets.<br>5. Raise victim's legs 8 to 12 inches (keep legs straight).<br>6. Cool the victim, but not as aggressively as for heatstroke.<br>7. If no improvement is seen within 30 minutes, seek medical care. |
| Painful muscle spasms that happen suddenly<br>Affects muscle in the back of the leg or abdominal muscles<br>Occurs during or after physical exertion | Suspect **heat cramp:**<br>Relief may take several hours.<br>1. Rest in a cool area.<br>2. Drink lightly salted cool water (dissolve ¼ teaspoon salt in 1 quart of water) or a commercial sports drink. Do not give salt tablets.<br>3. Stretch the cramped calf muscle or try acupressure method of pinching the upper lip just below the nose. |
| Victim is dizzy or faints | Suspect **heat syncope:**<br>1. If unresponsive, check ABCs. Person usually recovers quickly.<br>2. If victim fell, check for injuries.<br>3. Have victim rest and lie down with legs raised in cool area.<br>4. Wet skin by splashing water on face.<br>5. If not nauseated, drink lightly salted cool water (dissolve ¼ teaspoon salt in 1 quart of water) or a commercial sports drink. Do not give salt tablets. |
| Ankles and feet swell<br>Occurs during first few days in a hot environment | Suspect **heat edema:**<br>1. Wear support stockings.<br>2. Elevate legs. |
| Itchy rash on skin wet from sweating | Suspect **prickly heat:**<br>1. Dry and cool skin.<br>2. Limit heat exposure. |

Relative Humidity (%)

| °F | 40 | 45 | 50 | 55 | 60 | 65 | 70 | 75 | 80 | 85 | 90 | 95 | 100 |
|-----|-----|-----|-----|-----|-----|-----|-----|-----|-----|-----|-----|-----|-----|
| 110 | 136 | | | | | | | | | | | | |
| 108 | 130 | 137 | | | | | | | | | | | |
| 106 | 124 | 130 | 137 | | | | | | | | | | |
| 104 | 119 | 124 | 131 | 137 | | | | | | | | | |
| 102 | 114 | 119 | 124 | 130 | 137 | | | | | | | | |
| 100 | 109 | 114 | 118 | 124 | 139 | 136 | | | | | | | |
| 98 | 106 | 109 | 113 | 117 | 123 | 128 | 134 | | | | | | |
| 96 | 101 | 104 | 108 | 112 | 116 | 121 | 126 | 132 | | | | | |
| 94 | 97 | 100 | 101 | 106 | 110 | 114 | 118 | 124 | 129 | 135 | | | |
| 92 | 94 | 96 | 99 | 101 | 105 | 108 | 112 | 116 | 121 | 125 | 131 | | |
| 90 | 91 | 93 | 95 | 97 | 100 | 103 | 106 | 109 | 113 | 117 | 122 | 127 | 132 |
| 88 | 88 | 89 | 91 | 93 | 95 | 98 | 100 | 100 | 106 | 110 | 113 | 114 | 121 |
| 86 | 85 | 87 | 88 | 89 | 91 | 93 | 95 | 97 | 100 | 102 | 105 | 108 | 112 |
| 84 | 83 | 84 | 85 | 86 | 88 | 89 | 90 | 92 | 94 | 96 | 98 | 100 | 103 |
| 82 | 81 | 82 | 83 | 84 | 84 | 85 | 86 | 88 | 89 | 90 | 91 | 93 | 95 |
| 80 | 80 | 80 | 81 | 81 | 82 | 82 | 83 | 84 | 84 | 85 | 86 | 86 | 87 |

Air Temperature

Heat Index (Apparent Temperature)

**With Prolonged Exposure and/or Physical Activity**

**Extreme Danger**
Heatstroke or sunstroke highly likely

**Danger**
Sunstroke, muscle cramps, and/or heat exhaustion likely

**Extreme Caution**
Sunstroke, muscle cramps, and/or heat exhaustion possible

**Caution**
Fatigue possible

**Figure C.1**

The heat index (or apparent temperature) shows how heat and humidity affect the human body. (*Source:* National Weather Service. http//www.crh.noaa.gov/ict/heat.htm.)

## Sunburn

Sunburn, with its ultraviolet radiation burns, can significantly retard the skin's ability to shed excess heat.

See Table C.15 for information on how to determine and treat sunburns.

| Table C.15 | Determining and Treating Sunburns |
|---|---|
| **If…** | **Then…** |
| Skin that has been exposed to the sun later becomes:<br>• Red<br>• Mildly swollen<br>• Tender and painful | Suspect **first-degree (superficial) sunburn:**<br>1. Immerse burned area in cold water or apply a wet, cold cloth until pain free, both in and out of the water (usually 10–45 minutes). If cold water is unavailable, use any cold liquid available.<br>2. Give ibuprofen (for children, give acetaminophen).<br>3. Have victim drink as much water as possible without becoming nauseous.<br>4. Keep burned arm or leg raised.<br>5. After burn has been cooled, apply aloe vera gel or inexpensive moisturizer.<br>First-degree burns do **not** have to covered. |
| Skin that has been exposed to the sun later becomes:<br>• Blistered<br>• Swollen<br>• Weeping of fluids<br>• Severely painful | Suspect **second-degree (partial-thickness) sunburn:**<br>• If skin affected is less than 20% of the body surface (victim's palm, not including fingers and thumb, equals 1% of body surface area):<br>  1. Follow same procedures (steps 1–4) as for a first-degree burn, with these additions:<br>    a. After burn has been cooled, apply thin layer of antibacterial ointment (eg., bacitracin, Neosporin).<br>    b. Cover burn with a dry, nonsticking, sterile dressing or clean cloth.<br>• If skin has a large second-degree burn over more than 20% of the body surface area:<br>  1. Follow steps 2–4 of first-degree burn care.<br>  2. Seek medical care.<br>Do **not** apply cold because it may cause hypothermia. |

# Cold-Related Injuries

## Hypothermia

Hypothermia happens when the body's temperature (98.6 °F, 37 °C) drops more than 2 degrees ( Table C.16 ). Hypothermia does not require subfreezing temperatures. Severe hypothermia is life threatening. Check also for possible frostbite.

| Table C.16 | Determining and Treating Hypothermia |
|---|---|
| **If…** | **Then…** |
| Shivering uncontrollably<br>Has the "umbles"—grumbles, mumbles, fumbles, and stumbles<br>Has cool abdomen when felt with a warm hand | Suspect **mild hypothermia:**<br>1. Stop heat loss:<br>  • Get victim out of the cold.<br>  • Handle victim gently.<br>  • Replace wet clothing with dry clothing.<br>  • Add insulation (e.g., blankets, towels, pillows, sleeping bags) beneath and around victim. Cover victim's head (50%–80% of body's heat loss is through the head).<br>2. Keep in flat (horizontal) position.<br>3. Allow the victim to shiver—do not stop the shivering by adding heat. Shivering, which generates heat, will rewarm mildly hypothermic victims. DO NOT use the following procedures because they stop shivering:<br>  • Warm water immersion<br>  • Body-to-body contact<br>  • Chemical heat pads<br>Warm drinks are unable to rewarm sufficiently. However, warm sugary liquids can provide calories for shivering to continue and may provide a psychological boost.<br>DO NOT give alcohol to drink. |
| Muscles are rigid and stiff<br>No shivering<br>Skin feels ice cold and appears blue<br>Altered mental status<br>Slow pulse<br>Slow breathing<br>Victim appears to be dead | Suspect **severe hypothermia:**<br>1. Follow steps 1 and 2 from mild hypothermia for all hypothermic victims.<br>2. Check ABCs and give CPR as necessary. Check the pulse for 30 to 45 seconds before starting CPR.<br>3. Gently evacuate victim to medical help for rewarming. Rewarming in a remote location is difficult and rarely effective. However, when the victim is far from medical care, the victim must be warmed by any available external heat source (e.g., body-to-body contact, warm water immersion). |

**C**

## Frostbite and Frostnip

Frostbite happens only in below-freezing temperatures (less than 32 °F) Figure C.2 . Mainly the feet, hands, ears, and nose are affected. The most severe results are gangrene requiring surgical amputation. See Table C.17 for symptoms and treatment. Check for hypothermia, as it may also be present.

Frostnip is caused when water on the skin's surface freezes Table C.18 .

**Wind Chill Chart**

Wind (mph)

| Calm | 5 | 10 | 15 | 20 | 25 | 30 | 35 | 40 | 45 | 50 | 55 | 60 |
|------|-----|-----|-----|-----|-----|-----|-----|-----|-----|-----|-----|-----|
| 40 | 36 | 34 | 32 | 30 | 29 | 28 | 28 | 27 | 26 | 26 | 25 | 25 |
| 35 | 31 | 27 | 25 | 24 | 23 | 22 | 21 | 20 | 19 | 19 | 18 | 17 |
| 30 | 25 | 21 | 19 | 17 | 16 | 15 | 14 | 13 | 12 | 12 | 11 | 10 |
| 25 | 19 | 15 | 13 | 11 | 9 | 8 | 7 | 6 | 5 | 4 | 4 | 3 |
| 20 | 13 | 9 | 6 | 4 | 3 | 1 | 0 | −1 | −2 | −3 | −3 | −4 |
| 15 | 7 | 3 | 0 | −2 | −4 | −5 | −7 | −8 | −9 | −10 | −11 | −11 |
| 10 | 1 | −4 | −7 | −9 | −11 | −12 | −14 | −15 | −16 | −17 | −18 | −19 |
| 5 | −5 | −10 | −13 | −15 | −17 | −19 | −21 | −22 | −23 | −24 | −25 | −26 |
| 0 | −11 | −16 | −19 | −22 | −24 | −26 | −27 | −29 | −30 | −31 | −32 | −33 |
| −5 | −16 | −22 | −26 | −29 | −31 | −33 | −34 | −36 | −37 | −38 | −39 | −40 |
| −10 | −22 | −28 | −32 | −35 | −37 | −39 | −41 | −43 | −44 | −45 | −46 | −48 |
| −15 | −28 | −35 | −39 | −42 | −44 | −46 | −48 | −50 | −51 | −52 | −54 | −55 |
| −20 | −34 | −41 | −45 | −48 | −51 | −53 | −55 | −57 | −58 | −60 | −61 | −62 |
| −25 | −40 | −47 | −51 | −55 | −58 | −60 | −62 | −64 | −65 | −67 | −68 | −69 |
| −30 | −46 | −53 | −58 | −61 | −64 | −67 | −69 | −71 | −72 | −74 | −75 | −76 |
| −35 | −52 | −59 | −64 | −68 | −71 | −73 | −76 | −78 | −79 | −81 | −82 | −84 |
| −40 | −57 | −66 | −71 | −74 | −78 | −80 | −82 | −84 | −86 | −88 | −89 | −91 |
| −45 | −63 | −72 | −77 | −81 | −84 | −87 | −89 | −91 | −93 | −95 | −97 | −98 |

Temperature (°F)

Note: Frostbite occurs in 15 minutes or less.

$$\text{Wind Chill (°F)} = 35.74 + 0.6215T - 35.75(V^{0.16}) + 0.4275T(V^{0.16})$$

Where  T = Air Temperature (°F)

V = Wind Speed (mph)

**Figure C.2**

Wind chill chart. (*Source:* National Weather Service. http://www.erh.noaa.gov/er/iln/tables.htm.)

| Table C.17 | Determining and Treating Frostbite | |
|---|---|---|
| **If…** | **Then…** | |
| Skin color is white, waxy, or grayish yellow<br>Affected part is cold and numb<br>Tingling, stinging, or aching sensation is felt<br>Skin surface feels stiff or crusty, and underlying tissue feels soft when depressed gently | Suspect **superficial frostbite** | All frostbite injuries require the same first-aid treatment:<br>1. Get victim to a warm area.<br>2. Replace wet clothing or constricting items that could impair blood circulation (e.g., rings).<br>3. Do not rub or massage the area.<br>4. For deep frostbite, seek medical care.<br>5. When more than 1 hour from medical facility, place part in warm water (test by pouring some over the inside of your arm to test that it is warm, not hot). For ear or face, it is best but may be difficult to apply warm moist cloths, changing them frequently. May have to cover with warm hands. Give pain medication (preferably aspirin or ibuprofen). Rewarming may take 20 to 40 minutes or when parts become soft.<br>**DO NOT:**<br>• Rub or massage part.<br>• Rewarm with stove, vehicle's tailpipe exhaust, or over a fire.<br>• Break blisters. |
| Affected part feels cold, hard, and solid, and cannot be depressed—feels like a piece of wood or frozen meat<br>Affected part is pale, and skin may appear waxy<br>A painfully cold part suddenly stops hurting<br>Blisters appear after rewarming | Suspect **deep frostbite** | • Allow victim to smoke or drink alcohol.<br>• Rewarm if there is any possibility of refreezing.<br>• Allow thawed part to refreeze.<br>After thawing:<br>• Place dry, sterile gauze between toes and fingers to prevent sticking.<br>• Elevate part to reduce pain and swelling.<br>• Give aspirin or ibuprofen for pain and inflammation. Do not give to children.<br>• Apply thin layer of aloe vera on area.<br>• Seek medical care. |

| Table C.18 | Determining and Treating Frostnip |
|---|---|
| **If…** | **Then…** |
| Skin appears red and sometimes swollen<br>Painful | Suspect **frostnip** (it is difficult to tell the difference between frostnip and frostbite):<br>1. Gently warm area against a warm body part (e.g., armpit, stomach, bare hands) or by blowing warm air on the area.<br>2. Do not rub area. |

# Knowledge Check Answers

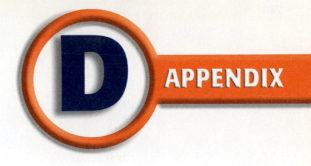

## Chapter 1

1. B
2. D
3. D
4. B

5. C
6. B
7. D
8. C

## Chapter 2

1. D
2. B
3. D
4. A
5. B

6. C
7. B
8. A
9. D
10. D

## Chapter 3

1. A
2. B
3. B
4. A
5. C

6. B
7. B
8. B
9. B
10. B

## Chapter 4

1. A
2. B
3. C
4. A
5. B

6. A
7. A
8. C
9. B
10. C

## Chapter 5

1. C
2. B
3. D
4. C
5. B

6. A
7. C
8. C
9. A
10. C

## Chapter 6

1. A
2. A
3. A
4. C
5. D

6. B
7. D
8. D
9. A
10. C

**D**

## Chapter 7

1. A
2. C
3. C
4. B
5. B

6. C
7. C
8. A
9. C
10. B

## Chapter 8

1. A
2. E
3. C
4. A
5. C

6. D
7. A
8. A
9. C
10. B

## Chapter 9

1. B
2. D
3. C
4. B
5. A

6. B
7. D
8. C
9. D
10. D

## Chapter 10

1. B
2. B
3. A
4. D
5. A

6. B
7. D
8. C
9. D
10. C

## Chapter 11

1. B
2. C
3. A
4. B
5. D

6. A
7. B
8. D
9. D
10. C

## Chapter 12

1. C
2. A
3. B
4. D
5. D

6. A
7. C
8. B
9. C
10. D

## Chapter 13

1. B
2. B
3. A
4. B

5. A
6. B
7. C
8. B

# Glossary

## A

abstinence  Complete refrain from sexual activity.

acquired immunodeficiency syndrome (AIDS)  Late-stage development of HIV infection.

addiction  Physiological and/or psychological need to perform a certain behavior.

adenosine triphosphate (ATP)  The only form of energy used in the human body.

adrenaline  A hormone that prepares the body to react during times of stress or in an emergency.

aerobic energy system  System that provides energy for activities lasting longer than 2 minutes. This system requires oxygen.

aerobic exercise  Exercise that depends on oxygen for energy production.

allostatic load  The ongoing demand on the body from long-term exposure to stress hormones.

amenorrhea  Absence of normal menstruation.

anabolic steroids  Synthetic male hormones that increase muscle size and strength.

anaerobic  Without using oxygen.

anaerobic energy system  System that creates energy for activities that last less than 2 minutes or have frequent rest periods.

anemia  A reduction in the number of red blood cells in the blood. Anemia is not a disease but a symptom of various diseases, including iron deficiency.

angina pectoris  Chest pain caused by the early stages of cardiovascular disease.

angioplasty  Technique used to open arteries blocked by plaque buildup.

anorexia nervosa  Extreme restriction of food intake.

antioxidants  A substance that can combine with or neutralize free radicals, and thus prevent oxidative damage to cells and tissues.

apoB  A small, dense form of cholesterol.

atherosclerosis  Plaque buildup inside the arteries.

asanas  Various postures used in doing yoga exercises.

atrophy  Progressive loss (wasting) of muscle mass.

autonomic nervous system  Part of the nervous system that controls automatic body functions, such as blood pressure, heart rate, and breathing. Subdivided into sympathetic and parasympathetic.

# B

**bacteria** Microscopic organisms that cause disease.

**ballistic stretching** Bouncing, repetitive movement during stretching.

**basal cell carcinoma** Form of skin cancer easily removed through surgery.

**basal metabolic rate (BMR)** Energy consumed (measured in calories) by the body at rest to keep vital functions going.

**benign** A noncancerous tumor that does not invade nearby cells.

**benzodiazepines** Central nervous system depressants used to reduce anxiety and induce sleep.

**binge drinking** Having five or more drinks for men, or four or more drinks for women, in a single occasion.

**binge eating** Uncontrolled eating during a short time period.

**bioelectrical impedance** Measurement of the strength and speed of an electrical signal sent through the body.

**blaming** Placing the responsibility of an unmet goal on someone else.

**blood alcohol concentration (BAC)** The concentration of alcohol found in the bloodstream; expressed as a percentage.

**blood clot** Blockage that results from coagulation of blood.

**body composition** Proportion of fat, muscle, bone, and other tissues in the body.

**body mass index (BMI)** A measure of body fatness, calculated by dividing your weight in pounds by your height in inches; divide that answer by your height in inches; and multiply by 703.

**botulism** Poisoning by the toxin of the microorganism *Clostridium botulinum*.

**bulimia** Periodic bingeing followed by purging, or alternate days of bingeing and fasting.

# C

**calorie** Unit of energy supplied by food; equals 1 kilocalorie (1 kcal), the amount if heated required to raise the temperature of 1 kilogram of water 1° C.

**cancer** A family of diseases characterized by rapid, uncontrolled growth of abnormal cells.

**carbo loading** Stuffing yourself with complex carbohydrates during the days before an endurance event.

**carbohydrates** Nutrient that is the body's main source of energy; consists of sugars and starches found in grains, vegetables, and fruits; two types are simple and complex.

**carbon monoxide** Most significant poisonous gas related to smoking.

**cardiac catheterization** Passage of a thin, flexible tube into the heart to provide treatment for heart disease.

**cardiorespiratory endurance activity** Exercise that contracts large muscle groups and increases breathing and heart rate.

**cardiovascular disease** Series of diseases affecting the heart and blood vessels.

**cellulite** Adipose tissue surrounded by stretched connective tissue.

**chancre** A predominantly painless open sore occurring in the early stages of syphilis.

**chew** Shredded tobacco leaves placed between the cheek and gum.

**chlamydia** A bacterial infection caused by *Chlamydia trichomatis*.

**cholesterol** Wax-like substance made by the body's liver and found in animal and plant foods.

**chronic disease** Disease that takes many years to develop.

**chronic obstructive pulmonary disease (COPD)** Family of breathing disorders most commonly contracted from smoking; includes emphysema and bronchitis.

**collars** Devices used to secure weights to a barbell or dumbbell. Without collars the weights on one side of the bar will slip off.

**complete protein** A protein that contains all the essential amino acids.

**compulsion** An increase in the amount of time spent on an activity.

**consistency** The constant activity level needed to maintain fitness.

**contusions** Bruising of tissue.

**cool-down** The 5–10 minutes at the end of a workout involving light movement and stretching.

**coronary bypass surgery** Procedure used to reroute blood flow around a damaged or blocked artery.

**CPR (cardiopulmonary resuscitation)** Clearing air passages to the lungs, giving mouth-to-mouth respiration, and massaging the heart to restore normal breathing after cardiac arrest.

**cramping** Muscular tightness and abdominal or limb pain from dehydration and high body temperature.

**creatine phosphate (CP)** Chemical present in muscles that makes ATP rapidly for 30 seconds' worth of exercise. Creatine phosphate is produced in the body from the digestion of meat. It can also be found as a supplement. Research is inconclusive as to its benefits or long-term risks.

**cross-training** Combining the components of fitness in a workout program, instead of focusing on only one area.

# D

**death rate** Statistical representation of the significance of a disease or disorder in society.

**delirium tremens** DTs; withdrawal symptom characterized by uncontrollable shaking and hallucinations.

**diabetes** Disease characterized by the body's inability to manage insulin.

**diastolic pressure** Lower blood pressure reading; measured when the heart relaxes between beats.

**dietary fiber** Nondigestible carbohydrates found in plants; two types are soluble and insoluble.

**dislocations** Bones are displaced from their normal joint alignment, out of their sockets, or out of their normal positions.

**distress** Harmful or bad response to a stressor.

**drug** Any nonfood substance that alters thought and/or behavior.

**dynamic or active stretching** Muscle is taken beyond its normal range of motion with help from a partner.

# E

**eating disorder** A spectrum of abnormal eating patterns that eventually may endanger a person's health or increase the risk for other diseases. Generally, psychological factors play a key role.

**endocrine system** Consists of glands that produce hormones that control body functions.

**endorphins** Proteins produced in your brain that serve as your body's natural painkiller. Endorphins also reduce stress, depression, and anxiety.

**endurance** Ability to work out for a period of time without fatigue.

**essential amino acids** The nine protein amino acids that the body cannot make and, therefore, must come from foods you eat.

**essential body fat** Minimum amount of body fat needed for good health.

**ethanol** Grain alcohol; consumable form of alcohol in alcoholic beverages.

**euphoria** The effect associated with being "high."

**eustress** Helpful or good response to a stressor.

**exercise** Planned, structured, and repetitive physical activity done to improve or maintain one or more components of physical fitness.

**exercise log** A record of your activity that includes the type, duration, and intensity of each exercise each day.

# F

**female athlete triad** Combination of eating disorders, amenorrhea, and osteoporosis.

**fitness** The body's response to physical effort.

**flexibility** Ability to move a joint smoothly through a full range of motion.

**free radicals** A short-lived chemical that can have detrimental effects on cells.

**frequency** How often; the number of times an exercise or group of exercises is performed within a certain time frame.

# G

**general adaptation syndrome** A series of body changes that result from stress. The syndrome occurs in three stages: alarm, resistance, and exhaustion.

**genetic modification** Manipulating the DNA of an organism to change some of its characteristics.

**genetic testing** Procedure used to investigate the pattern of human genes to determine the likelihood of disease development.

**genital herpes** Sexually transmitted disease caused by the herpes simplex virus.

**genital warts** One of many strains of human papillomavirus (HPV) transmitted through sexual contact, causing hard, round bumps on the skin surrounding the genitalia.

**gland** A group of cells that secretes hormones.

**glucose** Simple sugar circulating in the blood.

**glycogen** Complex carbohydrates stored primarily in the skeletal muscles and liver. When energy is needed, glycogen is converted to glucose.

**gonorrhea** A bacterial infection caused by *Niesseria gonorrhoeae.*

# H

**hallucinogens** Drugs that distort the senses and emotions, mimicking psychosis.

**health** The World Health Organization's 1946 definition of health has been used as a foundation for the contemporary term of wellness: "Health is a state of complete physical, mental, and social well-being and not merely the absence of disease or infirmity."

**heart attack** Damage or death of all or part of the heart due to insufficient blood supply.

**heavy drinkers** Individuals who consume five or more drinks on one occasion, five or more times in a 30-day period.

**hemorrhagic stroke** Disruption of blood flow to the brain caused by leaking of a blood vessel.

**hepatitis B** One of a family of diseases that slowly destroy the functioning ability of the liver.

**high-density lipoprotein (HDL)** Carries cholesterol from the blood back to the liver, which processes the cholesterol for elimination from the body. It is often referred to as *good* cholesterol.

**homeostasis** Stability and consistency of a person's physiology.

**hormone** Chemical messenger released into the bloodstream that controls many body activities.

**human immunodeficiency virus (HIV)** The virus that causes AIDS.

**hydrostatic (underwater) weighing** Measuring a person's weight while he or she is suspended in water.

**hypertension** High blood pressure.

**hypertrophy** Increase in bulk or size by thickening of muscle fibers.

# I

**immediate energy system** System using existing cellular ATP during first 10 seconds of activity.

**incomplete protein** A protein lacking one or more of the essential amino acids.

**individual differences** The variables in our physical ability.

**insoluble fiber** Does not dissolve in water.

**insomnia** Inability to sleep.

**intensity** How hard; the amount of energy exerted while performing an exercise.

**intravenous drug use** Drug use occurring by injecting the drug directly into the bloodstream using a needle and syringe.

**irradiation** Treatment with gamma rays, x rays, or high-voltage electrons to kill pathogens and, in the case of food, to increase shelf life.

**ischemic stroke** Disruption of blood flow to the brain caused by blockage of an artery (clot).

**isokinetic** Muscle contraction where the maximum tension is generated in the muscle as it contracts at a constant speed over the full range of motion of the joint.

**isometric** Muscle contraction without movement at the joint.

**isotonic** Muscle contraction where tension is constant while length increases.

# L

**lactic acid**  Chemical formed when muscles must use stored glucose or blood-sugar to produce ATP.

**lacto-ovo-vegetarian**  Person who includes milk, dairy products, and eggs in his or her diet.

**lacto-vegetarian**  Person who includes some or all dairy products in his or her diet.

**lipids**  Fats or fatlike substances characterized by their insolubility in water or solubility in fat.

**lipoprotein**  Allows cholesterol to dissolve in the blood and carries it through the bloodstream to all parts of the body; two main types are high-density lipoprotein (HDL) and low-density lipoprotein (LDL).

**locus of control**  The figurative place where a person locates the source of responsibility for the events in his or her life.

**lordosis**  Excessive pelvic tilt.

**low-density lipoprotein (LDL)**  Carries cholesterol from the liver to the rest of the body. When there is too much LDL cholesterol in the blood, it can be deposited on the walls of the coronary arteries. It is often referred to as *bad* cholesterol.

# M

**macrominerals**  Minerals needed by the body in amounts greater than 100 milligrams.

**macronutrients**  Nutrients needed by your body in relatively large amounts.

**malignant**  A cancerous tumor that invades other cells and inhibits their ability to function properly.

**malignant melanoma**  Dangerous form of skin cancer.

**mall-walking**  Walking a circuit around the lobby floors of an enclosed shopping mall in the morning before the stores open.

**mammography**  x ray procedure of the breast to determine if tumors are present.

**maximal oxygen uptake (VO$_{2max}$)**  How efficiently the cardiorespiratory system uses oxygen.

**menopause**  The time when a woman's body stops producing ova and hormones related to fertility and menstruation.

**metabolism**  The rate at which your body uses energy.

**microminerals (trace minerals)**  Minerals needed by the body in amounts less than 100 milligrams.

**micronutrients**  Nutrients needed by your body in relatively small amounts.

**minerals**  Inorganic nutrients that regulate many chemical reactions in the body.

**monounsaturated**  High concentrations of unsaturated fat in canola, peanut, and olive oils.

**motivation**  The underlying drive behind making changes.

**multiple-joint exercise**  An exercise in which two or more joints move together.

**muscular endurance**  The ability of muscles to apply force repeatedly.

**muscular strength**  The force muscles can exert against resistance.

**myocardial infarction (MI)**  Heart attack.

# N

**nicotine**  The addictive drug in tobacco products.

**nutrients**  Substances in food the body needs for normal function and good health.

# O

**obesity**  Excessive amounts of body fat.

**opioids**  Narcotics; used as pain relievers.

**osteoporosis**  Disease related to calcium deficiency in which bones become thin and brittle and fracture easily.

**overload**  Placing a greater-than-normal amount of stress (within reason) on the body in an attempt to make it function at a higher capacity.

# P

**pathogens**  Microorganisms causing disease.

**pelvic inflammatory disease (PID)**  Complication in women caused by untreated chlamydia or gonorrhea.

**pH (powerHydrogen)**  Condition of a solution represented by a number on a scale of acidity to alkalinity.

**physical activity**  Bodily movement produced by skeletal muscles that increases energy expenditure.

**physical fitness**  Set of attributes that people have or achieve that relates to the ability to perform physical activity.

**phytochemical**  Substance in plants (*phyto* = plant) that may have beneficial effects on the body.

**plaque**  Artery-blocking deposits impeding blood flow.

**plug**  Shredded tobacco leaves that are pressed into a hard block.

**plyometrics**  A form of training where muscles are subjected to rapid alternation of lengthening and shortening while resistance is continuously applied.

**polyunsaturated**  High concentrations of unsaturated fat in sunflower, corn, soybean oils, and fish.

**procrastination**  Pushing a task to a later point in time.

**progression**  The gradual increase of the level and intensity of exercise.

**progressive muscular relaxation**  Systematically tensing and relaxing the body's muscles from the feet to the head.

**progressive overloading**  Increasing, from one session to another, the amount of weight you lift during a set.

**proof**  Two times the percentage of alcohol in an alcoholic beverage.

**prostate**  Male gland responsible for producing seminal fluid.

**prostate-specific antigen (PSA)**  Blood test that detects a protein associated with prostate cancer.

**protein**  Nutrient made up of amino acids that is needed for growth to build, repair, and maintain body tissues.

**psychoneuroimmunology**  Study of nervous, endocrine, and immune system interaction.

**pulmonary circulation**  Circulation between the heart and the lungs.

**pulse**  The surge of blood that can be felt on certain points on the body each time the heart pumps blood into the arteries.

# R

**rate of perceived exertion (RPE)**  A person's own perception of the intensity of his or her exercise.

**rationalization**  Making excuses for not carrying out a task.

**reinforcement**  External support for a behavior.

**relaxation response**  Reversal of stress symptoms.

**repetition (rep)**  A single lifting and lowering of a weight.

**repetition maximums (RM)**  The maximum weight you can lift successfully once while using proper form.

**resistance training**  Building muscle by working against the resistance of weights.

**rest**  A period of inactivity to allow your body to recover from strenuous exercise.

**reversibility**  The principle that states that the results of physical fitness are not permanent.

# S

**safety**  Awareness of all aspects of your exercise routine to protect yourself from injury.

**saturated fat**  Fat from meat, poultry, dairy products, and hardened vegetable fat.

**scrotum**  Flesh-covered sac that hangs outside the male body and holds the testicles.

**sedatives**  Sleep and anxiety reduction drugs with small margin of safety.

**sedentary**  Little or no physical activity.

**semi- or partial vegetarian**  Person who eats no red meat, but may include chicken or fish, dairy products, and eggs in his or her diet.

**set**  Number of reps performed without stopping to rest.

**sexually transmitted infections (STIs)**  Infections and diseases transferred through intimate contact.

**snuff**  Ground-up moist tobacco placed between the bottom lip and gum.

**soluble fiber**  Partially dissolves in water.

**specificity**  The type of physical changes you desire in your body relates directly to the type of exercise you choose.

**spotter**  Another person who can help if the weight tilts or can help move a weight into position before or after a lift.

**sprains**  Tearing or stretching of the joints that causes mild to severe damage to the ligaments and joint capsules.

**squamous cell carcinoma**  Cancer in the top layer of skin; highly curable when detected early.

ST2  Stress-related protein that may be a predictor of how well an individual will recover from heart attack.

static or passive stretching  Muscle is stretched naturally without force being applied.

stent  A mesh coil used to open blocked arteries.

stimulants  Drugs used to increase activity in the central nervous system, causing increased energy and a sense of well-being.

storage fat  Excess fat deposited in adipose tissue (fat cells) that protects organs and insulates the body.

strains  Muscles are stretched or torn.

stress  The physical and emotional tension that comes from situations the body perceives as threatening.

stressor  A source or cause of stress; it may be physical, mental, social, or environmental.

stretch reflex  An involuntary muscle contraction against a quick stretch.

stretching  Primary method of improving flexibility.

sympathetic nervous system  Subsystem of the autonomic system that triggers your body's response to stress; known as the fight-or-flight response.

syphilis  Sexually transmitted disease caused by spirochete bacteria.

systemic circulation  Circulation between the heart and the rest of the body.

systolic pressure  Higher blood pressure reading; measured when the heart contracts.

# T

T cells  The immune system's primary defense system to fight disease.

t'ai chi  Thirteenth-century Chinese exercise routine involving graceful dancelike movements.

tar  Black, sticky substance from tobacco smoke that builds up in the lungs and promotes cancer development.

target heart rate zone  A range of heart rates used to maintain optimal effects during aerobic exercise.

tendinitis  Inflammation of a tendon from overuse.

tetrahydrocannabinol (THC)  The active drug in marijuana.

time  How long; the duration an exercise or group of exercises takes to complete.

tolerance  The condition where more of a drug or activity is required to reproduce the initial sensation.

trans fat  Chemically derived fat present in hydrogenated foods; promotes plaque development and high cholesterol.

trans fatty acids  Fats produced by heating liquid vegetable oils in the presence of hydrogen, a process called hydrogenation.

transient ischemic attack (TIA)  Warning sign of possible stroke.

tumor  A mass of cancer cells.

type  The classification of exercise.

type 2 diabetes  A disease that involves the inability to produce an adequate amount of insulin.

**type A** An individual exhibiting a sense of time urgency ("hurry sickness"), aggressiveness, and competitiveness, usually combined with hostility. Describes the majority of Americans.

**type B** An individual displaying no sense of time urgency, no hostility, noncompetitiveness, patience, and a secure sense of self-esteem.

# U

**underweight** A BMI less than 19.

**unsaturated fat** Type of fat obtained from plant sources and fish; two types are monounsaturated and polyunsaturated.

# V

**vegan** Person who eats only foods of plant origin.

**vegetarian diet** Diet in which vegetables are the foundation and meat products are restricted or eliminated.

**virus** Smallest of all disease-causing pathogens.

**vitamin** Nutrient necessary for normal functioning of the body; two types are water soluble and fat soluble.

**VO$_{2max}$** Amount of oxygen the body uses when it reaches its maximum ability to supply oxygen during exercise.

# W

**warm-up** The 5–10 minutes of low-intensity movement at the beginning of a workout that prepares the body for activity by increasing muscle temperature and metabolism.

**wasting** Occurs when the diet lacks protein; the body breaks down body tissue (e.g., muscle) and uses it as a protein source.

**weight management** The adoption of healthful and sustainable eating and exercise behaviors indicated for reduced disease risk and improved feelings of energy and well-being.

**wellness** An active process of becoming aware of and making choices toward a more successful existence.

**withdrawal** Symptoms related to the removal of a drug or activity.

# Index

# Photo Credits

## Contents

p. v © Ablestock; p. vi © LiquidLibrary; p. vii, top © LiquidLibrary; p. vii, bottom © Berta A. Daniels; viii, top © Photodisc; p. viii, bottom © Berta A. Daniels; p. ix © Photodisc; p. x, Courtesy of Bill Branson/National Cancer Institute; p. xi © LiquidLibrary; p. xii © Thinkstock/Index Stock Imagery; p. xiii © Photos.com; xiv © Jostein Hauge/ShutterStock, Inc.; p. xv © Ablestock; p. xvi © David Buffington/Photodisc/Getty Images

## Introduction

p. xvii © Ryan McVay /PhotoDisc/Getty Images; p. xviii © Photos.com; p. xix © Photodisc; p. xx © Keith Brofsky/PhotoDisc/Getty Images

## Chapter 1

Chapter Opener © Photodisc; Figure 1.1 Courtesy of the CDC; Figure 1.2, © Prochaska J. O., DiClemente C. O., and Norcross J. C. In search of how people change: Applications to addictive behaviors. American Psychologist 47 (1992): 1102-1114. Copyright © 1992 by the American Psychological Association. Reprinted by permission, Figure 1.3 Adapted from Prochaska J. O., Norcross J. C., and DiClemente C. O. Changing for Good. New York: Quill 2002; p. 4, © Photos.com; p. 5 © Ryan McVay/Photodisc; p. 7 © Ryan McVay/Photodisc; p. 10 © LiquidLibrary; p. 11 © Photos.com

## Chapter 2

Chapter Opener © Ron Chapple/Thinkstock/Almay Images; p. 17 top © BananaStock/age fotostock; Figure 2.1 National Center for Health Statistic (NCHS) Vital Statistics System. 10 Leading Causes of Deaths, United States, 2002. www.cdc.gov/ncipc; p. 17 bottom © LiquidLibrary; Figure 2.2 National Center for Chronic Disease Prevention and Health Promotion (NCCDPHP). U.S. Physical Activity Statistics: 2001 state summary data, 2001; p. 19 top © AbleStock; p. 19 middle © LiquidLibrary; Figure 2.3 © Jones and Bartlett Publishers; p. 20 middle © LiquidLibrary; p. 20 top © LiquidLibrary; p. 20 bottom © Ryan McVay/Photodisc/Getty Images; Figure

2.4 The Activity Pyramid © 2003 Park Nicollet Health Innovations, Minneapolis, U.S.A. 1-888-637-2675. Reprinted with permission; p. 23 top © Karl Weatherly/Photodisc/Getty Images; p. 23 middle © AbleStock; p. 23 bottom © LiquidLibrary; p. 24 © Polo Productions/Brand X Pictures/Almay Images; p. 25 © AbleStock; p. 26 © AbleStock; p. 27 top © Jones and Bartlett Publishers; Figure 2.6 © Jones and Bartlett Publishers

## Chapter 3

Chapter Opener © LiquidLibrary; p. 33 © Robert Brenner/PhotoEdit; Figure 3.1 © Jones and Bartlett Publishers; p. 36 top © Photodisc; p. 36 bottom © Frank Siteman/PhotoEdit; p. 37 © Berta A. Daniels, 2000; p. 38 © Photodisc; Figure 3.2 Source: For correct usage of the scale, the user must go to the instruction and administration given by Borg, se Borg, G. 1998. Borg's Perceived Exertion and Pain Scales. Champaign, IL: Human Kinetics, or to the folder published by Borg on the RPE scale or the CR10 scale, Borg Perception, Furuholmen 1027, 762 91 Rimbo, Sweden; p. 40 bottom © Photodisc/Getty Images; p. 43 top © Photos.com; p. 43 middle © LiquidLibrary; p. 43 bottom © LiquidLibrary; p. 44 top © E. Dygas/Photodisc/Getty Images; p. 44 middle © LiquidLibrary; p. 44 bottom © AbleStock; p. 45 top © LiquidLibrary; p. 45 bottom © Keith Brofsky/Photodisc/Getty Images; p. 46 top © Luca DiCecco/Almay Images; p. 46 bottom © Photodisc

## Chapter 4

Chapter Opener © Photodisc; p. 53 © Photos.com; p. 54 left © Berta A. Daniels, 2000; p. 54 right © Berta A. Daniels, 2000; p. 56 Courtesy of Danny Meyer/U.S. Air Force; p. 58 top left © Berta A. Daniels, 2000; p. 58 top middle © Berta A. Daniels, 2000; p. 58 top right © Berta A. Daniels, 2000; p. 58 middle left © Berta A. Daniels, 2000; p. 58 middle middle © Berta A. Daniels, 2000; p. 58 middle right © Berta A. Daniels, 2000; p. 58 bottom left © Berta A. Daniels, 2000; p. 58 bottom middle © Berta A. Daniels, 2000; p. 58 bottom right © Berta A. Daniels, 2000; p. 59 top left © Berta A.

Daniels, 2000; p. 59 top right © Berta A. Daniels, 2000; p. 59 top middle left © Berta A. Daniels, 2000; top middle right © Berta A. Daniels, 2000; p. 59 middle © Berta A. Daniels, 2000; p. 59 bottom left © Berta A. Daniels, 2000; p. 59 bottom middle © Berta A. Daniels, 2000; p. 59 bottom right © Berta A. Daniels, 2000; p. 60 top left © Berta A. Daniels, 2000; p. 60 top right © Berta A. Daniels, 2000; p. 60 middle left © Berta A. Daniels, 2000; p. 60 middle middle © Berta A. Daniels, 2000; p. 60 middle right © Berta A. Daniels, 2000; p. 60 bottom left © Jones and Bartlett Publishers; p. 60 bottom right © Jones and Bartlett Publishers; p. 61 top © Berta A. Daniels, 2000; p. 61 middle © Berta A. Daniels, 2000; p. 61 bottom © Berta A. Daniels, 2000; p. 62 top © Berta A. Daniels, 2000; p. 62 middle © Berta A. Daniels, 2000; p. 62 bottom © Berta A. Daniels, 2000; Figure 4.1 © Jones and Bartlett Publishers; Figure 4.2 © Jones and Bartlett Publishers; Figure 4.3 © Jones and Bartlett Publishers

## Chapter 5

Chapter Opener © Berta A. Daniels, 2000; p. 69 © Photos.com; Figure 5.1 © Jones and Bartlett Publishers; Figure 5.2 © Jones and Bartlett Publishers; Figure 5.3 © Jones and Bartlett Publishers; Figure 5.4 © CSMI; Figure 5.5 © Jones and Bartlett Publishers; p. 76 © Berta A. Daniels, 2000; p. 77 © Berta A. Daniels, 2000; Figure 5.6 © Berta A. Daniels, 2000; Figure 5.7 © Jones and Bartlett Publishers; Figure 5.8 © Jones and Bartlett Publishers; Figure 5.9 © Jones and Bartlett Publishers; Figure 5.10 © Berta A. Daniels, 2000; Figure 5.11 © Jones and Bartlett Publishers; Figure 5.12 © Jones and Bartlett Publishers; Figure 5.13 © Berta A. Daniels, 2000; Figure 5.14 © Jones and Bartlett Publishers; Figure 5.15 © Jones and Bartlett Publishers; Figure 5.16 © Jones and Bartlett Publishers; Figure 5.17 © Jones and Bartlett Publishers; Figure 5.18 © Jones and Bartlett Publishers; Figure 5.19 © Berta A. Daniels, 2000; p. 83 bottom ©LiquidLibrary; p. 84 © SW Productions/Photodisc/Getty Images

## Chapter 6

Chapter Opener © Photodisc; p. 89 top © Ryan McVay/Photodisc/Getty Images; p. 89 bottom left © Jess Alford/PhotoDisc; p. 89 bottom middle © Jules Frazier/Photodisc; p. 89 bottom right © PhotoLink/Photodisc; p. 90 Courtesy of National Cancer Institute; p. 91 © Berta A. Daniels, 2000; p. 93 © AbleStock; Figure 6.1 © Jones and Bartlett Publishers; p. 98 © LiquidLibrary; p. 99 © Ron Chapple/Thinkstock/Almay Images; Figure 6.2 © AbleStock; p. 100 bottom © AbleStock; Figure 6.3 Source: U.S. Department of Agriculture, Agriculture Research Service, Dietary Guidelines Advisory Committee. Nutrition and Your Health: Dietary Guidelines for Americans, 2000, 5th ed. Home

and Garden Bulletin No. 232. Washington, DC: 2000; Figure 6.4 Source: U.S. Department of Agriculture/U.S. Department of Health and Human Services; p. 109 top © Photodisc; p. 109 bottom © Ken Sherman/Phototake/Alamy Images; p. 110 © Photodisc; Figure 6.5 © Jones and Bartlett Publishers; Figure 6.6 © Jones and Bartlett Publishers; Figure 6.7 © Jones and Bartlett Publishers; Figure 6.8 © Jones and Bartlett Publishers; p. 114 bottom © LiquidLibrary

## Time Out #1

p. 120 © Jones and Bartlett, p. 121 © LiquidLibrary

## Chapter 7

Chapter Opener © Rubberball Productions; Figure 7.1 Data compiled from Nutrition for physical fitness and athletic performance for adults—Position of ADA and the Canadian Dietetic Association (1993). Journal of the American Dietetic Association 93: 691-697. Reprinted with permission from the American Dietetic Association; Figure 7.2 © Jones and Bartlett Publishers; p. 126 bottom © Roy Morsch/age fotostock; Figure 7.3 © Jones and Bartlett Publishers; p. 127 © Ed Reschke; Figure 7.4 fist: © Photos.com; cassette: © Ana Vasileva/ShutterStock, Inc.; soap © Lara Barrett/ShutterStock, Inc.; p. 129 © Stock Connection Distribution/Alamy Images; Figure 7.5A © Prado, Madrid, Spain/The Bridgeman Art Library; Figure 7.5B © Max Nash/AP Photo; Figure 7.6 © Jones and Bartlett Publishers; p. 133 top © David Young-Wolff/PhotoEdit; p. 133 bottom © Jones and Bartlett Publishers; p. 134 top Courtesy of Life Measurements, Inc.; p. 134 middle © SPL/Custom Medical Stock Photo; p. 134 bottom © SPL/Custom Medical Stock Photo; Figure 7.7 © Jones and Bartlett Publishers; Figure 7.8 © Jones and Bartlett Publishers; p. 138 Robert W. Ginn/ PhotoEdit; Figure 7.9 Source: CDC/NCHS, NHES, and NHANIES; p. 139 bottom © David Young-Wolf/PhotoEdit; p. 140 top © Photodisc; p. 140 bottom left © Photodisc; p. 140 bottom right © AbleStock; p. 142 © AbleStock; Figure 7.10A © Jones and Bartlett Publishers; Figure 7.10B © John Bolivar/Custom Medical Stock; Figure 7.11 © Jones and Bartlett Publishers; Figure 7.12 © Jones and Bartlett Publishers; Figure 7.13 © Jones and Bartlett Publishers; Figure 7.14 © Jones and Bartlett Publishers; photo © Jack Star/PhotoLink/ Photodisc/Getty Images

## Chapter 8

Chapter Opener © John Foxx/Alamy Images; Figure 8.1 © Jones and Bartlett Publishers; p. 154 top © AbleStock; p. 154 bottom © LiquidLibrary; p. 155 © Thinkstock/Getty Images; p. 156 top © Sheila Terry/Science Source/Photo Researchers; Figure 8.2 © Jones and Bartlett Publishers; Figure 8.3 © Jones and

Bartlett Publishers; Figure 8.4 © REUTERS/Jeff Christensen/Landov; p. 160 © Photos.com; p. 161 top © AbleStock; p. 161 middle © Creatas; p. 161 bottom © AbleStock; p. 163 bottom © AbleStock; Figure 8.5 © Jones and Bartlett Publishers; p. 164 top © Photos.com; Figure 8.6 © Jones and Bartlett Publishers; p. 165 top © AbleStock; p. 165 bottom © Jones and Bartlett Publishers; p. 166 © LiquidLibrary; p. 167 © Photos.com

## Chapter 9

Chapter Opener © Photodisc; p. 171 top © Yoav Levy/Phototake/Alamy Images; p. 171 bottom © Ryan McVay/Photodisc/Getty Images; p. 172 © SW Productions/PhotoDisc/Getty Images; Figure 9.1 © Jones and Bartlett Publishers; Figure 9.2 © Jones and Bartlett Publishers; Figure 9.3 © Jones and Bartlett Publishers; Figure 9.4 © Jones and Bartlett Publishers; p. 178 top © Muriel Lasure/ShutterStock, Inc.; p. 178 bottom © Photodisc; p. 179 top © Photodisc; p. 179 middle © Corbis; p. 179 bottom © Jack Starr/PhotoLink/Photodisc

## Chapter 10

Chapter Opener © Bernd Thissen/Landov; Figure 10.1 © Jones and Bartlett Publishers; p. 186 top © EyeWire, Inc.; Figure 10.2 © Jones and Bartlett Publishers; p. 190 top left Courtesy of National Cancer Institute; p. 190 bottom © Photodisc; p. 190 top middle Courtesy of National Cancer Institute; p. 190 top right Courtesy of National Cancer Institute; p. 191 middle © Photodisc; p. 191 top right © Photodisc; p. 191 top left © Photodisc; p. 191 bottom © Photodisc; p. 192 © Photodisc

## Time Out #3

p. 196 top © Photodisc; p.196 bottom © Photos.com; p. 197 middle © Andres Rodriguez/ShutterStock, Inc.; p. 197 top © Photodisc; p. 197 bottom © Howard Sandler/ShutterStock, Inc.

## Chapter 11

Chapter Opener © BananaStock/age fotostock; p. 199 top © EyeWire, Inc.; p. 199 middle © Photodisc; p. 199 bottom © Stewart Cohen/Getty Images; Figure 11.1 © Jones and Bartlett Publishers; Figure 11.2 Source: Office of Applied Studies (OAS), Substance Abuse and Mental Health Services Administration (SAMHSA), The NHSDA Report: Alcohol Use. Rockville, MD: Substance Abuse and Mental Health Services Administration (SAMHSA), 2003. http://www.drugabusestatistics.samhsa.gov; Figure 11.3 Courtesy of SAMHSA; p. 209 middle © Morris Huberland/Science Source/Photo

Researchers, Inc.; Figure 11.4 Courtesy of JAMA;1993;270;2207-12; p. 209 bottom © Biophoto Associates/Photo Researchers, Inc.; p. 210 bottom © Patrick Sheandell O Carroll/PhotoAlto/PictureQuest; Figure 11.6 Source: The National Household Survey on Drug Abuse, United States, 1991. Office of Smoking and Health, Centers for Disease Control and Prevention; p. 212 © Science Photo Library/Photo Researchers, Inc.; p. 213 © Richard Levine/Alamy Images

## Chapter 12

Chapter Opener © Photos.com; p. 218 © REUTERS/Jamil Bittar/Landov; Figure 12.1 Courtesy of Centers for Disease Control and Prevention; Figure 12.2 Courtesy of Centers for Disease Control and Prevention; Figure 12.3 Courtesy of Centers for Disease Control and Prevention; p. 221 bottom © Science VU/Visuals Unlimited; p. 222 top Courtesy of Dr. Wiesner/CDC; p. 222 middle Courtesy of Joe Millar/CDC; p. 222 bottom © Dr. M.A. Ansary/Photo Researchers, Inc.; p. 223 © logical Images/Custom Medical Stock Photo; p. 224 bottom Courtesy Susan Lindsley, VD/CDC; Figure 12.4 Courtesy of World Health Organization

## Time Out #4

p. 231 © Michael Lotenero/Photodisc/Getty Images

## Chapter 13

Chapter Opener © PhotoDisc; p. 233 top left © LiquidLibrary; p. 233 top right © Photodisc/Getty Images; 233 bottom © LiquidLibrary; p. 234 top © Robert Brenner/PhotoEdit; p. 234 bottom © LiquidLibrary; p. 235 top © AbleStock; p. 235 bottom © Photos.com; p. 236 top © AbleStock; p. 236 bottom © Photos.com; p. 237 © LiquidLibrary; p. 238 © LiquidLibrary; p. 239 © Michael Newman/PhotoEdit; p. 241 © Jones and Bartlett Publishers

## Time Out #5

p. 244 © David Buffington/Photodisc/Getty Images

## Appendix B

pp. 256-257 Canada's Food Guide to Healthy Eating, Health Canada, 2005. Reproduced with the permission of the Minister of Public Works and Government Services Canada, 2005; pp. 258-259 Canada's Physical Activity Guide to Healthy Active Livinghttp://www.phac-aspc.gc.ca/pau-uap/paguide/index.html, Public Health Agency of Canada, (2005) Reproduced with the permission of the Minister of Public Works and Government Services Canada, 2005; p. 260 © Jones and Bartlett Publishers; p. 261 © Jones and Bartlett Publishers